SURGERY
for the
MORBIDLY OBESE PATIENT

SURGERY
for the
MORBIDLY OBESE PATIENT

Editor

Mervyn Deitel, M.D.

Professor of Surgery,
Professor of Nutritional Sciences,
University of Toronto;
Surgeon,
St. Joseph's Health Centre

Lea & Febiger   Philadelphia ● London   1989

Lea & Febiger
600 Washington Square
Philadelphia, PA   19106-4198
U.S.A.
(215) 922-1330

Library of Congress Cataloging-in-Publication Data

Surgery for the morbidly obese patient / [edited by] Mervyn Deitel.
   p. cm.
  Includes bibliographies and index.
  ISBN 0-8121-1136-2
  1. Obesity—Surgery. 2. Gastrointestinal system—Surgery.
3. Jejunoileal bypass. I. Deitel, Mervyn.
  [DNLM: 1. Obesity, Morbid.   WD 210 S9595]
RD540.S87   1989
617'.43—dc19
DNLM/DLC
for Library of Congress   88-39994
                                      CIP

PRINTED IN THE UNITED STATES OF AMERICA

Print number: 5   4   3   2   1

FOREWORD

The title of this very practical book proclaims with enthusiasm *Surgery* for the morbidly obese, emphasizing the dedication of a vanguard of surgeons to bring relief from the bondage of weight.

What is it that drives surgeons so doggedly to pursue treatment of this obesity with its associated disease processes? Is the task analogous to climbing and conquering the highest peak that claims their allegiance by an unusual challenge? Could it be evangelistic zeal to help where medicine in general has worked, then abandoned with frustration and damning disgust those tortured ranks? One need not look beyond the gratitude of those liberated to a new life to give purpose to the surgeon's drive! It is like curing a neoplasm grown out of bounds.

The editor brings this zeal born of much experience face to face with the risk realities hanging in the balance for patient and surgeon. The intensity of his involvement has caused him to enlist others who have walked in these pathways, to help validate the innovative methods of surgery. His enthusiasm has brought new opportunity and new life to those in related fields to make significant contributions.

From this well-organized text one may comprehend the nature of the problem of morbid obesity and proven methods to deal with it. The balance of risk is exposed—so too is the unknown, the work of the future. While there is bias in this developing field, there is fairness shown by the editor. There is emphasis on the value of a team effort.

Finally, the reader is provoked to query:

Will the challenges to surgeons motivate them to understand the etiology of morbid obesity?

Is morbid obesity conquered or merely controlled by surgical procedures?

Will it be possible to eventually prevent morbid obesity rather than approach it by intervention?

Read and be stimulated.

Boyd E. Terry, M.D., F.A.C.S.
Columbia, Missouri

PREFACE

The commonest form of malnutrition in Western civilization is obesity. When the body weight approaches twice ideal, *morbid obesity* (i.e. obesity that results in progressive, serious, incapacitating physical disease) exists. An estimate of the true incidence of morbid obesity in the population is difficult to obtain, as these individuals very frequently withdraw from society and ultimately become secluded in a room.

The etiology of this massive obesity appears to originate in multiple, often poorly understood, factors. Ultimately, there is a vast increase in the adipose organ. Because of a very significant failure-rate of conservative regimens in these patients, surgeons have been called upon increasingly in the past 25 years to perform operations on medical "failures," as a last resort. The development of safe, lasting weight-reduction operations has taxed the courage and ingenuity of many research-oriented and dedicated surgeons. Operative technique and risk, postoperative sequelae, and patient surveillance have provided problems and challenges.

Bariatric surgery is no longer experimental but is *developmental*. As with the surgery for peptic ulcer disease, reflux esophagitis and hiatal hernia disorders, breast cancer, and the complications of portal hypertension, the surgery for morbid obesity has undergone development and metamorphosis. Operations have been developed which are appropriate and highly effective if employed cautiously. The vertical banded gastroplasty, silicone ring vertical gastroplasty, Roux-en-Y gastric bypass, gastric banding, bilio-pancreatic bypass, and jejunoileal bypass *with ileogastrostomy* are achieving considerable success in experienced hands.

In an attempt to present the current status to the practising surgeon, at a time when acceptable weight-loss operations with acceptable lasting results have been achieved, the authors offer this book as a contribution. The usual compilation is weighted in chapters discussing epidemiology, possible etiologies, medical and psychiatric treatments, and results of various clinics; this book aims principally at the *surgeon's role*, while providing a *basic* appreciation of the concepts of obesity. The book opens with a discussion of the offending cell, the peculiar adipocyte, followed by a chapter detailing the consequences of massive obesity. Conservative treatments and their results in the morbidly obese patient are presented. A chapter follows on risks, considerations, and principles which apply to *any* operation in the obese patient. The next section illustrates the development of bariatric operations, including patient selection and the current procedures, with an emphasis on those operations which have now proved effective and relatively safe. In the final section, a chapter on anesthetic management details the protocol in the operating-room; although many of these patients will tolerate a general anesthetic, thoracic epidural is highly advantageous in the extremely massively obese with major respiratory dysfunction, both for anesthesia and postoperative analgesia—and as a means of enabling the patients to move themselves without burdening the hospital staff. The nursing care is detailed, and sequelae are discussed. A chapter presents important principles of plastic surgery after massive weight-reduction, which contributes very significantly to the final rehabilitation of these patients; a part on suction lipectomy is included as a final step towards acceptable body contour.

The authors thank Medi-Edit Limited of Toronto for efficient and pleasant editorial assistance.

Mervyn Deitel, M.D.
Toronto, Canada
Editor

vii

SPONSORS

3M Medical/Surgical Division—3M Surgical Staplers
Auto Suture Canada Ltée/Ltd. United States Surgical Corporation
ETHICON Ltd. (a Johnson & Johnson Company)
Cook (Canada) Inc. Wilson-Cook Medical Inc.
PILLING Company
HDC Corporation
The Hans and Josephine Boerghers Family
The Weston/Loblaw Group of Companies
The Annie Walsh Family
Department of Surgery, University of Toronto
The Nelson Arthur Hyland Foundation
St. Joseph's Health Centre Research Foundation
Mentor Corporation—Heyer-Schulte Products
Pharmacia (Canada), Inc.
IVH Services, Inc.
Ross Laboratories, Division of Abbott Laboratories Ltd.
Kendall McGaw Canada
Alpha Therapeutic Corporation

CONTRIBUTORS

Zohair Y. Al-Halees, M.D., F.R.C.S.(C)
Consultant Cardiovascular Surgeon,
King Faisal Specialist Hospital and
Research Centre, Riyadh, Saudi Arabia

**Sundaram V. Anand, M.B., F.R.C.S.(C)
F.R.C.S.(Eng), M.P.H. (Johns Hopkins)**
Lecturer, Departments of Surgery and
Epidemiology, Queen's University,
Kingston, Ontario; Surgeon, Lennox
and Addington County General Hospital,
Napanee, Ontario, Canada

**Aubie Angel, M.D., B.Sc.(Med), M.Sc.,
F.R.C.P.(C)**
Professor of Medicine, Department of
Medicine, University of Toronto; Director,
Institute of Medical Science, School of
Graduate Studies, University of Toronto;
Director, Clinical Science Division,
Faculty of Medicine, University of Toronto;
Staff Physician, Toronto General Hospital,
Division of Endocrinology and Metabolism,
Toronto, Ontario, Canada

**Samuel B. Bashour, M.D., D.A.B.S., F.A.C.S.,
F.I.C.S.**
Clinical Instructor, Department of Surgery,
University of Texas Health Science Center,
Dallas; Past President, Medical Staff, G.C.
Morton Hospital, Dallas, and Past Attending
Staff, Pioneer Park Hospital Center, Irving,
Texas

Hu A. Blake, II, M.D.
Instructor in Surgery, University of Pennsylvania
School of Medicine; Clinical Instructor in
Surgery, Graduate Hospital and Pennsylvania
Hospital, Philadelphia, Pennsylvania

**Iain G.M. Cleator, M.B., Ch.B., F.R.C.S.(Edin.),
F.R.C.S.(Lond.), F.R.C.S.(C.), F.A.C.S.**
Professor of Surgery, University
of British Columbia; Surgeon, St. Paul's
Hospital, Vancouver; Chairman, Gastrointestinal
Clinic, St. Paul's Hospital, Vancouver, British
Columbia, Canada

**Stephen M. Collins, M.B.B.S., M.R.C.P.(UK),
F.R.C.P.(C)**
Associate Professor of Medicine (Division
of Gastroenterology), Director, Intestinal
Disease Research Unit, McMaster University;
Staff Physician, McMaster University Medical
Centre, Hamilton, Ontario, Canada

George S.M. Cowan, Jr., M.D.
Associate Professor, Department of Surgery,
The University of Tennessee Health Sciences
Center, Memphis, Tennessee

Douglas E. Crowell, M.D.C.M., F.R.C.P.(C)
Chief, Department of Anaesthesia,
St. Joseph's Health Centre, Toronto,
Ontario, Canada

**Mervyn Deitel, M.D., F.R.C.S.(C), F.A.C.S.,
F.I.C.S., F.A.C.G., F.A.C.N.**
Professor of Surgery and Professor of
Nutritional Sciences, University of Toronto;
Surgeon, St. Joseph's Health Centre, Toronto,
Ontario, Canada

Gifford V. Eckhout, M.D., F.A.C.S.
Associate Clinical Professor of Surgery,
University of Colorado School of Medicine;
Attending Surgeon, St. Joseph Hospital,
Denver, Colorado

Joel B. Freeman, M.D., F.R.C.S.(C), F.A.C.S.
Professor of Surgery, University of Ottawa;
Staff Surgeon, Ottawa General
Hospital, Ottawa, Ontario, Canada

Arnis Freiberg, M.D., F.R.C.S.(C), F.A.C.S.
Associate Professor of Surgery, University
of Toronto; Chief of Division of Plastic
Surgery, Toronto Western Hospital; Active
Staff, Hillcrest Hospital, Toronto,
Ontario, Canada

Glenna French, R.N.
Assistant Nursing Co-ordinator,
Operating-Room, St. Joseph's Health
Centre, Toronto, Ontario, Canada

J.L. Galbraith, R.N.
Acute Care Nurse, St. Joseph's Health Centre,
Toronto, Ontario, Canada

Paul E. Garfinkel, M.Sc., M.D., F.R.C.P.(C)
Professor of Psychiatry,
University of Toronto; Psychiatrist-in-Chief,
Toronto General Hospital; Vice Chairman,
Department of Psychiatry, University of
Toronto, Toronto, Ontario, Canada

David S. Goldbloom, A.B., M.A., M.D.,
F.R.C.P.(C)
Centennial Fellow, Medical Research Council
of Canada; Assistant Professor of
Psychiatry, University of Toronto; Staff
Psychiatrist, Toronto General Hospital,
Toronto, Ontario, Canada

Gerald N. Goodman, M.D., F.A.C.S.
Clinical Instructor in Surgery, University
of Utah School of Medicine; Surgical Staff,
LDS Hospital, Primary Children's Medical
Center, Salt Lake Surgical Center and
Intermountain Surgical Center and St. Marks
Hospital, Salt Lake City, Utah

Robert H. Gourlay, M.D.C.M., M.Sc.
(Experimental Surgery), F.A.C.S., F.R.C.S.(C)
Senior Surgeon, St. Paul's Hospital, Vancouver;
Clinical Professor of Surgery, University of
British Columbia; Senior Consultant,
Shaughnessy Hospital, Vancouver and Mount St.
Joseph Hospital, Vancouver, British Columbia,
Canada

D. Michael Grace, M.D., D. Phil., F.R.C.S.(C),
F.A.C.S.
Associate Professor of Surgery, University of
Western Ontario; attending staff, University
Hospital, London, Ontario, Canada

Darwin K. Holian, B.A., M.B., M.D., F.A.C.S.
Surgical Staff, Santa Barbara Cottage Hospital;
Coleta Valley Community Hospital, Santa
Barbara, California

Beverly A. Jones, M.D., F.R.C.S.(C)
Staff Surgeon, Oakville Trafalgar Hospital,
Oakville, Ontario, Canada

John G. Kral, M.D., Ph.D.
Professor of Surgery, State University of New
York Health Science Center at Brooklyn; Director
of Surgery, Kings County Hospital Center,
Brooklyn, New York

Lubomyr I. Kuzmak, M.D., Sc.D., F.I.C.S.
Attending Surgeon, St. Barnabas Medical
Center, Livingston, New Jersey; Attending
Surgeon and Former Chairman, Department of
Surgery, Irvington General Hospital, Irvington,
New Jersey; Medical Director and Surgeon,
Surgical Center for Obesity, Livingston,
New Jersey

Claude P. Lieber, M.D., F.A.C.S.
Assistant Professor of Surgery, Thomas Jefferson
University; Clinical Associate in Surgery,
University of Pennsylvania School of Medicine;
Attending Surgeon, Graduate Hospital
and Pennsylvania Hospital; Consultant Surgeon,
Inglis House, Philadelphia, Pennsylvania

William R.N. Lindsay, B.Sc., M.D., F.R.C.S.(C),
M.S.(Tor)
Assistant Professor of Surgery, University
of Toronto; Division of Plastic Surgery,
Wellesley Hospital, Toronto, Ontario, Canada

Edward Eaton Mason, M.D., Ph.D., F.A.C.S
Professor and Chairman, Division of General
Surgery, The University of Iowa Hospitals and
Clinics, Iowa City, Iowa

David K. Miller, M.D., F.A.C.S.
Clinical Instructor in Surgery, University of
Utah School of Medicine; Surgical Staff,
LDS Hospital, Primary Children's Medical
Center, Salt Lake Surgical Center and IHC
Surgical Center, Salt Lake City, Utah

Robert L. Milne, M.D., F.A.C.S.
Clinical Assistant Professor of Surgery,
University of New Mexico Medical School; Active
Staff, Presbyterian Hospital Center and St.
Joseph Hospital, Albuquerque, New Mexico

Ole A. Peloso, M.D., F.A.C.S.
Clinical Associate Professor of Surgery,
University of New Mexico Medical School; Active
Staff, Presbyterian Hospital Center and St.
Joseph Hospital; Consultant, Veterans
Administration Hospital, Albuquerque, New
Mexico

Thomas G. Peters, M.D.
Professor, Department of Surgery, The
University of Tennessee Health Sciences
Center, Memphis, Tennessee

Pauline S. Powers A.B.(Math), M.D.
Professor of Psychiatry and Behavioral Medicine,
University of South Florida College of Medicine,
Tampa; Director, Division of Psychosomatic
Medicine, University of South Florida; Director,
Department of Psychiatry Eating Disorders
Clinic, University of South Florida Medical
Center; Staff, Tampa General Hospital; Attending
Physician, VA Medical Center, Tampa, Florida

Daniel A.K. Roncari, M.D., M.Sc. Ph.D.,
F.R.C.P.(C), F.A.C.P.
Professor of Medicine, University of Toronto;
Physician-in-Chief, Department of Medicine,
Sunnybrook Medical Centre, Toronto, Ontario,
Canada

Alexander S. Rosemurgy, M.D.
Assistant Professor of Surgery, Department
of Surgery, University of South Florida College
of Medicine, Tampa, Florida

Peter F. Rovito, M.D.
Chief Surgical Resident, Department of Surgery, Lehigh Valley Hospital Center, The Allentown Hospital, Allentown Affiliated Hospitals, Allentown, Pennsylvania

Dahlia Mishell Sataloff, M.D.
Clinical Associate in Surgery, University of Pennsylvania School of Medicine; Clinical Instructor in Surgery, Graduate Hospital and Pennsylvania Hospital, Philadelphia, Pennsylvania

Ursula L. Seinige, M.D.
Clinical Associate in Surgery, University of Pennsylvania School of Medicine; Clinical Instructor in Surgery, Pennsylvania and Graduate Hospitals; Consultant in Breast Cancer, Cancer Prevention Center, Philadelphia, Pennsylvania

Richard E. Seppala, M.D., F.R.C.P.(C)
Staff Radiologist, Ottawa General Hospital; Clinical Lecturer in Radiology, University of Ottawa, Ottawa, Ontario, Canada

Elaine Stone, M.D., F.R.C.P.(C)
Lecturer, Department of Internal Medicine (Endocrinology), University of Toronto; Attending Staff, Department of Medicine, St. Joseph's Health Centre, Toronto, Ontario, Canada

Richard Jay Strauss, M.D., F.A.C.S.
Associate Professor of Clinical Surgery, The State University of New York (Stony Brook); Surgeon, Long Island Jewish-Hillside Medical Center, New Hyde Park, New York; Assistant Clinical Professor of Surgery, Cornell Medical School

Boyd E. Terry, B.S., M.D., F.A.C.S.
Associate Professor of Surgery, University of Missouri Medical School, Columbia; Attending Surgeon, University of Missouri Health Science Center; Director, George David Peak Memorial Burn Center, University of Missouri Health Science Center, Columbia, Missouri; Secretary-Treasurer, American Society for Bariatric Surgery

Toan B. To, M.D.
Research Associate, St. Joseph's Health Centre Research Foundation, Toronto, Ontario, Canada

Harvey P. Weingarten, B.Sc., M.Sc., M.Phil., Ph.D.
Associate Professor, Department of Psychology, McMaster University: Associate Member, Department of Medicine (Intestinal Disease Research Unit), McMaster University Medical Centre, Hamilton, Ontario, Canada

Lawrence H. Wilkinson, M.D., F.A.C.S.
Clinical Professor of Surgery, University of New Mexico Medical School; Honorary Staff, St. Joseph Hospital and Presbyterian Hospital Center, Albuquerque, New Mexico

Otto L. Willbanks, B.S., M.A., M.D., F.A.C.S.
Attending Staff, Baylor University Medical Center, Dallas, Texas

Janis T. Winocur, M.Sc., R.P.Dt.
Nutritionist, Eating Disorders Clinic, Toronto General Hospital, Toronto, Ontario, Canada

Leslie Wise, M.D., F.A.C.S.
Professor of Surgery, The State University of New York (Stony Brook); Chairman, Department of Surgery, Long Island Jewish-Hillside Medical Center, New Hyde Park, New York

CONTENTS

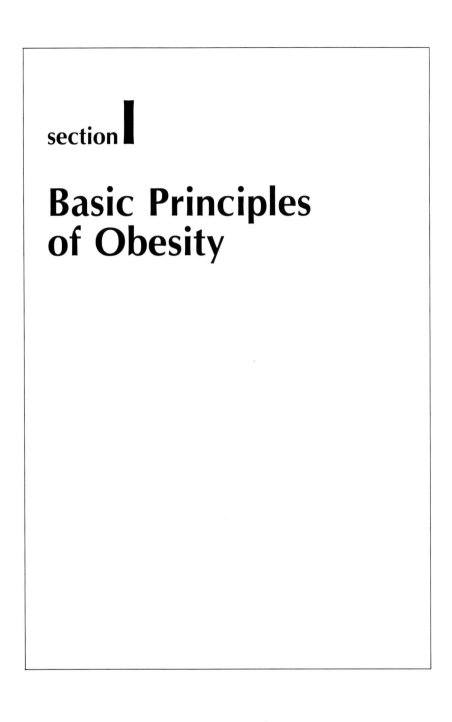

section I

Basic Principles of Obesity

1

The Fat Cell

DANIEL A. K. RONCARI
AUBIE ANGEL

The fat cell is ultimately the site where the morphologic changes of obesity occur.[1] Indeed, the invariant cytologic characteristic of obesity is manifested by expanded fat cells (adipocytes). Their total number either remains normal, as in moderate obesity, or becomes excessive, as in massive obesity.[1] Moderate obesity may be defined by body weights greater than 120% and less than 170% of reference; the usual standards of desirable body weights for adults are the Metropolitan Life Insurance Company tables, which were revised and became available in 1983.[2] Massive obesity may be defined by body weights greater than 170% of reference.

During evolution, mechanisms developed for the efficient storage of chemical energy, in the form of triglyceride, in fat cells. While in "affluent" societies we are concerned with excessive deposition ("overshoot of the mark"), the fuel reserve had, and in extensive areas of the globe still has, survival value. Indeed, a lean person can survive without food for about 2 months, while a massively obese person, who may store as many as $1\frac{1}{2}$ million kilocalories (1 kilocalorie, or 1 Calorie is equivalent to 4.186 kilojoules), has a chance to survive for at least 1 year, provided appropriate fluids, minerals and vitamins are taken. Oxidation of the fatty acids released from adipocyte triglycerides generates not only life-preserving energy, but also considerable water, of obvious value in certain situations.

STRUCTURE AND FUNCTION OF FAT CELLS

Fat cells are the characteristic elements of adipose tissue, although it is comprised of a number of other constituents. Adipocytes are derived from embryonic secondary mesenchyme. While closely related to fibroblasts, adipoblasts and pre-adipocytes (the latter will be referred to as adipocyte precursors in ensuing sections) are mesenchymal cells endowed with the unique ability to differentiate into fat cells.[3-5] From its earliest development, the appearance and growth of adipocyte progenitors proceeds concurrently and interdependently with those of capillary networks, and later with innervation, particularly by sympathetic nerve endings.

When replete with triglyceride, the differentiated white fat cell (white adipocyte) is normally a large spherical cell (70–120 μm in diameter, containing 0.2–0.7 μg of lipid) (Fig. 1.1).[4,5] The central, vast lipid globule, comprised predominantly of triglyceride, compresses the cytoplasm and nucleus against the plasma membrane, resulting in a flimsy cytoplasmic rim and a flattened nucleus that bulges the limiting membrane to manifest the characteristic "signet-ring" appearance (Figs. 1.1 and 1.2). In view of its spherical shape, a given change in diameter results in a 100-fold greater alteration in volume and, hence, triglyceride content. Thus, the flexible fat cell is remarkably adapted to accommodate large quantities of reserve fuel during nutritional plenitude, and to contract during starvation. The profuse vascular and neural supplies mediate these adaptations.

The brown fat cell is smaller (at 25 to 40 μm in diameter) than the white adipocyte and is polygonal in shape.[4,5] Instead of a central lipid globule, numerous small, triglyceride-enriched inclusions are present. Quite characteristic for brown adipocytes are the abundant (brownish) mitochondria, which are deeply invaginated, giving rise to many characteristic cristae.[4,5] Brown adipose tissue is even more profusely vascularized and innervated than its white counterpart, allowing ready access of catecholamines, which trigger reactions in mitochondria resulting in non-shivering thermogenesis. This process is critical at birth and during early neonatal life. However, in human beings, brown adipose tissue is practically absent after the first year of life, and will not be considered further.[1] From this point on the term fat cell (adipocyte) or adipose tissue will refer exclusively to the "white" form.

In addition to its vital role in energy storage and release of energy-yielding fatty acids, the adipocyte subserves other interesting functions. Indeed, fat tissue is important for thermal and mechanical insulation, body configuration with its cosmetic effects, and buoyancy. Additional functions, which will be described in later sections, comprise low-density lipoprotein (LDL) and high-density lipoprotein (HDL) metabolism, with storage of excessive cholesterol, and formation of estrogens from androgens. Further, fat cells take up and store to variable degrees lipid-soluble vitamins as well as hydrophobic drugs (hence, tissue distribution of anesthetics and other pharmacologic agents may require consideration when determining dosage in appreciably obese persons) and environmental toxins.

It should be emphasized that in vivo (as opposed to cell culture) the fat cell is structurally and functionally closely linked to cap-

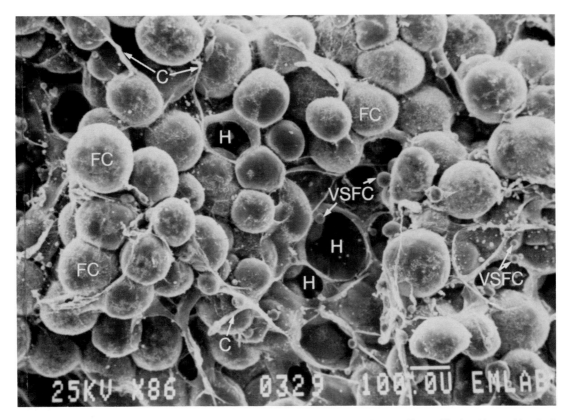

FIGURE 1.1. A Scanning Electron Microscopic View of Human Subcutaneous Adipose Tissue Obtained from a Massively Obese 34-Year-Old Woman Undergoing Gastroplasty. Small fragments (2 × 2 mm) were prefixed in 4% formaldehyde-5% glutaraldehyde (pH 7.4), then washed and fixed in 2% osmium tetroxide. The fixed tissue fragments were dehydrated in graded ethanol and subjected to critical point drying. The specimens were then gold-coated and examined. Note the large mature fat cells (FC) separated by collagen fibers (C) which serve as a support matrix. Many very small fat cells (VSFC) are also evident. Honeycomb cavities (H) are spaces once occupied by fat cells that were dislodged while processing. Magnification × 85, and a 100 μm marker is shown (P. Julien and A. Angel, unpublished).

illaries (at least one per adipocyte), which supply nutrients, other growth factors, and hormones, and is connected to nerve endings, particularly those from the sympathetic nervous system, critical for lipid mobilization. Thus, the fat cell-capillaries-nerve endings should be considered the "Functional Unit."

GROWTH AND DEVELOPMENT OF ADIPOSE TISSUE

Mature fat cells are derived from fibroblast-like cells, termed adipocyte precursors.[3-5] These have the ability to multiply, and the potential to differentiate into mature adipocytes. These triglyceride-laden cells no longer can replicate. Recent studies have indicated that adipocyte precursors are present not only up to completion of puberty, but throughout life.[1,3,6-8]

Appreciable accumulation of triglyceride takes place during the third trimester in differentiating adipocyte precursors, many of which mature completely (hence the extreme leanness of premature infants).[1] The body fat content of full-term neonates is about 1/25 that of normal adults, i.e., about 1/5 the number of adipocytes containing 1/5 the quantity of fat.

Normally, a rise in the total *number* of adipocytes takes place from late fetal life up to completion of puberty, when adult values are attained.[1] Recent evidence has refuted previous suggestions of intense replication of adipocyte precursors during the first postnatal year as a result of overeating.[1] Rather, precursor replication may be accelerated shortly before birth and, particularly in girls, at puberty.[1]

As far as *size* is concerned, substantial en-

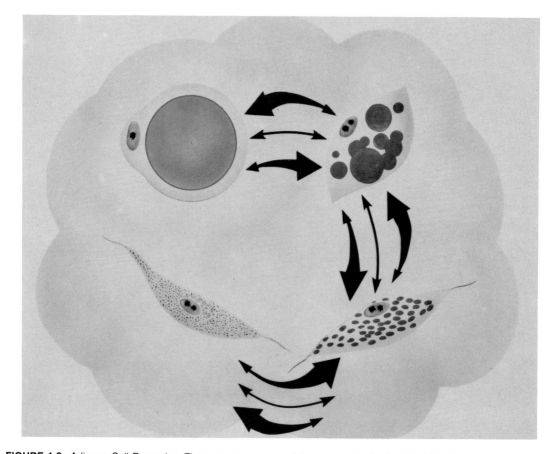

FIGURE 1.2. Adipose Cell Dynamics. The ↔ arrows represent the proposed situation in which the rates of replication and differentiation of adipocyte precursors (depicted by the fibroblast-like cell at lower left) are balanced by reverse processes, notably reversion of mature fat cells (depicted by the "signet-ring" cell at upper left) described in text. This situation would apply to an adult with steady body fat content in which a normal total number of adipocytes is maintained by a dynamic equilibrium between the mentioned processes. The arrows with thick ends pointing counterclockwise represent the proposed situation in which exaggerated degrees of replication and differentiation of adipose precursors result in adipocyte hyperplasia, as might occur in a person susceptible to the development of massive obesity, under conditions of energy excess. The arrows with the thick ends pointing clockwise represent the hypothetical situation in which sustained energy deficiency induces exaggerated reversion of mature fat cells and suppresses replication and differentiation of adipocyte precursors; thus, the adipocyte hyperplasia of massive obesity is potentially reversible by prolonged compliance to dietary and exercise programs. (Modified from Roncari DAK, Van RLR (6): Clin Invest Med 1:71–79, 1978, by permission.)

largement of fat cells does occur during the first year of life.[1] As mentioned, further enlargement normally occurs up to the end of puberty. Up to this point, adipocytes and their precursors have been considered as if they behaved uniformly throughout the various fat tissue regions comprising the "adipose organ." On the contrary, regional specialization conferring structural and functional flexibility is a distinction of the "adipose organ." For example, the size of gluteal fat cells enlarges, particularly in pubertal girls.[9] The hormonal basis for this topologic selectivity will be described.

HORMONAL AND GROWTH FACTOR CONTROL OF ADIPOSE CELL NUMBER

A novel group of anterior pituitary proteins, which stimulate the replication of cultured adipocyte precursors, has been recently recognized and characterized.[3,10,11] These factors might function as primary messengers (hormones) in a brain (hypothalamic)-pituitary-adipose axis, regulating adipose tissue mass through their influence on cell number. (Of course, appreciable influence on mass only occurs after the newly-formed precursors differentiate or mature into triglyceride-laden fat cells.) We have termed these pituitary proteins ''adipocyte (mesenchymal) growth factors,'' because they stimulate the replication of not only adipocyte precursors, but also such other mesenchymal cells as cultured fibroblasts and chondrocytes.[3] Pituitary fibroblast growth factor(s), previously shown to be also mitogenic on adipocyte precursors, might be related to the recently recognized pituitary proteins.[10] Our research should soon determine whether the ''adipocyte (mesenchymal) growth factors'' play a pathogenetic role in certain categories of obesity.

17-β-estradiol is the only ''classical'' hormone known to result in promotion of cultured adipocyte precursor replication.[9] It is probable that this effect of 17-β-estradiol contributes to the pubertal changes in adipose tissue distribution occurring in girls. It is possible that estrogens are not directly mitogenic, but induce the synthesis in adipose cells of paracrine/autocrine factors stimulating the multiplication of adipocyte precursors. Indeed, we have discovered recently that 17-β-estradiol promotes the production of the human adipose cell paracrine/autocrine trophic proteins.

Pancreatic polypeptide suppresses the replication of adipocyte precursors in vitro.[10] Very recently, we have confirmed this effect in vivo, indicating the probably profound significance of this phenomenon. Thus, pancreatic polypeptide might oppose the influence of mitogenic factors, and its sustained elevation might lead to contraction of body fat content through inhibition of adipocyte precursor multiplication. It is intriguing that pancreatic polypeptide levels may be decreased in some obese subjects, and that this hormone is not appreciably released in response to nutritional stimuli in genetic types of rodent obesity and in children with the Prader-Willi syndrome.[1]

HORMONAL AND GROWTH FACTOR CONTROL OF ADIPOSE CELL SIZE

To expand adipose tissue mass, differentiation or maturation of adipocyte precursors or lipid-depleted adipocytes must occur. Insulin plays the predominant role in the enlargement of adipocytes and their precursors, both in the normal size range and the marked further expansion achievable in obesity.[1] Glucose-dependent insulinotropic polypeptide (gastric inhibitory polypeptide, GIP) and in-

sulin-like growth factor I may also modulate adipocyte enlargement through their influence on lipoprotein lipase, as will be described.

Culture systems have recently indicated that growth hormone is a potent inducer of adipocyte differentiation in fetal cells.[12,13] This effect is not evident in cultured adipocyte precursors from post-natal fat tissue. The absence of an appreciable influence of growth hormone in early in vivo studies in rats may support the fact that this hormone could only induce differentiation during fetal life.[14] Additional factors are undoubtedly involved in promoting adipocyte differentiation, including paracrine/autocrine substances recently recognized by us, and as yet uncharacterized circulating compounds.

In addition to their effect on the replication of adipocyte precursors, estrogens affect the size of fat cells.[9,15] However, this influence is relatively selective, being most prominent in depots around the pelvic girdle. Thus, estrogens lead to pubertal alterations in adipose tissue distribution by increasing both cell number and adipocyte size in certain depots.

Glucocorticoid hormones have opposite effects on adipose cell size, depending on the anatomic site of a particular depot.[16] As exemplified dramatically by Cushing's syndrome, facial, nuchal, periscapular and truncal adipose tissue regions expand, while those in the limbs contract. This redistribution of lipid is an extreme demonstration of topologic specialization of adipose tissue.

While insulin is the major hormone responsible for enlargement of adipocytes, catecholamines (norepinephrine from the sympathetic nervous system and the adrenal medulla and epinephrine from the adrenal), through their β-adrenergic influence, are the predominant effectors of fat cell contraction.[1] The varying strengths of the effects of insulin and catecholamines in different adipose depots will be described in an ensuing section.

In contrast to hormones that promote differentiation, culture systems have indicated that oxytocin, a hormone circulating even in non-parturient women and in men in whom its function is not known, inhibits adipocyte maturation.[17] Oxytocin has specific receptors on adipose cells and it had been previously demonstrated that it has both insulin-like (e.g., stimulation of glucose transport and utilization) and anti-insulin metabolic effects. The potentially great significance of inhibition by oxytocin of adipocyte maturation requires exploration in vivo.

NEWER CONCEPT WHICH INVOKES DYNAMIC ADIPOSE CELL KINETICS IN ADULTS

The realization that adipocyte precursors capable of multiplication and maturation into fat cells in culture are present in fat tissue of adults, inspired the development of a newer concept invoking dynamic adipose cell kinetics throughout life (Fig. 1.2).[1,6-8] This concept is now widely accepted and is receiving increasing corroboration from in vivo studies.[1]

Not only can adipocyte precursors replicate and differentiate into mature fat cells, but the latter can also revert to elongated, triglyceride-depleted cells which have regained the ability to multiply, and resemble adipocyte precursors (Fig. 1.2).[7,18] We have proposed that, as also appears to be the case for such other mesenchymal cells as chondrocytes, adipocytes might not engage in terminal differentiation.[1,7,18] Rather, during sustained energy deficiency, the total number of mature fat cells might decrease on a longterm basis by reversion to fibroblast-like cells (Fig. 1.2). Such reversibility would confer onto adipose tissue an extra dimension of plasticity, superimposed upon the more rapid responses of expansion and contraction of adipocytes resulting from short-term energy overload or insufficiency.

According to the newer concept, during maintenance of a steady body fat content, the processes of adipocyte precursor replication and differentiation are balanced by reversion of mature fat cells to elongated, triglyceride-depleted forms and possibly by a limited degree of necrosis (Fig. 1.2).[1,6-8] Thus, the total number of mature adipocytes would remain the same, but as a consequence of a dynamic equilibrium.

Under conditions of prolonged energy deficiency, in addition to the early contraction of pre-existing mature fat cells, the nutrient energy restriction suppresses the replication of adipocyte precursors.[1,14] In addition, and making the reasonable assumption that the relevant animal experiments can be extrapolated to humans, regular exercise inhibits the formation of new fat cells.[1] Further, and as already referred to, sustained energy restriction may lead to accelerated reversion of differentiated adipocytes. The overall result of suppressed precursor replication and augmented reversion would be protracted decrease in the total number of mature fat cells (Fig. 1.2).

Most persons exposed to relative (i.e., there is wide inter-individual variability in the "energy threshold" beyond which obesity develops) energy overload develop moderate obesity, in which fat cells are enlarged, but not excessive in number.[1] A fraction of the obese population, after an initial hypertrophic response, form supernumerary adipocytes, i.e., develop the adipocyte hyperplasia typical of massive obesity, as follows.[1,3] Genetic factors are almost certainly operative in this abnormal proliferative response.

CELLULAR ABNORMALITIES IN MASSIVE OBESITY

Subjects with massive obesity characteristically have an excessive total number of mature fat cells.[1] What is the basis for this hypercellularity? Our cell culture system has revealed that omental adipocyte precursors from massively corpulent persons replicate to a significantly greater extent than cells from either lean or moderately obese subjects (Fig. 1.2).[1,8,19] Cells from almost all the 140 massively obese individuals studied had this property. The excessive multiplication persists in successive subcultures, indicating that this phenomenon is not due to any alterations in circulating or other factors external to adipose cells. Furthermore, the inordinate proliferation is not secondary to any factors associated with the development of massive corpulence, because the exaggerated multiplication of precursors in vitro persisted even in cells derived from the few subjects whose massive adiposity was corrected. As expected, this inordinate proliferation is accounted by the existence of clones of adipocyte precursors with the inherent capacity for excessive multiplication (Fig. 1.2).[8] In addition, fat tissue in massive obesity contains precursor clones with the unusual property of spontaneous differentiation (Fig. 1.2).[8]

What mediates exaggerated replication and differentiation of adipocyte precursors from massively obese persons? Our discovery of paracrine/autocrine adipose tissue growth factors may provide at least a partial explanation.[3] We have recently found that cultured adipose cells derived from massively obese individuals produce these paracrine/autocrine proteins in much greater abundance (or potency) than analogous cells from lean subjects.[3,19a] These mitogenic substances may explain, at least partly, the excessive proliferation of adipocyte precursors in massive corpulence. This abnormality may well be linked to inordinately high production of adipose tissue paracrine/autocrine factors that promote adipocyte differentiation, probably explaining the unusual propensity to maturation of precursors. The sequence in which excessive adipocyte precursor replication is coupled to inordinate differentiation would lead to the hyperplasia of mature fat cells characteristic of massive obesity (Fig. 1.2). The paracrine/autocrine trophic effects of substances produced in fat tissue itself, acting excessively on neighboring adipocyte precursors, would confer onto adipose tissue of the massively corpulent, partial autonomy (from circulating and other factors external to this tissue), conspiring with environmental stimuli to amplify the adiposity. Since massive obesity is more common in women, do estrogens, which appear to induce the production of the paracrine/autocrine factors, play a contributory role in susceptible subjects?

The newer concept invoking a dynamic cellular state in adipose tissue throughout life readily explains the development of massive obesity during adult life. While marked corpulence onsets most commonly during childhood or puberty, some persons do not become exposed to the necessary environmental triggers until adulthood. Then, adoption of pronounced overeating and physical underactivity would trigger the probably genetically programmed cellular abnormalities required for the transition from hypertrophic to hypertrophic-hypercellular obesity.

Replication of cultured fibroblast-like, triglyceride-depleted cells that had reverted from mature fat cells is also unusual in the case of cells obtained from the massively corpulent. Indeed, these reverted cells proliferate to a significantly greater extent, in successive subcultures, than either reverted cells from lean or moderately obese individuals, or the latter's adipocyte precursors.[18] Thus, the mature adipocytes in massive adiposity, which like the differentiated fat cells from any other person have lost the ability to multiply, have retained the "memory" related to excessive growth, because after regaining replicative capacity, they proliferate excessively.

Extrapolation of these findings to in vivo situations might partly explain the development of progressively more severe corpulence through cycles of compliance to appropriate nutrient energy intake coupled to regular exercise, and relapse, i.e., energy overload. During prolonged compliance, not only would the enlarged mature fat cells contract (a relatively earlier event), but reversion to fibroblast-like forms would proceed more rapidly (Fig. 1.2). However, each relapse to overeating and sedentariness would trigger the probably genetically programmed excessive replication and maturation of adipocyte precursors. Thus, cycles of compliance-relapse would eventuate in a progressively greater complement of supernumerary, enlarged adipocytes, accommodating the enormous quantities of triglyceride stored in massive corpulence (Fig. 1.2). On the hopeful side, sustained compliance to healthful eating and exercise habits might even lead to eventual reversion of the adipocyte hyperplasia (Fig. 1.2).

REGIONAL VARIATION IN ADIPOSE TISSUE GROWTH

In experimental animals and most probably in humans as well, different adipose tissue regions reveal varying capability for growth.[20,21] Thus, in addition to the regionally diverse responsivity to hormones already described, precursors from different sites are endowed with inherent variability in capacity for replication and differentiation. This topologic disparity is due to differences in clonal composition. Thus, some depots contain adipocyte precursor clones with much greater potential for proliferation and maturation. Such properties probably contribute to dissimilar expansion of different depots within a subject. In addition, clonal variations between subjects may explain inter-individual variability upon exposure to the same energy load, both in terms of specific regions and total body fat content.[20,21]

Indeed, it has been proposed that some subjects have precursors that not only proliferate and mature excessively, but that these, and their derivatives, the young fat cells (in analogy to young erythrocytes) also function with unusual efficiency.[20–22] For example, they might have inordinately high lipoprotein lipase activity, thus "pulling in" excessive quantities of circulating triglycerides, with a consequent susceptibility to develop regional adiposity or obesity. The function of lipoprotein lipase and its possible relation to corpulence will now be described.

CONTROL OF TRIGLYCERIDE CONTENT IN FAT CELLS

In an appropriately nourished person, most of the fat cell is comprised of triglyceride. Thus, cell size is mainly determined by the content of this storage lipid. This section will outline the physiologic mechanisms mediating A) triglyceride accretion, and B) mobilization of lipid. Relevant pathophysiologic events will also be pointed out.

A. TRIGLYCERIDE ACCRETION

i. Assimilation of Exogenous Lipids

Most dietary lipids, after absorption in the small intestine, are packaged into chylomicrons. While these particles consist of a variety of lipids and of apolipoproteins, triglyceride is the main component. Chylomicrons eventually gain access to the capillary bed of adipose tissue (as well as skeletal and heart muscle), where most triglycerides are cleaved by lipoprotein lipase (Fig. 1.2).[1] This interesting enzyme is formed in and released by mature and differentiating adipocytes, reaching neighboring capillaries, to whose endothelial wall lipoprotein lipase becomes attached through (endothelial) heparan sulfate stalks. At this site, lipoprotein lipase catalyzes hydrolysis of lipoprotein-triglycerides (Fig. 1.3). The freed fatty acids traverse the membranes of endothelial cells, pericytes and adipocytes. Contrary to previous notions of passive diffusion, recent evidence indicates that long-chain fatty acids permeate adipocytes through the specific mediation of protein transporters.[23]

ii. Assimilation of Endogenous Lipids

When the energy available to an individual exceeds the metabolic and other needs, it is converted mainly to chemical storage in the form of glycogen and triglyceride.[1] During fasting, glycogen (mainly in liver, but small quantities are also stored in adipocytes) can only satisfy energy needs for little longer than 24 hours, whereas adipocyte triglyceride is the predominant reserve fuel, as described. For such eventual storage, surfeit energy is channeled to hepatic production of triglycerides. These and other endogenous lipids, as well as specific apolipoproteins, are packaged into very-low-density lipoproteins (VLDL), which are secreted into the circulation to reach fat tissue as well as skeletal and heart muscle. The VLDL-triglycerides are

then cleaved by lipoprotein lipase, and the freed fatty acids taken up by adipocytes, as described for chylomicrons, and most are eventually stored as components of triglycerides (Fig. 1.3).[1]

iii. Physiologic and Pathophysiologic Role of Lipoprotein Lipase

Thus, lipoprotein lipase plays a critical role in the assimilation of lipid, from the circulation into fat cells, as also indicated by the severe hypertriglyceridemia that characterizes syndromes of congenital and acquired (e.g., renal failure) depression of this enzyme's activity.[1,3,22] At the physiologic level, lipoprotein lipase is dependent on appropriate nutrition and insulin levels for its normal synthesis and activity. The marked hypertriglyceridemia associated with diabetic ketoacidosis is not only due to excessive production of VLDL, but also to lipoprotein lipase deficiency.[1] For "fine-tuning" of lipid assimilation from the circulation, the intestinal hormone, glucose-dependent insulinotropic polypeptide (gastric inhibitory polypeptide, GIP), which is secreted in response to dietary fat, also enhances lipoprotein lipase activity.[1,22] Very recently, evidence has been adduced suggesting that an insulin-like growth factor, produced in adipose tissue itself, may promote the synthesis of lipoprotein lipase in neighboring adipocyte cells (i.e., through a paracrine mechanism).[24] Disparities in lipoprotein lipase activity in different adipose tissue regions, and in different organs, in response to prolactin, will be discussed in an ensuing section.

Lipoprotein lipase activity is elevated in adipocytes of obese subjects.[25] It was thought that this deviation, like most of the other metabolic abnormalities associated with adiposity, is reversible upon correction of the obesity. On the contrary, weight loss resulted in even further elevation of lipoprotein lipase activity (per adipocyte) in most of the group of obese subjects.[25] It was postulated that this finding may indicate a primary abnormality mediating the development of obesity, and rendering these subjects particularly vulnerable to its recurrence after weight loss resulting from nutrient energy restriction.[25]

iv. Plasma Glucose is the Major Source of the Glycerol Backbone of Triglycerides

Just as circulating lipoprotein-triglycerides are the main source of the fatty acyl ("fatty

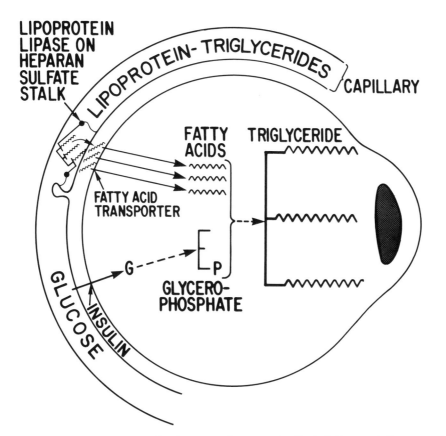

FIGURE 1.3. Lipid Assimilation, Triglyceride Synthesis, and Storage in the Fat Cell. Lipoprotein lipase, synthesized and released by the fat cell, becomes affixed to heparan sulfate "stalks" on the endothelium of neighboring capillaries, where it cleaves the triglyceride ( ) components of chylomicrons and very-low-density lipoproteins. The freed fatty acids ( ) gain access to the interstitial fluid, and are carried through the plasma membrane of the adipocyte by a specific transporter. Thus, circulating lipoprotein-triglycerides are the major source of the fatty "acid" (acyl) chains of adipocyte triglycerides. Plasma glucose, which depends on insulin for transport across the plasma membrane of the fat cell, is the predominant source of the glycerol backbone of adipocyte triglycerides.

Glycerophosphate derived by glycolysis is esterified by the "activated" fatty acids (fatty acyl-CoA), and the series of subsequent reactions yield triglyceride, which is eventually stored in the central globule of the fat cell, under conditions of nutritional plenty and appropriate insulin action.

acid") components of adipocyte triglycerides, plasma glucose is the predominant source of the glycerol backbone of these triglycerides.[1,3] After binding to specific receptors on the cell surface of fat cells, insulin triggers chains of events responsible for this hormone's life-sustaining functions, some in the cell interior and others on the cell surface. Among the latter, insulin stimulates glucose transport into adipocytes (Fig 1.3).[1,3] Inside the cell, this hormone promotes the activity of a number of ezymes involved in triglyceride formation.

Through glycolysis, glycerophosphate is eventually derived from glucose.[1,3] By esterification of "active" fatty acids (fatty acyl-CoA) with glycerophosphate, dephosphorylation and another esterification step, triglyceride is

eventually formed.[26] Under conditions of nutritional and insulin adequacy, most of the newly-formed triglycerides are incorporated into the central lipid storage globule of adipocytes (Fig. 1.3).

Glucose is also the source of acetyl-CoA, the precursor for fatty acid synthesis.[1,3] Under most conditions, de novo fatty acid synthesis in adipocytes and their precursors is of only minor quantitative significance, since most fatty acyl moieties of stored triglycerides are derived from circulating lipoprotein-triglycerides.[1,3] However, under such rare situations as in subjects with severe deficiency of lipoprotein lipase activity, this accessory mechanism for providing fatty acids to the adipocyte probably becomes quantitatively important.[1,3]

This fact is indicated by the normal adipocyte triglyceride content of these markedly hypertriglyceridemic patients, despite their inability to assimilate circulating lipoprotein-triglycerides into their fat cells. Moreover, since de novo fatty acid synthesis appears to be exaggerated in massive obesity, this pathway might also contribute to the excessive triglyceride accumulation in this state.[27]

B. MOBILIZATION OF LIPID FROM ADIPOCYTES

Mechanisms have evolved for prompt mobilization of stored lipid from fat cells under conditions of negative energy balance, and during acute emergency situations. Indeed, the mobilized fatty acids provide, through oxidation in such organs as liver, heart and skeletal muscle, life-sustaining energy.[1,22,28]

In humans, the principal lipolytic (triglyceride-cleaving) hormones are the catecholamines, epinephrine and norepinephrine.[1] The lipolytic hormones bind to specific receptors on the cell surface of adipocytes (Fig. 1.4).[28] This hormone-receptor interaction triggers a series of events, mediated by the complex of guanine nucleotide-binding regulatory (coupling or G) proteins, the second messenger, cyclic AMP, and a specific protein kinase, resulting in the activation, by phosphorylation, of a unique lipase,"hormone-stimulated lipase."[1,28] The activated lipase catalyzes the hydrolysis of adipocyte triglycerides. The released fatty acids are transported in the circulation bound to albumin, thus reaching several tissues. Through a number of mechanisms, including lipase inactivation by direct dephosphorylation, insulin inhibits lipolysis.[1,22,28]

Since insulin is the dominant hormone responsible for triglyceride formation and storage, a decrease in insulin level is the main influence responsible for lipid mobilization.[1,22] Thus, as insulin levels decline during starvation, the energy stored in the form of triglycerides during times of plenty, is utilized through lipolysis and availability of oxidizable fatty acids.

Under "fight-and-flight" conditions, in addition to inhibition of insulin secretion, catecholamines intensify lipolysis and the consequent fat mobilization.[1,28] Norepinephrine is derived not only from the adrenal medulla, but in even greater abundance from the rich supply of sympathetic nerve terminals impinging upon adipocytes. The lipolytic effect of catecholamines is mediated by the β-adrenergic receptors on the cell surface of fat cells.[1,28] In contrast, α_1 and α_2 adrenergic receptors present in appreciable quantities on adipocytes of some fat tissue regions, and interacting with the same hormones, inhibit lipolysis, a braking mechanism superimposed upon the dominant anti-lipolytic influence of insulin.[1,22,28] Stimulation of α_2 receptors (as by prostaglandin E_2) leads to decreased levels of cyclic AMP, and thus to inhibition of lipolysis.[1,22,28] Stimulation of α_1-adrenergic receptors has an anti-lipolytic effect through complex intracellular interactions including phosphoinositides, inositol triphosphate, diglyceride, and Ca^{++}.[1]

Adenosine, which exerts insulin-like effects, attenuates lipolysis by inhibiting β-adrenergic-stimulated lipolysis.[29,30] After binding to specific receptors (R_i) on fat cells, adenosine acts by stimulating the activity of a specific cyclic AMP phosphodiesterase(s), an enzyme that cleaves the second messenger for β-adrenergic agonists, cyclic AMP.[29] Like the receptor-coupling (G) protein systems, the adenosine receptor is modulated (its affinity is decreased) by guanine nucleotides.

Thyroid hormones (T_3) and glucocorticoid hormones (cortisol) facilitate lipolysis.[28] In view of these facts and those described in the previous sections, the pathophysiologic mechanisms responsible for the dampened fatty acid mobilization in hypothyroidism (and in adrenocortical insufficiency) are becoming clearer. There is depressed activity of coupling (G) proteins and of other transmitters of β-adrenergic action, partly related to and amplified by "dominance" of α_1-adrenergic activity in certain adipose tissue regions.[22] Augmented adenosine levels in adipocytes might also contribute to the attenuation of catecholamine-stimulated lipolysis in hypothyroidism.[30]

During starvation, "physiologic" hypoinsulinemia is mainly responsible for fat mobilization; sympathetic nervous system activity is actually decreased.[1,22] Clinically significant ketoacidosis (in the absence of associated substantial ethanol intake) does not occur. By comparison, during acute insulin deficiency, the "stress" associated with this setting, including the contraction of body fluid compartments, results in marked sympathoadrenal stimulation and much more intense lipolysis and mobilization of fatty acids from adipose tissue.[1] This massive release of acids, in concert with high glucagon/insulin

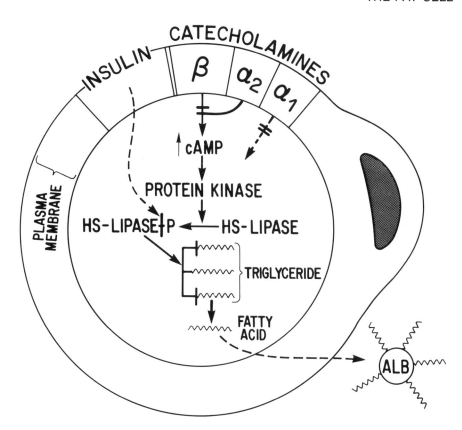

FIGURE 1.4. Lipid Mobilization from the Fat Cell. Epinephrine and norepinephrine, through their β-adrenergic effects, are the most potent lipolytic (triglyceride-cleaving) agents in humans. Acting through the plasma membrane β-receptor, coupling (G) proteins, cyclic AMP (cAMP), and protein kinase(s), these catecholamines lead to the activation, by phosphorylation, of hormone-sensitive (HS)-lipase. Insulin exerts the predominant anti-lipolytic influence, partly by leading directly to dephosphorylation of HS-lipase-P. α_2-adrenergic (by decreasing cAMP levels) and α_1-adrenergic stimuli inhibit lipolysis.

After catalysis of triglyceride hydrolysis by the active hormone-sensitive lipase, the free fatty acids are mobilized from the fat cell and gain access to the plasma, where they are carried by albumin to such sites of oxidation as liver (the partial hepatic oxidation products, β-hydroxybutyrate and acetoacetate, are indispensable to the brain during prolonged starvation), as well as cardiac and skeletal muscle, where they provide life-sustaining energy under conditions of energy deprivation.

ratios in liver, results in life-threatening ketoacidosis in untreated insulin-dependent (Type I) diabetes.

Since insulopenia and the resulting accentuation of fat mobilization result in contraction of adipose tissue, one might expect that lipolysis is inhibited as fat tissue expands during the development of obesity. This is not the case. As obesity develops or persists, both triglyceride formation and hydrolysis are exaggerated, i.e., triglyceride turnover is accelerated.[1] During expansion, triglyceride synthesis obviously exceeds breakdown. The relative acceleration of lipolysis prevents even greater degrees of adiposity. Incidentally, it is characterisitic for such other functions as lipid assimilation, as well as basal and insulin-stim-

ulated glucose transport and utilization, to be augmented proportionally with the size of the fat cell.[15] But with the already described exception of lipoprotein lipase, correction of the adipocyte enlargement during successful treatment of obesity reverses these metabolic abnormalities.[1,25]

Parenthetically, and as an introduction to the discussion of anti-lipolysis, the pathophysiology of non-insulin-dependent (Type II) diabetes associated with obesity is of course quite different from that of Type I diabetes. In Type II diabetes associated with adiposity, hyperinsulinemia and resistance to certain actions of insulin prevail.[1,31] A prominent example is the resistance by insulin-sensitive target cells to insulin-stimulated glucose transport into adipocytes and myocytes.[1,31] Since adipose tissue is only responsible for a small fraction of glucose disposal, the resistance of liver (uncontrolled glycogenolysis and gluconeogenesis) and skeletal muscle (depressed utilization) is mainly responsible for the glucose intolerance or frank Type II diabetes triggered or aggravated by obesity.[1,31] (In this type of diabetes, in addition to a decrement in insulin receptor number which is characteristic of obesity, post-receptor defects, including insufficient insulin-stimulated recruitment of intracellular glucose transporters, occur.)

At least two features of the anti-lipolytic effect of insulin differ from those pertaining to glucose transport. First, only about 1/10 as much insulin is required for inhibition of fat mobilization.[1,31] Secondly, the resistance to insulin actions is not as severe for this hormone's anti-lipolytic effect.[1,31] Thus, increasing impairment of glucose tolerance and progressive obesity proceed concurrently.

During appropriate treatment, the resistance to such actions as insulin-stimulated glucose transport is relieved relatively rapidly.[1] Nutrient energy deficiency promotes, of course, fat mobilization effected mainly by decreased levels of the anti-lipolytic hormone, insulin.[1,22] In addition, exercise has complementary influences that enhance lipid mobilization. Appropriate physical activity may accentuate the depression of insulin levels affected by caloric restriction. Lipolysis may be stimulated further by the exercise-induced rise in catecholamine levels.[1] In fact, adipocytes isolated from physically trained persons respond more briskly to these lipolytic hormones.[1]

FORMATION OF ESTROGENS IN FAT CELLS

In addition to its vital role in lipid metabolism, adipocytes have acquired the interesting property of forming potentially large quantities of estrogens.[1] Indeed, both adipocyte precursors and mature fat cells are capable of converting (aromatizing) androgens to estrogens; i.e., adipose tissue is an important site of extragonadal ("extraglandular") production of female sex-steroid hormones.[32] The main reaction involves aromatization of 3,17-androstenedione, which is of adrenal and ovarian origin, to estrone. While some estrogens are formed in lean, premenopausal women, extragonadal production is the main source in postmenopausal women, and in men of all ages.[1]

Production of estrogens from androgens in fat tissue rises with aging and, increasingly, with progressively greater degrees of obesity, in which it is the predominant site of formation.[1,33] In massive obesity, production of estrone is augmented at least 10-fold, the excessive number of adipocyte precursors and mature fat cells being the additional aromatizing units.[1,33] An amplifying sequence can be envisioned: estrogen production is augmented in fat tissue of obese subjects; the estrogens, partly through increased production of paracrine/autocrine growth factors, exaggerate the formation of precursors and mature fat cells, in turn supplying additional sites for estrogen formation. This sequence would contribute to the aggravation of corpulence in susceptible subjects. The excessive, unregulated formation of estrogen perturbs the hypothalamic-pituitary-ovarian axis, resulting in the increasing incidence of gynecologic problems observed with progressively more severe degrees of corpulence. (Exceptionally obese men have testicular hypofunction for similar reasons.[1])

Recently, a new syndrome characterized by excessive conversion of androgens to estrogens at a number of extragonadal sites, has been described.[34] In addition to the characteristic gynecomastia, some of the men of the reported family manifested the "female pattern" of adipose tissue distribution, a consequence of the systemic, and probably more significantly, the in situ estrogen excess.

The excessive, unregulated production of estrogens has been causally implicated in the genesis and progression of endometrial hyperplasia and neoplasia, conditions strongly associated with obesity, particularly postmenopausally.[1] Similar considerations apply to the weaker association between obesity and carcinoma of the breast.[1]

In adipocyte precursors and mature fat cells, androgens are converted not only to estrogens, but to a lesser extent also to other, at times more potent, androgens.[1] Different subjects vary in the relative degrees to which androgens are channeled to either estrogens or to other pathways, e.g., forming testosterone and dihydrotestosterone.[1] Disproportionate channeling to these potent androgens may lead to the varying degrees of virilization (usually mild) observed in a fraction of obese women.

CONTROL OF CHOLESTEROL CONTENT IN FAT CELLS

Adipose tissue is a major cholesterol storage organ in human subjects and lower animals.[35] While the concentration of cholesterol in fat tissue is in the order of 0.1 to 0.2% of the triglyceride present, the total mass of cholesterol is large because the "organ" normally represents 15 to 20% of body weight. Thus, in normal persons, up to 25% of total body cholesterol is in adipose tissue, and in obesity it is increased proportionally. In massively obese subjects, 50% or more of the total body cholesterol is found in the adipose stores. Adipose cholesterol exists in a dynamic state of turnover with a half-life less than that of triglyceride. In humans, almost all the cholesterol is present in the free, unesterified form and almost all of it is associated with the central oil droplet. In human subjects and in experimental animals, the content of adipose cholesterol is largely determined by fat cell size, but it is also affected by age and dietary cholesterol load;[35] however, the major determinant appears to be fat cell size. Larger fat cells contain more cholesterol than do their smaller counterparts. The adipose cholesterol pool is labile and most readily mobilized by weight loss and mobilization of lipid stores. The rate of triglyceride mobilization from fat tissue exceeds that of cholesterol, resulting in an increase in cholesterol/triglyceride ratio. Cholesterol mobilized from adipose tissue during weight loss is transported to the liver for excretion in bile. This excess cholesterol excretion explains in part the high risk of cholelithiasis observed in massively obese patients following gastrointestinal surgery for weight reduction.

Human adipose tissue derives its cholesterol almost entirely from circulating lipoprotein particles, because the fat cell cannot synthesize cholesterol *de novo* to any significant extent. There appears to be a biosynthetic arrest at the level of squalene, the hydrocarbon precursor which is found in adipose tissue in very high concentrations. The reason for this arrest in human as compared to rat adipose tissue has not been explained.

In studies designed to determine which lipoproteins are involved in cholesterol flux from adipose tissue, it became apparent that the major interstitial lipoproteins, low-density lipoproteins (LDL) and high-density lipoproteins (HDL), could bind and interact with isolated fat cells and purified plasma membranes studied in vitro. Thus, both LDL and HDL specifically bind and interact with human fat cells in a saturable and specific manner.[36] Human LDL is readily bound, internalized and degraded by human fat cells freshly obtained from volunteers, explaining how lipoprotein-cholesterol is delivered to the fat cell. The mode of LDL recognition by the human fat cell is distinct from the classical LDL pathway of Brown and Goldstein, in that it is not regulated by cellular cholesterol content, and does not require prior upregulation for its expression in vitro. LDL-cholesterol is presented primarily in its esterified form, but the adipocyte has a potent cholesterol ester-hydrolase activity which converts the cholesterol ester to its free form. Human fat cells also bind HDL with high affinity[37] and specificity, but this binding appears to be reversible and the HDL apoprotein components are not degraded. These observations suggest that HDL particles serve as acceptors for cholesterol efflux from adipose cells and then as transporters of cholesterol to the liver for excretion.

PLASTICITY AND REGIONAL SPECIALIZATION OF ADIPOSE TISSUE

As already pointed out when discussing replication and differentiation of adipocyte precursors, adipose tissue is endowed with remarkable regional specialization, i.e., different depots reveal varying properties. In 1915, J. Strandberg reported the case of a 12-year-old girl who received a transplant of abdominal "skin" at the site of injury to a wrist; after going through puberty and later developing obesity, the transplant also revealed a marked expansion in adipose tissue mass, forming a large pad over the back of her hand.[38] Another pertinent historic recount relates to the findings in 1938 of F.X. Hausberger, one of the principal pioneers in the field of adipose tissue. Hausberger observed that transplanted fetal tissues in animals would retain their adipose tissue for later development, which would recapitulate what would have occurred at the original location.[38]

In addition to the diversity at the cellular level, different adipose tissue regions disclose striking biochemical and metabolic variation. In women, lipoprotein lipase activity in adipocytes derived from femoral fat tissue is higher than that of cells from subcutaneous abdominal adipose regions.[15] During lactation, this disparity no longer exists, mainly because of a decrease in femoral adipocyte lipoprotein lipase activity. This decrement is related to the influence of prolactin, which suppresses lipoprotein lipase activity in certain adipose depots, while enhancing it in mammary cells, thus channeling energy to the site where it is required for lactation.[1,15]

Glucose metabolism also varies in different adipose tissue regions. For example, femoral fat cells of women have a greater number of insulin receptors, and more active post-receptor machinery.[39] Thus, the greater transport and, of even higher significance, utilization of glucose in femoral as compared to abdominal adipose tissue regions, mainly through the provision of more abundant supplies of the glycerol backbone of triglycerides, would contribute to the relatively greater deposition of fat in the femoral region of women, an accumulation further accentuated in obesity.[39] It is pertinent that adipocytes from certain depots of females respond to insulin to a greater extent than those from males, partly because of higher affinity of the insulin receptor and more efficient post-receptor mechanisms.[40]

The extent of lipolysis also varies considerably in different adipose regions. While topologic variation probably occurs in the number and affinity of β-adrenergic receptors, as well as the plasma membrane transduction and intracellular mediation of their signal, regional disparities have been best studied for adrenergic receptors (both α_1 and α_2), and by reasonable inference, their post-receptor machinery.[22,41] As described, α-adrenergic influences put a brake on lipolysis triggered by β-adrenergic stimulation. Further, regional disparities in the facilitative effect of glucocorticoid hormones on β-adrenergic-stimulated lipolysis probably contribute to the topologic variability, which is expressed dramatically in Cushing's syndrome.[16]

Complementing the alterations in assimilation of lipid from the circulation, already described, are topologic disparities in lipolytic activity. Both in nonpregnant and pregnant (early gestation) women, β-adrenergic-stimulated lipolysis is significantly greater in abdominal than in femoral adipocytes.[15] However, during lactation, the extent of lipolysis is similar in both depots, because of augmented basal and stimulated triglyceride hydrolysis in femoral adipocytes.[15] Thus, the promotion of lipid assimilation and attenuation of lipolysis in femoral adipocytes favor selectively greater triglyceride accumulation in femoral relative to abdominal fat depots. During lactation, decreased assimilation and augmented lipolysis in femoral adipose tissue contribute to diversion of the energy required for milk production and secretion.

The usual metabolic regional differences are probably altered in women with "abdominal obesity," i.e., that characterized by a high "waist/hip circumference ratio."[1] This form of adiposity may be due, at least partly, to "relative androgenicity," as indicated in these women by lowered plasma sex steroid-hormone-binding globulin and raised free testosterone levels.[1] While "truncal" adiposity is common in men, women manifest "peripheral" obesity more commonly, and thus usually have appreciably lesser association with cardiovascular risk factors than men, at comparable degrees of obesity.

SUMMARY AND PROSPECTIVE

The fat cell is remarkably adapted, both structurally and functionally, for energy storage in the form of triglyceride under conditions of nutritional plenty and appropriate insulin availability and action, and for mobilization of lipid under conditions of energy deficiency, a life-sustaining process.

Adipocytes are dependent for growth and function on profuse vascular and neural networks which supply indispensable or regulatory factors, including nutrients, hormones, growth factors, and neurotransmitters.

Throughout life, a dynamic state prevails in adipose tissue: adipocyte precursors can replicate or differentiate, while differentiated fat cells can probably revert to less mature forms. These dynamics are distorted in subjects with massive obesity, resulting in an excessive number of enlarged fat cells. While the cellular abnormalities most probably have a genetic basis, such environmental factors as overeating and sedentariness act as triggers.

In terms of both growth and metabolic behavior, adipose tissue is endowed with conspicuous regional diversity or specialization.

In our opinion, the fundamental question

to be resolved is whether the fat cell, and hence adipose tissue, is primarily responsible for the development of obesity. In other words, are adipocytes of most obese persons unusually efficient in the extraction of circulating lipid and its storage, and is the formation of supernumerary fat cells in massive obesity a primary phenomenon ("pull" concept)? Such active role of adipose tissue should be resolved from the possibility that in most cases of obesity, a primary disorder of energy utilization and interconversion exists, resulting in energy excess, with consequent or secondary accumulation of triglyceride in the fat cell, which would then play a passive role ("push" concept). Resolution of this problem has fundamental scientific and therapeutic implications.

REFERENCES

1. Roncari DAK: Obesity and lipid metabolism. In Spittell JA, Jr, Volpé R (eds): Clinical Medicine. Philadelphia, Harper & Row, 1986, vol 9, chapter 14, pp 1–57.
2. 1983 Metropolitan Height and Weight Tables. Stat Bull Metropol Life Insur Co, 1 Madison Av, New York, NY 10010, 64:2–9, 1983.
3. Roncari DAK: Pre-adipose cell replication and differentiation. Trends Biochem Sci 9:486–489, 1984.
4. Napolitano L: The fine structures of adipose tissues. In Cahill GF, Jr, Renold AE (eds): Adipose Tissue. Handbook of Physiology. Washington, DC, American Physiological Society, 1965, section 5, chapter 12, pp 109–123.
5. Greenwood MRC, Johnson PR: The adipose tissue. In Weiss L (ed): Histology. Cell and Tissue Biology, 5th ed. New York, Elsevier Biomedical, 1983, pp 178–199.
6. Roncari DAK, Van RLR: Adipose tissue cellularity and obesity: New perspectives. Clin Invest Med 1:71–79, 1978.
7. Van RLR, Bayliss CE, Roncari DAK: Cytological and enzymological characterization of adult human adipocyte precursors in culture. J Clin Invest 58:699–704, 1976.
8. Roncari DAK, Lau DCW, Djian P, et al: Culture and cloning of adipocyte precursors from lean and obese subjects: Effects of growth factors. In Angel A, Hollenberg CH, Roncari DAK (eds): The Adipocyte and Obesity. New York, Raven Press, 1983, pp 65–73.
9. Roncari DAK, Van RLR: Promotion of human adipocyte precursor replication by 17-β-estradiol in culture. J Clin Invest 62:503–508, 1978.
10. Roncari DAK: Hormonal influences on the replication and maturation of adipocyte precursors. Int J Obesity 5:547–552, 1981.
11. Lau DCW, Roncari DAK, Yip DK, et al: Purification of a pituitary polypeptide that stimulates the replication of adipocyte precursors. FEBS Lett 153:395–398, 1983.
12. Morikawa M, Nixon T, Green H: Growth hormone and the adipose conversion of 3T3 cells. Cell 29:783–789, 1982.
13. Morikawa M, Green H, Lewis UJ: Activity of human growth hormone and related polypeptides on the adipose conversion of 3T3 cells. Molec Cellular Biol 4:228–231, 1984.
14. Hollenberg CH, Vost A: Regulation of DNA synthesis in fat cells and stromal elements from rat adipose tissue. J Clin Invest 47:2485–2498, 1968.
15. Rebuffe-Scrive M, Enk L, Crona N, et al: Fat cell metabolism in different regions in women. Effect of menstrual cycle, pregnancy, and lactation. J Clin Invest 75:1917–1976, 1985.
16. Lau DCW, Roncari DAK: Effects of glucocorticoid hormones on lipid-synthetic enzymes from different adipose tissue regions and from liver. Can J Biochem Cell Biol 61:1245–1250, 1983.
17. Wilson EJ, Hollenberg MD: Effects of oxytocin and vasopressin on the preadipocyte 3T3-F442A cell line. Biochem Cell Biol 65:211–218, 1987.
18. Roncari DAK, Kindler S, Hollenberg CH: Excessive proliferation in culture of reverted adipocytes from massively obese persons. Metabolism 35:1–4, 1986.
19. Roncari DAK, Lau DCW, Kindler S: Exaggerated replication in culture of adipocyte precursors from massively obese persons. Metabolism 10:425–427, 1981.
19a. Lau DCW, Roncari DAK, Hollenberg CH: Release of mitogenic factors by cultured preadipocytes from massively obese subjects. J Clin Invest 79:632–636, 1987.
20. Djian P, Roncari DAK, Hollenberg CH: Influence of anatomic site and age on the replication and differentiation of rat adipocyte precursors in culture. J Clin Invest 72:1200–1208, 1981.
21. Djian P, Roncari DAK, Hollenberg CH: Adipocyte precursor clones vary in capacity for differentiation. Metabolism 34:880–883, 1985.
22. Hollenberg CH, Roncari DAK, Djian P: Obesity and the fat cell: Future prospects. In Angel A, Hollenberg CH, Roncari DAK (eds): The Adipocyte and Obesity: Cellular and Molecular Mechanisms. New York, Raven Press, 1983, pp 291–300.
23. Abumrad NA, Park JH, Park CR: Permeation of long-chain fatty acids into adipocytes. J Biol Chem 259:8945–8953, 1984.
24. Kern PA, Marshall S, Eckel RH: Regulation of lipoprotein lipase in primary cultures of isolated human adipocytes. J Clin Invest 75:199–208, 1985.
25. Schwartz RS, Brunzell JD: Increase of adipose tissue lipoprotein lipase activity with weight loss. J Clin Invest 67:1425–1430, 1981.
26. Roncari DAK, Hollenberg CH: Esterification of free fatty acids by subcellular preparations of rat adipose tissue. Biochim Biophys Acta 137:446–463, 1967.
27. Angel A, Bray GA: Synthesis of fatty acids and cholesterol by liver, adipose tissue and intestinal mucosa from obese and control patients. Eur J Clin Invest 9:355–362, 1979.
28. Steinberg D, Khoo JC: Hormone-sensitive lipase of adipose tissue. Fed Proc 36:1986–1990, 1977.
29. de Mazancourt P, Giudicelli Y: Guanine nucleotides and adenosine "R_1"-site analogues stimulate the membrane-bound low-K_m cyclic AMP phosphodiesterase of rat adipocytes. FEBS Lett 173:385–388, 1984.
30. Fedholm BB, Vernet L: Accumulation and inactiva-

tion of adenosine by fat cells from hypothyroid rats. Acta Physiol Scand 121:155–163, 1984.

31. Howard BV, Klimes I, Vasques B, et al: The antilipolytic action of insulin in obese subjects with resistance to its glucoregulatory action. J Clin Endocrinol Metab 58:544–548, 1984.

32. Perel E, Killinger DW: The interconversion and aromatization of androgens by human adipose tissue. J Steroid Biochem 10:621–627, 1979.

33. Cleland WH, Mendelson CR, Simpson ER: Effects of aging and obesity on aromatase activity of human adipose cells. J Clin Endocrinol Metab 60:174–177, 1985.

34. Berkovitz GD, Guerami A, Brown TR, et al: Familial gynecomastia with increased extraglandular aromatization of plasma carbon$_{19}$-steroids. J Clin Invest 75:1763–1769, 1985.

35. Angel A, Farkas J: Regulation of cholesterol storage in adipose tissue. J Lipid Res 15:491–499, 1974.

36. Fong B, Rodrigues PO, Angel A: Characterization of low density lipoprotein binding to human adipocytes and adipocyte membranes. J Biol Chem 259:10168–10174, 1984.

37. Fong B, Rodrigues PO, Salter AM, et al: Characterization of high density lipoprotein binding to human adipocyte plasma membranes. J Clin Invest 75:1804–1812, 1985.

38. Cahill GF, Jr, Renold AE: Adipose tissue: a brief history. In Angel A, Hollenberg CH, Roncari DAK (eds): The Adipocyte and Obesity: Cellular and Molecular Mechanisms. New York, Raven Press, 1983, pp 1–7.

39. Bolinder, J, Engfeldt P, Ostman J, et al: Site differences in insulin receptor binding and insulin action in subcutaneous fat of obese females. J Clin Endocrinol Metab 57:455–461, 1983.

40. Guerre-Millo M, Leturque A, Girard J, et al: Increased insulin sensitivity and responsiveness of glucose metabolism in adipocytes from female versus male rats. J Clin Invest 76:109–116, 1985.

41. Burns TW, Langley PE, Terry BE, et al: Pharmacological characterization of adrenergic receptors in human adipocytes. J Clin Invest 67:467–475, 1981.

2

Morbid Obesity—The Problem and Its Consequences

AUBIE ANGEL
JANIS T. WINOCUR
DANIEL A.K. RONCARI

DEFINITION

Obesity is best defined as an abnormal state of health in which there is an excess of body fat. This is a common disorder in the United States and Canada where over 30% of the adult population over age 30 weighs more than the optimum for their height.[1,2] The most serious form of obesity which affects about 3 to 5% of the adult population occurs when the amount of surplus body weight reaches more than 170% above ideal.[3]* This degree of overweight is called massive or morbid obesity to emphasize the serious hazard to physical health and social well-being.

CAUSES AND MECHANISMS

Because of widespread concern about its prevalence, there have been many attempts to clarify the metabolic, psychologic and genetic factors leading to the development of obesity. There is general agreement that it is a complex disorder with multiple etiologies. The simplest explanation of weight gain and adiposity is that it occurs when the calorie (energy) or nutrient intake by an individual is greater than the expenditure of calories to maintain body functions and perform physical activity. These excess calories are stored by the body as fat in the adipose tissue. The traditional view that obese people have gained weight because they either eat more or exercise less than normal-weight individuals is only part of the explanation of the development of obesity. There is remarkable variability in the energy requirements of individuals—some people are able to eat twice as much as others with no weight gain. A study of young thin men who had thin families showed that they could overeat to the extent of doubling their normal caloric intake for a period of many months and show only a small weight gain; as well, the substantial amount of calories required to maintain this weight gain was more than could be explained simply by the increase in body size.[4] In a similar experiment, a group of normal-weight students overfed an extra 1400 calories per day for 4 weeks gained only one-fifth of the amount of weight that would be expected if all of the extra calories were converted to fat.[5] It appears that some individuals have the capacity to use this excess energy by producing increased heat which is then lost to the environment. Thus certain individuals are not

*Calculation of "ideal weight" is discussed in Chapter 7.

obliged to store unneeded calories in the form of fat deposits.[5]

The striking differences in the ability of different individuals to lose weight have also been shown. A group of 29 women with a history of difficulty in losing weight was given a 1500-calorie diet in a closely monitored situation.[6] Twenty of the women lost weight as expected, but nine did not. This latter group of women had lower basal metabolic rates, indicating that their bodies were able to function on less energy than the others.[6] Although most obese people do not have reduced basal metabolic rates, this factor can explain the resistance to weight loss that sometimes occurs. The differences between individuals begin very early in life. Studies of energy expenditure in infants under 6 months of age found no relationship between the amount of milk taken by an infant and size, rate of weight gain, or amount of fat that is deposited.[7] While there is pronounced individual variation in susceptibility to develop obesity, some massively obese persons require a large nutrient energy intake to sustain their corpulence. In these, metabolic studies have indicated that in order to maintain a weight of 160 kg (350 lb), an intake of at least 4500 calories is required. This is more than twice what the average adult would consume.[8]

GENETIC, SOCIAL AND ECONOMIC FACTORS

It has long been obvious that there is a strong familial factor in the development of obesity. For example, 50% of the offspring in families with two obese parents will be overweight.[9] These overweight children have a much greater chance of becoming obese adults than do normal-weight children. On looking back, the early weights of obese adults suggest that they are likely to have begun life as obese infants.[10] Of 6-month-old babies who were among the heaviest 10% in the population, 36% were subsequently found to be overweight in their twenties and thirties, compared to only 14% of the average-weight babies. This is a 2.6-fold difference. It is important, however, to note that the majority of these overweight infants grew to be normal-weight adults.[10] Furthermore, 80% of obese children become obese adults,[11] indicating that obesity in childhood is predictive of adult obesity. The disheartening statistic is that the odds of an overweight adolescent becoming an average-weight adult are 28 to 1.[12]

Evidence supporting genetic determinants of weight and particularly excess weight mounts. Twin studies have suggested that genetic factors override environmental experiences in predicting the development of obesity.[13] These findings have been substantially confirmed in a recent study comparing the adult weights of adopted children to weight profiles of biologic and adoptive parents (N). Overweight adoptees were the issue of overweight biologic parents, and there was no relationship between the body mass index of adoptees and their adoptive parents. The strength of the genetic influence on body fatness is thus emphasized, as the findings indicated that the relationship was present at all levels of body fatness—from the very lean to the very fat.[14]

The development of obesity is also strongly influenced by social, economic, racial and ethnic factors.[15] The relationship between socioeconomic status and the prevalence of obesity, particularly in women, has been noted repeatedly.[15] An examination of the American population reveals that women are more likely than men to be obese. During their early twenties, there are slightly fewer massively obese women than men; during the thirties, the numbers are similar for both sexes, but during the fifth and sixth decades, approximately twice as many women as men are severely obese. In the U.S. the estimated number of severely obese males between the ages of 35 and 74 was 1,600,000, compared to 3,300,000 females between the same ages.[3] One possible factor contributing to the greater tendency of women to obesity may be the higher percentage of fat that women have in their bodies (25%) compared to men, who have approximately 15% of their total body weight as fat.

What is the impact of socio-economic status? In affluent societies, both children and adults from the lower classes are more likely to be overweight.[16] As income increases, the young men are more overweight, while the women, particularly if they marry into higher income families, are thinner. Successive generations of immigrant families also tend to be less obese than the first generation that came to the U.S. Black women are more at risk than white women, while the reverse is true for males. Cultural factors are also important in that different ethnic groups can have different ideals regarding body size and in their attitudes about the denial of pleasure that comes with eating generous quantities of food.

Although obesity is frequently associated with a variety of psychologic problems, it appears that the obese as a group are no more prone to emotional disturbances than are normal-weight individuals.[1] However, the stigma of obesity, in a society which values leanness, places an extra burden on the obese. This burden may involve relatively mild feelings of inferiority for the moderately overweight, but for many of the massively obese, opportunities for normal work and social life are inhibited because of rejection by society. This may become a source of tremendous frustration, anxiety and emotional turmoil.

Indolence has been discussed as an important contributor to obesity. There is a strong correlation between the percentage of men in sedentary occupations and the occurrence of obesity, and this is true in many countries.[17] Also, both obese adults and adolescents are less active than normal weight people under a variety of conditions.[18] However, this decreased activity could be a cause or a result of obesity.

EFFECTS OF PREGNANCY

Pregnancy is a common precursor of obesity. One of the results of pregnancy is a further increase in body fat. The average woman deposits about 9 lb (4 kg) of body fat during her pregnancy.[19] This increased store can be of great value during breast feeding when large amounts of energy are needed for milk production. Many women do in fact lose this excess body fat after delivery, but it is also true that for many women, the onset of obesity coincides with a pregnancy. In general, women who become pregnant tend to be heavier than those who do not have children, and more weight tends to be gained with successive pregnancies.[20] The precise reason for the fat accumulation is not yet known, but there appears to be an increase in food intake during early pregnancy and a decrease in physical activity during the latter period.[21] As well, there may also be an increased efficiency of the metabolic processes during pregnancy. Finally, hormone levels (estrogen and prolactin) increase sharply in mother's blood during pregnancy, and these hormones are known to favor fatty tissue growth.

It has also been shown that the menstrual cycle affects appetite.[22] Food intake increases by about 10% during the postovulatory phase of the cycle, and increased hunger is also reported by many women in the premenstrual phase. These regular periods of increased intake may well contribute to the obese condition of many women.

ADIPOSE TISSUE CHANGES IN OBESITY

Morbidly obese people generally have a greatly increased amount of body fat, comprising 50 to more than 75% of their total body weight.[23] As well, with increasing weight gain, the size of the fat cells increases to an upper limit which occurs when the individual reaches approximately 170% of ideal weight. With further increases in weight, the number of fat cells increases. However, it appears that there is also a minimum size for each fat cell, which tends to be maintained despite efforts at weight loss. In a study of 26 women who had varying numbers of fat cells of different sizes, all of whom were on reduced calorie diets, body weight did not continue to decrease once normal fat cell size was achieved.[24] These increased numbers persist for a long time, despite weight loss. This may explain the ease with which obese people tend to regain lost weight.

The expanded adipose mass has itself been implicated in the pathophysiology of clinical complications. Certain cardiovascular risk factors, notably hypertension, are more commonly associated with 'truncal' or 'abdominal' obesity, a common form of adult-onset obesity, particularly in men.[25] Abdominal adipose tissue is more reactive than gluteal fat and may contribute to hypertriglyceridemia because of increased lipolysis and free fatty acid flux to the liver. Thus regional distribution of adipose accumulation may be an important clinical predictor of future metabolic/cardiovascular complications.[25]

MEDICAL AND SOCIAL COMPLICATIONS

Obesity is associated with a number of serious medical complications which are detrimental to health and longevity. These include cardiovascular and pulmonary disease, obstructive sleep-apnea, stroke, diabetes, gallbladder disease, psychosocial impairment and musculoskeletal disorders affecting the weight-bearing joints.* Massive obesity (body weight greater than 170% of reference values) is particularly hazardous. Of 16 patients whose maximal weight averaged 369 kg, average age at time of death was 35 years.[26] Another report indicates that massively obese men 25–35 years of age suffer from a mortality ratio 12 times greater than that of their lean contemporaries.[27] While remaining excessive, this ratio decreases with age. Massively obese women are also prone to considerable morbidity and mortality, but to a lesser extent.[26]

Obesity has, for some time, been recognized as a factor in the development of coronary heart disease, but its impact was thought to be indirect. However, it now has been shown that longstanding obesity itself increases the risk of coronary disease, congestive heart failure and coronary death.[28] Furthermore, many illnesses that enhance the risk for coronary disease and stroke are aggravated with increasing degrees of overweight. These include hypertension, hypercholesterolemia, hypertriglyceridemia, and hyperglycemia.[1] Persons 20% or more overweight develop high blood pressure ten times more often than do normal-weight individuals.[29] A German study of massively obese individuals showed that 71% of them suffered from high blood pressure.[24] As well, the obese are more likely to have high triglyceride and high cholesterol levels in their blood.[30] There is some evidence which suggests that obesity acquired between the ages of 20 and 40 is more likely to result in development of subsequent cardiovascular disease than is obesity which occurs after 40, although the effect may not be evident until some time after the weight gain.[31]

There is a strong association between obesity and non-insulin dependent (Type II) diabetes, the prevalence of which rises with age, duration, and degree of obesity. Obese people tend to be resistant to both endogenous and exogenous insulin and to have an impaired ability to use circulating glucose.[32] In moderate obesity, the risk of diabetes is about ten times that which would be expected in normal-weight people. In those who are 45% or more overweight, the risk is increased by 30-fold.[33] As well, the severity of glucose intolerance increases with increasing age, duration of obesity, and increasing overweight.

Gallbladder disease occurs more frequently

---

*The complications of massive obesity are also discussed in Chapter 7.

with increasing body weight, e.g., more than one-third of a large group of women aged 45 to 55 who were ≥100% overweight had a history of gallbladder disease.[34] The obese, as well, are more resistant to drug therapy to dissolve gallstones than are normal-weight individuals.[35]

While many conditions appear to worsen with increasing weight levels, some medical complications seem to be related only to massive obesity. These include respiratory disorders (snoring and nocturnal oxygen desaturation)[36]* and liver dysfunction, especially fatty liver.[37]

Massively corpulent persons are prone to the development of mixed central and obstructive sleep-apnea and alveolar hypoventilation, progressing, if untreated, to the full syndrome of pulmonary hypertension (which can be aggravated by the not infrequent pulmonary embolization), right ventricular hypertrophy and failure, and erythrocytosis.[38] This hypoventilation syndrome is responsible for considerable morbidity and mortality. Recent studies have re-emphasized the importance of the central nervous system in this syndrome.[39]

Menstrual irregularities and relative infertility are very common in massive obesity.[40] Extremely obese men also reveal impairment of the hypothalamic-pituitary-testicular axis.[41] In both women and men, the gonadal dysfunction is due to excessive production of estrogens from androgens in the vastly expanded adipose tissue mass. Further, the elevated levels of estrone have been implicated in the increased incidence of endometrial hyperplasia and neoplasia in obese women.

Various dermatitides, notably fungal infections, commonly occur in the redundant, intertriginous regions of the massively obese. Moreover, because of mechanical reasons, they are particularly prone to serious accidents. Relatedly, they have an increased incidence of post-traumatic osteoarthropathy and intervertebral disc disease.

Probably the most painful impact of severe obesity is not the concern for medical risks which it inflicts, but rather the social, economic, and other discrimination which is suffered.[42] It is clear that massive obesity is a stigma in a society that places a high value on thinness and associates overweight with lack of self-control and other character dis-

orders. Overweight children in particular can suffer, as they are perceived by others to be responsible for their condition. By adolescence, many of them have a reduced self-esteem as a result of the rejecting and condemning attitudes of their peers.[43]

TREATMENT

The treatment of obesity must, in some manner, involve a change in the intake and output of energy (calories). In most cases, body weight is most effectively controlled by modifying food intake. However, it is important to emphasize that long-term control of obesity will require more than the mere prescription of a diet; it requires a basic and permanent change in eating behavior and exercise patterns.

Most individuals attempting to lose weight have used one of the multitude of diets or techniques described in the scientific literature and the popular press. These diets can be grouped and discussed according to the approach they advocate. Thus, there are very-low-calorie diets, fasting diets, and numerous combinations of low or high carbohydrate, protein, or fat diets.

The prolonged use of **starvation** or very-low-calorie diets, although effective in producing weight loss, can be dangerous or even deadly. During the late 1970's, the U.S Food and Drug Administration and the Centers for Disease Control investigated 58 deaths associated with the use of **very-low-calorie, protein diets.** The investigation revealed changes in the hearts of victims, similar to those which occur during starvation and protein-calorie malnutrition.[44,45] Even short-term fasting would present a risk to obese people with pre-existing heart disease, because of the danger of cardiac arrest. In addition, prolonged very low calorie regimens have no effect on teaching patients appropriate food habits, and therefore the weight losses are generally not well maintained.[46]

The **low-carbohydrate diet** is a recurring theme. It appears under various names, but its main focus is the elimination or restriction of carbohydrate foods, both sugars and starches. The original principle behind the diet is that food intake is automatically reduced to about 1500 Calories (6300 kJ) when the scheme is followed, because dieters do not substitute other foods to replace the carbohydrate foods which are restricted. These diets have serious shortcomings, however,

---

*Respiratory disorders are discussed in Chapter 6.

including inadequate fiber intake and a high fat content, which promotes coronary artery disease in individuals who already have an increased risk.

A popular notion has been that **high protein diets** are particularly effective in promoting weight loss because of the alleged thermal effect of this nutrient. However, there is no advantage in any weight loss program that promotes excessive amounts of protein.[47] Ideally, a weight loss diet should provide enough carbohydrate to minimize loss of body muscle tissue and enough protein to replace tissue losses and maintain reserves. Adequate amounts of all other essential nutrients such as vitamins and minerals and a decreased number of calories should be provided.

Behavior modification therapy is now commonly used and is based on the idea that obesity is the result of learned inappropriate eating and exercise behaviors, which can be changed by new learning. The standard program includes record keeping to help identify maladaptive eating behaviors, controlling the stimuli which initiate inappropriate eating behavior, modification of the actual act of eating so as to result in a reduced intake, and reinforcement or reward of desirable behaviors. The underlying principle is that an obese person needs to learn to reorganize eating behavior permanently in order to lose weight and maintain the loss. This approach results in modest weight losses during the treatment period, which usually lasts 2 to 3 months. However, maintenance of the weight loss beyond one year is less satisfactory. Over the longer term, weight regains are seen in the majority of patients.[48]

Regular physical exercise is useful in the treatment of obesity in that it uses food calories, facilitating weight loss, and it also appears to have a moderating effect on appetite.[49] More body fat and less lean tissue are lost when diet restriction is combined with exercise than when diet alone is used for weight loss. As well, the increase in basal metabolism produced by exercise helps to maximize weight loss.

Numerous **drugs** have been used in attempts to promote weight loss, but only a few have been found to have been of help, and these only in the initial stages of weight loss. Bulk fillers, such as methylcellulose, have been used on the premise that they increase the amount of bulk in the stomach and therefore reduce hunger. Most of this type of product available on the market, however, contain only a very small dose and there is no evidence that they are effective in reducing food intake.[50] Because of the potential danger of psychologic dependence, abuse, or other undesirable side-effects, drugs to inhibit appetite and bulk fillers should probably be used, if at all, only as short-term aids to assist in beginning a program of weight reduction for those who have great difficulty in adhering to a restricted calorie diet.[51]

Membership in **self-help groups** for the management of obesity such as Weight Watchers and TOPS provides many obese people with a support group to help them in the difficult task of weight loss. An assessment of these groups is difficult, since information about them is restricted by the groups themselves. Although members show weight loss, there is no evidence that these losses are maintained on a long-term basis.

SURGERY

For massively obese individuals who have failed to lose weight by the traditional treatments, and for whom obesity poses serious medical and psychosocial risks, surgery is considered to be an effective treatment.[52] Historically this involved intestinal bypass, an operation which limits the absorption of food which is eaten. Although weight losses with this procedure proved to be adequate, serious complications including severe diarrhea and liver disorders, resulted in the abandoning of this approach in favor of gastric partitioning. This type of surgery restricts the stomach's food capacity, thus effectively limiting the amount of food a person is able to eat at one sitting. A small pouch is created at the top of the stomach with an outlet into the rest of the stomach about the diameter of a pencil. In recent variations of this operation, the outlet is reinforced to prevent its enlarging. Overindulgence at any meal will result in discomfort, nausea and vomiting. This treatment, with its inherent long-term appetite suppression, has been found to result in a substantial weight loss in greater than two-thirds of the patients treated, with most maintaining their loss beyond 2 years.[52,53] As well, patients show very few adverse reactions to gastric staplings, the only one being vomiting, which is usually the result of ingestion of too large quantities of food. With appropriate medical and nutritional follow-up and long-term support, the gastric restrictive operations which have developed offer selected massively obese persons the greatest likelihood of a substantial, well-maintained weight loss of any therapy presently available.

SUMMARY

Obesity represents an adaptive state featuring enlarged adipose mass and conditioned by nutrient excess intake and inadequate energy expenditure. In a very significant proportion of affected people a host of metabolic, cardiovascular and psychosocial complications arise that interfere with well-being and that carry significant risk. Obesity is strongly predictive of future development of hypertension, diabetes mellitus, cholelithiasis, coronary heart disease and stroke. In massively obese persons the frequency of serious cardiopulmonary complications and premature death is staggering. Unfortunately, conventional approaches in the treatment of obesity are not a success story, and the medical management of massive obesity is totally frustrating to patients and their physicians alike. In these patients, gastric restrictive operations together with long-term follow-support by a group emphasizing the principles of behavior modification provide some hope for a salutary outcome. In the short term, gastric plication using the vertical banding procedure in properly selected patients will result in progressive and significant weight loss in the majority. The resultant decrease in nutrient intake that follows often improves the metabolic abnormalities, with amelioration of diabetes mellitus, dyslipoproteinemia and hyperuricemia. Hypertension may also regress dramatically. It would be anticipated that reduction or elimination of these risk factors will be attended by reduction of the development of coronary heart disease and stroke. In any event, improvements in patient compliance, psychosocial adaptation and management of metabolic disorders are often forthcoming. It is hoped that these short-term effects will predict long-term positive value of this approach. We await assessment of accumulating experience.

REFERENCES

1. Kannel WB: Health and obesity: An overview. In Kuo PT, Conn HL, Jr, DeFelice EA (eds): Health and Obesity. New York, Raven Press, 1983, pp 1–19.
2. Nutrition: A national priority. A report by Nutrition Canada to the Department of National Health and Welfare. Ottawa Information Canada, 1973.
3. Abraham S, Johnson CL: Prevalence of severe obesity in adults in the United States. Am J Clin Nutr 33:364–369, 1980.
4. Sims EAH: Experimental obesity, dietary-induced thermogenesis, and their clinical implications. Clin Endocrinol Metab 5:377–395, 1976.
5. Miller DS, Mumford P: Gluttony. 1. An experimental study of overeating low- or high-protein diets. Am J Clin Nutr 20:1212–1222, 1967.
6. Miller DS, Parsonage S: Resistance to slimming: Adaptation or illusion. Lancet 1:773–775, 1975.
7. Morgan J, Mumford P: Preliminary studies of energy expenditure in infants under six months of age. Acta Paediatr Scand 70:15–19, 1970.
8. Drenick EJ: Definition and health consequences of morbid obesity. Surg Clin North Am 59:963–976, 1979.
9. Mayer J: Correlation between metabolism and feeding behavior and multiple etiology of obesity. Bull NY Acad Med 33:744–761, 1957.
10. Charney E, Goodman HC, McBride M, et al: Childhood antecedents of adult obesity. Do chubby infants become chubby adults? N Engl J Med 295:6–9, 1976.
11. Abraham S, Nordsieck M: Relationship of excess weight in children and adults. Public Health Rep 75:263–273, 1960.
12. Stunkard A, Burt V: Obesity and the body image. II. Age at onset of disturbances in the body image. Am J Psychiatry 123:1443–1447, 1967.
13. Borneson M: The aetiology of obesity in children: a study of 101 twin pairs. Acta Paediatr Scand 65:279–287, 1976.
14. Stunkard AJ, Sorensen TIA, Hanis C, et al: An adoption study of human obesity. N Engl J Med 314:193–198, 1986.
15. Goldblatt PB, Moore ME, Stunkard AJ: Social factors in obesity. JAMA 192:1039–1044, 1965.
16. Garn SM, Clark DC: Trends in fatness and the origins of obesity, Ad Hoc Committee to review the ten-state nutrition survey. Pediatrics 57:443–456, 1976.
17. Keys A: Coronary heart disease in seven countries. Circulation 41 (Suppl I): 1–211, 1970.
18. Geliebter A: Exercise and obesity. In Wolmann BB (ed): Psychological Aspects of Obesity: A Handbook. New York, Van Nostrand Reinhold, 1982, pp 291–310.
19. A report of the Royal College of Physicians: Obesity. J R Coll Physicians Lond 17:5–65, 1983.
20. McKeown T, Record RG: The influence of reproduction on body weight in women. J Endocrinol 15:393–409, 1957.
21. Prentice AM: Variation in maternal dietary intake, birthweight and breast-milk output in the Gambia. In Aebi H, Whitehead R (eds): Maternal Nutrition during Pregnancy and Lactation. A Nestlé Foundation Workshop, Lutry/Lausanne, April 26 and 27, 1979. Berne, Switzerland, Huber, 1980, pp 167–183.
22. Dalvit SP: The effect of the menstrual cycle on patterns of food intake. Am J Clin Nutr 34:1811–1815, 1981.
23. Van Itallie TB, Kral JG: The dilemma of morbid obesity. JAMA 246:999–1003, 1981.

24. Björntorp P, Carlgren G, Isaksson B, et al: Effect of an energy-reduced dietary regimen in relation to adipose tissue cellularity in obese women. Am J Clin Nutr 28:445–452, 1975.

25. Björntorp P: Regional patterns of fat distribution. Ann Intern Med 103:994–995, 1985.

26. Van Itallie TB: Morbid obesity: a hazardous disorder that resists conservative treatment. Am J Clin Nutr 33:358–363, 1980.

27. Drenick EJ, Bale GS, Seltzer F, et al: Excessive mortality and causes of death in morbidly obese men. JAMA 243:443–445, 1980.

28. Hubert HB, Feinleib M, McNamara PM, et al: Obesity as an independent risk factor for cardiovascular disease: A 26-year follow-up of participants in the Framingham heart study. Circulation 67:968–977, 1983.

29. Kannel WB, Brand N, Skinner JJ, Jr, et al: The relation of adiposity to blood pressure and development of hypertension: The Framingham study. Ann Intern Med 67:48–59, 1967.

30. Bray GA, Dahms WT, Greenway FL, et al: Evaluation of the obese patient. 2. Clinical findings. JAMA 235:2008–2010, 1976.

31. Rabkin SW, Mathewson FA, Hsú PH: Relation of body weight to development of ischemic heart disease in a cohort of young North American men after a 26 year observation period. The Manitoba study. Am J Cardiol 39:452–458, 1977.

32. Genuth SM: Plasma insulin and glucose profiles in normal, obese, and diabetic persons. Ann Intern Med 79:812–822, 1973.

33. Weslund K, Nicolaysen R: Ten-year mortality and morbidity related to serum cholesterol. A follow-up of 3751 men aged 40–49. Scand J Clin Lab Invest 30 (Suppl 127): 1–24, 1972.

34. Rim AA, Werner LH, Yserloo BV, et al.: Relationship of obesity and disease in 73,532 weight-conscious women. Public Health Rep 90:40–54, 1975.

35. Iser JH, Maton PN, Murphy GM, et al: Resistance to chenodeoxycholic acid (CDCA) treatment in obese patients with gall stones. Br Med J 1:1509–1512, 1978.

36. Zurillich CW, Sutton FD, Pierson DJ, et al: Decreased hypoxic ventilatory drive in the obesity-hypoventilation syndrome. Am J Med 59:334–348, 1975.

37. Kral JG, Lundholm K, Björntorp P, et al: Hepatic lipid metabolism in severe human obesity. Metabolism 26:1025–1031, 1977.

38. Alexander JK, Amad KH, Cole VM: Observations on some clinical features of extreme obesity, with particular reference to cardiorespiratory effects. Am J Med 32:512–524, 1962.

39. Sampson MG, Grassinok L: Neutromechanical properties in obese patients during carbon dioxide rebreathing. Am J Med 75:81–90, 1983.

40. Garner P: Management of female hyperandrogenic states. Ann R Coll Phys Surg Can 18:458–489, 1985.

41. Glass AR, Swerdloff RS, Bray GA, et al: Low serum testosterone and sex hormone binding globulin in massively obese men. J Clin Endocrinol Metab 45:1211–1219, 1977.

42. Cahnman WJ: The stigma of obesity. Social Q 9:283–299, 1968.

43. Tobias AL, Gordon JB: Social consequences of obesity. J Am Diet Assoc 76:338–342, 1980.

44. Deaths associated with liquid protein diets. Morbidity Mortality Weekly Rep (CDC, US Dept HEW) 26:383, 1977.

45. Van Itallie TB: Liquid protein mayhem. JAMA 240:144–145, 1978.

46. Johnson D, Drenick EJ: Therapeutic fasting in morbid obesity: Long-term follow-up. Arch Intern Med 137:1381–1382, 1977.

47. Apfelbaum M: The effects of very restrictive high protein diets. Clin Endocrinol Metab 5:417–430, 1976.

48. Stunkard AJ, Penick SB: Behavior modification in the treatment of obesity: The problem of maintaining weight loss. Arch Gen Psychiatry 36:801–806, 1979.

49. Stuart RB, Davis B: Slim Chance in a Fat World. Champaign, Ill., Research Press Company, 1972.

50. Evans E, Miller DS: Bulking agents in the treatment of obesity. Nutr Metabol 18:199–203, 1975.

51. Dykes MH: Evaluation of three anorexiants: clortermine hydrochloride (Voranil), fenfluramine hydrochloride (Pondimin), and mazindol (Sanorex). JAMA 230:270–272, 1974.

52. Anderson T, Backer OG, Stokholm KH, et al: Randomized trial of diet and gastroplasty compared with diet alone in morbid obesity. N Engl J Med 310:352–356, 1984.

53. Deitel M., Jones BA, Petrov I, et al: Vertical banded gastroplasty: results in 233 patients, Can J Surg 29:322–324, 1986.

3

Conservative Treatments for Morbid Obesity

PAULINE S. POWERS

The conservative treatments of obesity include dietary regimens (both moderate calorie-restricted diets and various fasts), exercise, anorectic drugs, behavior therapy, psychotherapy, and self-help groups. Although certain of these treatments may be effective for mild obesity (for example, self-help groups or behavior modification) or moderate obesity (specifically, the protein-sparing fast), there are cogent arguments against their use in their current form in the morbidly obese patient. The problems with the conservative treatments fall into four main categories. 1) The weight loss achieved in patients who are more than 100% above ideal body weight (i.e., those who are morbidly obese) are often clinically irrelevant; e.g., although weight losses of 10 to 15 lb (4.5 kg to 6.8 kg) are frequently achieved in behavior therapy programs and may represent modest success in the mildly obese patient, this is a trivial weight loss in the seriously obese patient. 2) Although some regimens such as the protein-sparing fast (PSF) may produce clinically significant weight losses, the weight loss is not maintained and the patient may regain over the previous highest weight. 3) Although called "conservative" methods, by which is actually meant non-surgical methods, many of these treatments are associated with very significant psychologic sequelae. 4) Some of these regimens may predispose to even greater weight gains.

In this chapter, the psychologic and physiologic hazards of weight loss, and subsequent weight regain, with the conservative treatment methods will be discussed. Then the effectiveness and potential of the most common non-surgical treatment modalities will be addressed.

PSYCHOLOGIC HAZARDS OF CONSERVATIVE METHODS

The reasons for the failure of conservative regimens are multiple, but one shared reason may be that obese individuals are at a higher physiologic "set-point" in terms of fat content and that none of these regimens influence this basic physiologic abnormality. Attempts to change fat content without altering the set-point may set into motion powerful biologic regulatory mechanisms that account for some of the complications associated with these treatment modalities.

Patients who follow low calorie diets, even if obese, may actually be in a state of semi-starvation. Keys and colleagues[1] demonstrated in their experimental semi-starvation study that subjects who were starved were irritable, depressed, preoccupied with food and were likely to overeat if and when food was available. Over 30 years ago, the hazards of dieting were described by Hamburger, who noted that 6 of 18 patients developed emotional problems while dieting.[2] In 1952, Bruch carefully described psychotic episodes which occurred in three obese adolescents who were dieting.[3]

In 1957, Stunkard[4] described a "dieting depression" which had a characteristic temporal sequence: when the decision to diet was made, there were extravagant fantasies about the benefits of weight loss and feelings of euphoria and exultation; about 1 to 3 weeks after the diet began, there was the abrupt onset of anxiety; this was followed by significant symptoms of depression including crying spells, sleep disturbances, and difficulties in functioning. This pattern occurred most often in patients who were severely obese and who had been referred to a special clinic because their obesity was refractory to treatment. However, even among a moderately obese group referred to a general clinic, over 50% had experienced some untoward emotional responses during dieting.

In a study by Halmi and colleagues[5] the emotional responses to weight loss by the usual methods of diet, fasting and drugs were compared to those after gastric and jejunoileal bypass. With the conservative methods, 15% of patients had severe depressive episodes and another 26% were moderately depressed; more than 50% were very preoccupied with food and another 25% moderately preoccupied with food; more than half the patients experienced irritability and anxiety; fewer than one-fourth of the patients had no symptoms. In contrast, patients who had the gastric bypass compared their post-surgical emotional responses to their emotional responses during previous weight loss efforts; more than half were less or much less depressed, anxious, irritable or preoccupied with food after the surgery when losing more weight than when previously dieting. In addition, more than half the patients who had had the gastric bypass reported more feelings of well-being and self-confidence than during previous weight loss efforts. The improvement in body image after gastric bypass is even more striking. Body image is the inner mental view of oneself and the sum of attitudes toward that appearance. The perceptual aspect of body image has tactile, kinesthetic and visual components. Many obese patients overestimate their size and have very derogatory attitudes toward their bodies. In this study, there was a decrease in body image disparagement after surgery in 70% of the patients and it occurred when patients had lost only small amounts of weight. It is as yet unclear whether the perceptual aspect of body image also changes abruptly after surgery. In a small group of obese patients, Leon et al.[6] found that the change in the attitudinal aspect of body image preceded the improvement in the perceptual aspect of body image.

In a report by Anderson and colleagues,[7] 60 morbidly obese patients were randomly assigned to either the protein-sparing fast (a very low calorie diet) or horizontal stapling gastroplasty. Although the maximum weight losses did not differ significantly between groups (26.1 kg in the gastroplasty group and 22 kg in the diet alone group), patients treated with diet not only regained significantly more weight but one-third of these patients developed depressive symptoms. None of the gastroplasty patients had depressive symptoms. In this study, the actual incidence of psychiatric complications may have been underestimated, since follow-up was not by a psychiatrist and no standardized method for determining emotional complications was described.

The factors that determine which patients treated wth conservative methods will develop untoward psychologic responses have not been extensively studied. However, it is known that patients with childhood onset of obesity seem more vulnerable than those with adult onset obesity. Grinker and colleagues[8] reported on 15 obese patients on a very low calorie diet; all 10 with onset of obesity in childhood became sad, anxious and pessimistic during the diet, while none of the 5 whose obesity started in adulthood became depressed. Furthermore, as they lost weight, those who had become obese as children continued to misperceive their body size (i.e., the inaccuracy in the perceptual aspect of body image persisted), while those who became obese in adulthood accurately perceived the decreases in their sizes.

In another study by Rosen and Aniskiewicz,[9] significant differences were found between morbidly obese individuals who decided to have surgery and those who did not. Obese patients who elected surgery had a higher frequency of personality disorders, more psychosocial difficulties (e.g., marital discord, occupational difficulties, etc.), and more feelings of victimization and social isolation. These patients also felt hopeless about achieving weight loss on their own. Solow[10] has described this hopeless posture and posits that the success of surgery may introduce a sense of hope and achievement that generalizes to other areas of the patient's life. In contrast, patients who elected not to have the surgery had not given up hope of achieving weight loss through their own efforts. Thus, it may be that morbidly obese patients who are most likely to develop depression or other untoward psychologic reactions with conservative regimens can be identified; those who select the surgical procedures may be poor candidates for other modes of treatment.[11]

In summary, untoward emotional responses occur during weight loss regimens in the majority of morbidly obese patients, particularly those who have been obese since childhood or who have had previous psychologic complications with weight loss. Methods for identifying that minority of patients who are not at risk have yet to be fully developed. As noted by Stunkard,[12] these studies have also made it clear that in describing psychiatric side-effects of gastric surgery, the control period should not be the time prior to surgery but rather previous periods of weight loss efforts.

BEHAVIOR MODIFICATION

CURRENT STATUS

Classically, there are four parts to a behavioral program for obesity. *First,* the behavior to be controlled is carefully described and documented, often via a daily food intake and exercise diary. *Second,* the stimuli that precede eating are identified; certain situational cues come to be associated with a certain behavior and a certain reinforcing consequence, with the result that the cue influences behavior more each time. For example, turning on the television may be a cue to begin eating snack foods. There may be a chain of behaviors that result in eating. The *third* step is the development of techniques to control the act of eating. For example, patients may be taught to eat more slowly and to associate eating with highly specific stimuli (e.g., they may be asked to use a special place setting or to eat only in the dining room). The *fourth* step is to modify the consequences of eating; a system of formal rewards for changes in eating habits or weight is established.

The use of behavioral methods in the treatment of obesity generated tremendous interest 15 to 20 years ago, when early reports indicated that significant weight losses (4–7 kg) could be achieved in mildly obese patients in group settings in 2 to 3 months.[13,14] Unfortunately, moderately and morbidly obese patients did not lose much more weight than mildly obese individuals,[15] and the clinical significance of a 10 lb (4.5 kg) weight loss in a 300 lb (136 kg) patient is probably trivial. Furthermore, Stunkard and Penick in their classic follow-up study[16] found that after 5 years, most patients had regained the weight lost on a well-designed, carefully supervised program. This and other follow-up studies have clarified the difference between weight loss and maintenance of weight loss.

POTENTIAL APPLICATIONS OF BEHAVIORAL THERAPY

Although behavioral programs are not the primary modality of treatment for morbid obesity, certain behavioral strategies for modifying eating behavior might be effectively incorporated into either a pre-surgical or post-surgical treatment plan.

At the time of initial evaluation, certain eating behaviors may be identified which are poor prognostic signs in terms of adequate post-surgical weight loss. Patients who snack may be able to obviate the effectiveness of gastric restrictive procedures by repeated snacking. There is some preliminary evidence that patients who snack more than two or three times a day preoperatively do not lose as much weight as those who do not,[17] even though after the procedure there is some normalization of eating patterns.[5] It might be that these patients would benefit from a preoperative behavioral program aimed at decreasing snacking, even if significant weight were not lost.

There are some patients who do not comply with dietary restrictions after surgery. For example, one patient currently under our care consumed large quantities of spicy foods immediately after discharge from the hospital and developed a rupture of the suture-line and peritonitis which required several months' hospitalization. Identifying patients who are unable to comply with dietary restrictions may be difficult in one or two evaluation sessions but a required preoperative behavioral program might identify these patients. Lindner and Blackburn[18] required candidates for the protein-sparing fast to pass a behavioral program prior to starting their diet. A similar program in which patients are required to keep diaries of their food intake and exercise and modify the consequences of certain problematic eating behavior prior to surgery, might help identify patients who will not follow postoperative dietary restrictions.

Certain behavior techniques, such as the deposit-refund strategy in which the patient deposits money and receives a partial refund dependent on attendance or other behavior, might be used to improve compliance with diet or follow-up regimens in post-surgical patients. For example, before surgery, patients might be asked to make deposits which would be gradually refunded if dietary proscriptions were followed or appointments were kept. Other behavior strategies might be adapted to improve the effectiveness and safety of surgery.

DIETARY REGIMENS

TRADITIONAL DIETS

Traditional restricted diets in which calories are limited to 1,000 to 1,500 calories do produce weight losses in morbidly obese patients, but it is an unusual patient who continues to follow the regimen long enough to lose adequate weight to reduce the health hazards of serious obesity. Furthermore, nearly all patients regain the lost weight, and many gain more than was lost. Although rarely considered, the physiologic hazards of weight loss followed by weight gain may be greater than that with static obesity.[19] Perhaps most importantly, the psychologic consequences of repeated failure may be devastating. Therefore, traditional dietary regimens are rarely indicated for the morbidly obese patient.

PROTEIN-SPARING FAST

The very low calorie diets, also called the protein-sparing fast (PSF), are the most effective non-surgical treatment of obesity. A recent survery of seven studies by Wadden and colleagues[20] found average weight losses of 20 kg in 12 weeks. The PSF was an outgrowth of early studies on total fasting for obesity. Several investigators found that significant weight losses were achieved with total fasting. Drenick and Smith[21] reported 32 patients who lost 22 kg in 51 days. However, total fasts were associated with significant physiologic hazards, and five deaths were reported by 1970. Furthermore, weight losses were poorly maintained.

The very low calorie diets were designed to produce rapid weight loss while preserving lean body mass by providing dietary protein or protein with carbohydrates. It has been hypothesized that the resulting ketosis produces anorexia, which is therapeutic and allows the patient to comply with the diet more easily. Neither the assumption that lean body mass is preserved nor that the ketosis is therapeutic has been proven. Rosen and colleagues[22] found no relationship between ketosis and anorexia.

The preservation of lean body mass is determined indirectly by the method of measuring nitrogen balance. Howard and associates[23] found that nitrogen balance was not achieved until the sixth week on a diet with 33 g of protein and 44 g of carbohydrate (a dietary prescription similar to that in most regimens utilizing the PSF). In view of these and other findings Blackburn and colleagues[24] have recommended that relatively large amounts of protein be used—1.5 g of protein per kg of ideal body weight (IBW). Several mineral and vitamin supplements are prescribed. Salt is used to decrease diuresis and prevent hypotension. Electrolyte balance, especially potassium and calcium, is maintained with supplementation. Table 3.1 lists the dietary prescription for an obese man whose IBW is 70 kg.

Monitoring Patients on PSF

Patients must be carefully evaluated before the fast and monitored weekly. Before starting the PSF, a complete blood count, urinalysis, SMA6, fasting SMA18, chest X-ray (PA and lateral) and electrocardiogram (EKG) are obtained. Each 3 months on the fast the SMA6 and 18 are repeated. Serum uric acid is re-

TABLE 3.1. PRESCRIPTION FOR PSF FOR A MODERATELY OBESE MAN WITH IBW OF 70 KG

1. 105 g protein/day of animal meat. 1 ounce = 7 g protein. Thus, patient to consume 15 ounces animal meat in 3–5 servings.
2. Fluid intake of 1500–2000 mL (8 8-oz glasses)/day.
3. Table salt at each meal.
4. 3 g K^+ (25 mmol K^+ b.i.d.).
5. Multivitamin with iron and zinc daily.
6. Calcium supplement of 400–800 mg.

peated each week for the first 2 months and then monthly.

If uric acid levels rise above 10 mg% (normal 4–8 mg%) for 2 successive weeks, drug therapy is instituted until serum uric acid levels return to normal for 2 successive weeks.

Electrolytes (SMA6) are detemined monthly unless there are some signs or symptoms of electrolyte depletion, in which case they are monitored weekly. If serum potassium falls 10% below the lower limits of normal, potassium supplementation is increased, and if sodium falls 20% below the lower limits of normal, sodium chloride supplements are increased. If hypokalemia is suspected (even if serum potassium is normal), a strip EKG is obtained in which the most prominent T-waves occurred (usually standard lead 2) to determine if there has been a decrease in the amplitude of the T-waves. If potassium or sodium chloride supplementation is required, the supplementations may be decreased to the usual levels after 2 successive weeks of normal serum levels.

Fasting blood sugar, serum albumin/globulin (A/G) ratio, BUN, serum creatinine and a complete urinalysis should be obtained monthly. If serum A/G ratios fall, patients should be questioned to determine if they are taking the prescribed amount of protein, since some patients may attempt to speed up weight loss by consuming less protein. If they are consuming less than prescribed, they should be encouraged to follow the diet, and the A/G ratios are determined weekly until they return to normal; levels are then checked monthly.

If mean corpuscular hemoglobin concentration drops 10% below lower limits of normal, ferrous gluconate 300 mg t.i.d. is prescribed, and when this measure returns to normal, this additional supplementation is discontinued. If serum creatinine or BUN rises above 10% of the upper limits of normal, patients should be reminded to drink 8 to 10 8-oz glasses of fluid per day, and values usually return to normal.

At weekly visits, patients are weighed, lying and standing blood pressures are obtained, and urine is checked for ketones. During the weight loss phase, the patient is seen weekly, and during this time participates in individual or group nutritional counseling and education and begins to learn and practise the principles of behavior modification.

Contraindications to the PSF

Although most investigators recommend the PSF for patients with moderate obesity (i.e., 60–99% above ideal body weight) as detemined by standard actuarial tables,[25] it is not clear if morbidly obese subjects are suitable candidates. In the study by Anderson and colleagues[7] noted earlier, the morbidly obese patients lost as much weight with the PSF as with horizontal gastroplasty, but not only had a higher incidence of depressive reactions, but also regained significantly more weight after maximum weight loss had been achieved.

All the follow-up studies of the very low calorie diets have shown poor maintenance of weight loss achieved. Genuth and colleagues[26] found that 56% of patients had regained more than one-half the weight lost. Even the best reported results by Lindner and Blackburn[18] reported that patients had regained an average of one-third of the weight lost. Furthermore, the most careful follow-up studies have all been done on moderately obese patients. In view of the severity and chronicity of the problem in morbidly obese patients, it seems likely that relapse rates would be even greater. In addition, complications from the fast may be more likely among the morbidly obese, with their higher incidence of high blood pressure, diabetes, and cardiac disease.

Thus, the potential usefulness of the very low calorie diets in morbidly obese patients seems limited. It is possible that certain very high risk obese patients might be able to lose sufficient weight to qualify for surgery. Patients over 500 lb (227 kg) have an unacceptable predicted intra-surgical mortality rate and hence must lose weight prior to surgery. A carefully supervised very low calorie diet might allow the patient to lose sufficient weight to undergo the surgery.

PSYCHOTHERAPY

Although it has been postulated that obesity is the consequence of major psychologic abnormalities such as unmet oral dependency needs or personality disorders, this proposition has not been proven. The issue has been more carefully studied among morbidly obese patients who are candidates for a surgical procedure than for any other group of obese patients. Halmi and colleagues[27] studied 80 morbidly obese patients who had the gastric bypass operation and found that the lifetime prevalence of major psychiatric diagnoses was 47.5%, with depressive disorders occurring in 28.7% of the total sample. No other diagnoses exceeded 2.5% prevalence. Although this was not a controlled study, the authors cite the epidemiologic study of Weissman and Myers,[28] which found a prevalence of depression of 24.7% among the general population, a prevalence which did not differ significantly from the finding among morbidly obese patients. Of course, it is possible that in the general epidemiologic study, depression and obesity were correlated.

Nonetheless, other studies of morbid obesity suggest that there is no more psychopathology among morbidly obese patients than among matched normal weight controls. Several studies utilizing the Minnesota Multiphasic Personality Inventory have failed to identify significant or consistent abnormalities.[6,29] In view of the very negative attitude society has toward obesity (which begins as early as kindergarten[30]) and the stigmatization invariably experienced by morbidly obese patients, the absence of more significant psychopathology is remarkable.

Of course, since depression and other psychiatric disorders occur in this group as often as in the general population, treatment for specific psychiatric problems may facilitate weight loss. It has been our experience that depressed obese patients treated with antidepressants are able to follow any treatment plan better whether it is diet, exercise or surgery. Similarly, patients who have specific neurotic conflicts related to their obesity should be treated. One particularly common conflict relates to the use of obesity to ward off both sexual impulses and sexual advances. This problem may not be more common among morbidly obese patients than among the general population, but the use of obesity as a shield is unique and should be addressed in psychotherapy either before or during weight loss efforts. Rand and Stunkard[31] have described a group of moderately and mildly obese patients in psychoanalytic psychotherapy who lost weight and had improvement in their body images; these patients had presented for treatment for anxiety and depression rather than obesity.

Obese patients with the binge-eating syndome and the night-eating syndrome are two sub-groups of patients who usually need psychiatric treatment. In 1959, Stunkard[32] first described the binge-eating syndrome among obese patients, and in the last 10 or 15 years a very similar disorder, bulimia, has been described. Although the term, binge-eating syndrome, has been used most often to describe certain obese patients and bulimia has most often been used to describe normal-weight individuals who also purge by various methods, both conditions have three primary characteristics.[33] 1) There is episodic, uncontrolled, impulsive ingestion of large quantities of food within a short period of time. 2) The episode terminates when discomfort occurs (self-induced vomiting is common). 3) The episode is followed by guilt and self-condemnation. Although the binge-eating syndrome may account for only a small percentage of the obese population, it may account for a larger percentage of patients with refractory obesity. Stress frequently precedes episodes of binge-eating, and amongst patients with bulimia, more than 50% have been found to have a major depressive episode. Therefore, patients with the binge-eating syndome should be in psychiatric treatment.

Patients with the night-eating syndrome[34] consume more than 25% of their calories after the evening meal, have insomnia, and have morning anorexia. Although probably fewer than 10% of obese patients have this pattern of eating, it is probably a poor prognostic sign in terms of conventional treatment. Nearly half of the patients reported by Stunkard and colleagues had disabling emotional responses with dieting and only half were able to lose more than one-third of their excess weight with dieting. Periods of stress were found to precede night-eating and thus psychiatric treatment is probably needed.

EXERCISE

ENERGY BALANCE

The principle of homeostatic regulation of energy balance was described by André Mayer.[35] Essentially, he demonstrated that: energy in [intake] minus energy out [accounted for primarily by basal metabolic rate (BMR), activity level, and the thermic effect of food] is equal to the difference in energy reserves [i.e., fat content]. The thermic effect of food refers to the observation that resting oxygen consumption increases after each meal. This concept is illustrated by the following formula:

$$\underset{\text{(food intake)}}{\text{Energy in}} - \underset{\substack{\text{(BMR, activity,} \\ \text{thermic effect} \\ \text{of food)}}}{\text{Energy out}} = \underset{\text{(fat content)}}{\text{Differences in energy reserves}}$$

If food intake exceeds energy expenditure, the difference is stored as fat. If food intake is less than the energy expended, fat stores decrease. Until the last 10 years, the majority of treatment efforts for obesity have been aimed at lowering food intake. Recent work, however, suggests that increasing energy expenditure via exercise may hold more promise, especially for weight loss in mildly obese individuals, for maintenance of weight loss, and for the prevention of obesity.

EFFECT OF DIET ON ENERGY EXPENDITURE

Four assumptions underlie the expectation that restricting calories will result in a weight loss that is proportionate to the calorie deficit. The *first* assumption is that with a decrease in calorie intake, there will be no change in activity levels. There are several studies that suggest that this is not the case and that activity levels do decrease with decreases in food intake.[36,37] The *second* assumption is that basal calorie expenditure is unchanged during dieting. There are now numerous studies demonstrating a decrease in BMR from 10–30% on restricted calorie diets;[38–40] furthermore, the decrease in BMR is greater in chronic dieters, in hyperplastic obesity (i.e., those who have an increase in number of fat cells as well as an increased size of their fat cells), in women, and in the severely obese. The *third*, usually unstated, assumption is that there will be no change in the thermic effect of food. The thermic effect of food expends energy in a least two ways—via the work of intestinal absorption of the food consumed and via hepatic metabolism to amino acids. If less food is consumed, probably there will be a decrease in energy required for these processes. The *fourth* assumption is that the "efficiency" with which energy is supplied by metabolic processes does not change when food intake is restricted; this means that the fraction of total available energy which is converted to adenosine triphosphate (ATP) does not change. There are several studies which suggest that this assumption is also incorrect. Bray[39] has reported reduced activity of the glycerophosphate cycle in obese, non-dieting individuals and a further reduction in two enzymes of this cycle during calorie restriction. When the activity of these enzymes is reduced, it leads to greater efficiency in the formation of ATP, and consequently less weight is lost than predicted.

Thus, reducing calorie intake may result in decreased activity, decreased BMR, decreased thermic effect of food and enhanced efficiency of the glycerophosphate cycle; all these factors may result in less than predicted weight loss.

PROPOSED BENEFITS OF EXERCISE

These and other considerations have resulted in a renewed interest in exercise in the treatment of obesity. It has been proposed that exercise results in a decrease in food intake. In a classic, but now controversial, study by Mayer and colleagues,[41] sedentary individuals were found to consume more calories than moderately active individuals. In a study of eight normal-weight military cadets, exercise resulted in a decrease of calorie intake in the hours following exercise but was compensated for 2 days later.[42] In a study by Björntorp and colleagues[43] of myocardial infarction patients, there was a concomitant decrease in food intake with exercise. Unfortunately, a similar decrease in intake with exercise among severely obese individuals has not been demonstrated.

It has been suggested, but not proven, that exercise prevents the well-known decrease in BMR and decrease in tri-iodothyronine concentration that occurs in calorie restriction.[44] Strenuous exercise has been shown to raise metabolism by 25% above basal levels for 15 hours and 10% for as long as 24 hours in nondieting individuals. However, exercise has not been conclusively demonstrated to counter the low BMR that occurs during calorie restriction, especially among the severely obese.

Exercise has been demonstrated to increase the thermic effect of food by 10% in six normal-weight men who consumed a 1,000-calorie breakfast.[45] Whether exercise would increase the thermic effect of food in obese, dieting patients has not been demonstrated. Similarly, the effect of exercise on the glycerophosphate cycle has not been studied.

LEAN BODY MASS, BASAL METABOLIC RATE AND EXERCISE

Another related aspect of calorie restriction and exercise is lean body mass (LBM). Even moderate calorie restriction produces some loss in lean body tissue. Fasting produces a very significant loss of LBM, with initial losses totalling 75 g of protein per day in the first few days; in the first 30 days, 18–24 g of protein are lost per day.[46] Although designed to spare lean body mass, even the protein-sparing fast results in some loss of LBM, particularly during the first week. Howard and associates[23] have shown that on 33 g of protein and 44 g of carbohydrate, nitrogen balance was not achieved until 6 weeks. Most popular fad diets produce quick weight losses in the first week during which there is a significant loss of LBM. With all calorie-restricted diets, if weight gain follows the initial weight loss, the weight gain is stored primarily as fat rather than returning to lean body stores. Thus, an obese patient who regains weight after losing may be the same weight as prior to the diet, but fat content may be higher and LBM less.

Since BMR is closely related to LBM, a decrease in LBM will result in a decrease in BMR; the metabolic requirements of fat tissue are less than that of LBM. Thus, after weight regain, even at the same weight, the obese individual may require fewer calories to maintain the weight than prior to dieting. This may account for the tendency of obese patients to regain more than the original weight lost. The primary way of increasing LBM is exercise. Obese subjects who have been chronic dieters may have a significant decrease in LBM and hence, theoretically, might benefit from an elevation in their LBM to fat content ratio via exercise.

EXERCISE AND THE MORBIDLY OBESE

Unfortunately, exercise has not been shown to be an effective treatment for morbidly obese patients. In a very careful study of morbidly obese patients by Björntorp and colleagues,[47] exercise alone did not produce either weight loss or a decrease in fat content. Eight patients who had adipose tissue hypercellularity participated in a physical training program for 6 months consisting of 35 minutes three times a week, individualized so that the heart-rate was 10 to 15 beats below maximum for three 5-minute periods during each training session. After 3 months, fasting plasma insulin decreased, and by 6 months, glucose tolerance had also improved and there was a tendency for plasma triglycerides to be at lower levels. However, there was no change in body weight or fat content after 6 months. These findings are in marked contrast to the findings among other groups. In one study by Björntorp and colleagues,[43] a group of patients who had suffered a myocardial infarction showed decreases in body fat from 18.6 kg to 11.6 kg during a 9-month program consisting of 30-minute exercise sessions three times per week. This is a decrease of nearly 40% of original fat content without any decrease in food intake. In studies of normal-weight, middle-aged, sedentary men, training programs of walking[48] or running[49] produced a significant decrease in fat content. In another study of moderately obese middle-aged men, a training program similar to that used in the study of morbidly obese patients resulted in a weight loss of 4.5 kg.[50]

In a review of the studies utilizing exercise to treat obesity, Epstein and Wing[51] found that heavier subjects who exercised lost more weight than lighter subjects. However, most of the subjects described as "heavier" were mildly or moderately obese, and the weight losses were small. Furthermore, the weight losses with exercise were less than predicted, considering the energy requirements for the exercise performed.

Another problem noted by Epstein and Wing was that relatively long periods of strenuous exercise are required before there is a significant change in fat content even among normal-weight and moderately obese individuals. Two months of physical training of 30-minute sessions three times a week, during which near maximal heart rate is achieved during half the session, is required for fat content to change. Furthermore, fat content may change before weight loss occurs, since there may be a relative increase in muscle content which weighs more than fat.

Dropout rates will probably prove to be another important drawback to exercise programs. In a study of myocardial infarction patients by Sanne,[52] more than half dropped out of the program.

DRUG THERAPY

Various drug treatments have been tried in obese patients, but none have been demonstrated effective in producing significant weight loss that is maintained. For a comprehensive review of available drug treatments for obesity, see Powers.[53] Several groups of drugs have been considered, at least theoretically, for the treatment of obesity. These include drugs which decrease appetite or enhance satiety, drugs which increase basal metabolic rate of physical activity levels, and agents which alter intestinal absorption of nutrients. Drugs which interfere with the metabolism of lipid, either by decreasing lipid synthesis or increasing lipid utilization or mobilization, might theoretically be useful. Several hormones have been used in the treatment of obesity, including human chorionic gonadotropin (HCG), thyroid hormones, growth hormones and progesterone.

The best studied drugs are the anorectic agents, particularly amphetamine. Although amphetamines result in a decrease in appetite, the weight loss that follows is usually small, often less than 5 kg, and in a morbidly obese individual this is a trivial weight loss. Furthermore, there are a number of side-effects, including central nervous system stimulation and stimulation of the sympathetic nervous system which can be quite troublesome. Furthermore, the potential for abuse of amphetamine is significant and the cessation of the drug may result in severe depression. For these reasons, amphetamine has fallen into disrepute as an anti-obesity agent. Most other anorectic agents that have been developed and are still occasionally used are modifications of the chemical structure of d-amphetamine (a phenyl ring and side chain). These include fenfluramine (Pondimin), diethylpropion (Tenuate), mazindol (Sanorex), and phentermine resin (Ionamin). None, however, has been shown to be more effective in producing significant weight loss than the original d-amphetamine and all have side-effects. Fenfluramine has an unusual side-effect in that it may result in depression soon after it is discontinued, even in patients without a prior history of depression.

Other drugs, e.g., those which alter basal metabolic rate or influence fat metabolism, have generally been proven either ineffective or hazardous. HCG shots, which are still marketed as an effective treatment for obesity in some areas, have been demonstrated to be ineffective in producing weight loss; the 500-calorie diet which is usually part of the HCG regimen accounts for any weight loss achieved.[54,55] Thyroid hormones have been extensively studied in the treatment of obesity, but the weight loss that occurs is primarily lean body mass, is usually regained, and there are potentially very serious cardiovascular and other side-effects. Gwinup and

Poucher[56] conclude that the use of thyroid hormones "merely substitutes one clinical entity for another (thyrotoxicosis for obesity)."

CONCLUSION

In conclusion, the currently available nonsurgical treatments for morbid obesity are neither safe nor effective. The physiologic hazards of weight loss followed by weight regain are significant and may predispose to further weight gain. The psychologic complications include the loss of self-esteem due to repeated failure and the significant propensity for developing a "diet depression" during calorie restriction. Although exercise may be without certain of these hazards (e.g., untoward psychologic effects during physical training have not been described), it is ineffective in producing weight loss in the morbidly obese. All these methods may have potential as part of a comprehensive program for surgical patients.

REFERENCES

1. Keys A, Brozek J, Henschel A, et al: The Biology of Human Starvation. Minneapolis, University of Minnesota Press, 1950.
2. Hamburger WW: Emotional aspects of obesity. Med Clin North Am 35:483–499, 1951.
3. Bruch H: Psychological aspects of reducing. Psychosom Med 14:337–346, 1952.
4. Stunkard AJ: The dieting depression: incidence and clinical characteristics of untoward responses to weight reduction regimens. Am J Med 23:77–86, 1957.
5. Halmi KA, Stunkard AJ, Mason EE: Emotional responses to weight reduction by three methods: gastric bypass, jejunoileal bypass, diet. Am J Clin Nutr 33:446–451, 1980.
6. Leon GR, Eckert ED, Teed D, et al: Changes in body image and other psychological factors after intestinal bypass for massive obesity. J Behav Med 2:39–54, 1979.
7. Anderson T, Backer O, Stokholm KH, et al: Randomized trial of diet and gastroplasty compared with diet alone in morbid obesity. N Engl J Med 310:352–356, 1984.
8. Grinker J, Hirsch J, Levin B: The affective response of obese patients to weight reduction: a differentiation based on age of onset of obesity. Psychosom Med 35:57–62, 1973.
9. Rosen LW, Aniskiewicz AS: Psychosocial functioning of two groups of morbidly obese patients. Int J Obesity 7:53–59, 1983.
10. Solow C: Psychological aspects of intestinal bypass surgery for massive obesity: Current status. Am J Clin Nutr 30:103–108, 1977.
11. Danish Obesity Project: Randomized trial of jejunoileal bypass versus medical treatment in morbid obesity. Lancet 2:1255–1258, 1979.
12. Stunkard AJ: The current status of treatment for obesity in adults. In Stunkard AJ, Stellar E (eds): Eating and its Disorders. New York, Raven Press, 1984, pp 157–172.
13. Stuart RB: Behavioral control of overeating. Behav Res Ther 5:357–365, 1967.
14. Harris MB: Self-directed program for weight control: a pilot study. J Abnorm Psychol 74:263–270, 1969.
15. Leon GR: Personality and morbid obesity: Implications for dietary management through behavior modification. Surg Clin North Am 59:1007–1015, 1979.
16. Stunkard AJ, Penick SB: Behavior modification in the treatment of obesity: the problem of maintaining weight loss. Arch Gen Psychiatry 36:801–806, 1979.
17. Powers PS: Factors which predispose to optimal results with gastroplasty for morbid obesity. (In preparation.)
18. Lindner PG, Blackburn GL: Multidisciplinary approach to obesity utilizing fasting modified by protein sparing therapy. Obesity/Bariatric Med 5:198–216, 1976.
19. US Department of Health, Education and Welfare: Obesity and Health: A Sourcebook of Information for Professional Health Personnel. Arlington, VA, US Govt Printing Office, 1966.
20. Wadden TA, Stunkard AJ, Brownell KO: Very low calorie diets: Their efficacy, safety and future. Ann Intern Med 99:675–684, 1983.
21. Drenick EJ, Smith R: Weight reduction by prolonged starvation. Postgrad Med A93–100, 1964.
22. Rosen JC, Hunt DA, Sims EAH, et al: Comparison of carbohydrate-containing and carbohydrate-restricted hypocaloric diets in the treatment of obesity: effects on appetite and mood. Am J Clin Nutr 36:463–469, 1982.
23. Howard AN, Girant A, Edwards O, et al: The treatment of obesity with a very-low-calorie liquid-formula diet: an inpatient/outpatient comparison using skimmed milk as the chief protein source. Int J Obesity 2:321–332, 1978.
24. Blackburn GL, Bistrian BR, Flatt, JP: Role of a protein-sparing modified fast in a comprehensive weight reduction program. In Howard AN (ed): Recent Advances in Obesity Research. London, Newman, 1975, pp 279–281.
25. 1983 Metropolitan Height and Weight Tables, Stat Bull Metropol Life Insur Co, 1 Madison Av, New York, NY 10010, 64:2–9, 1984.
26. Genuth SM, Vertes V, Hazelton J: Supplemented fasting in the treatment of obesity. In Bray G (ed): Recent Advances in Obesity Research. London, Newman, 1978, pp 370–378.
27. Halmi, KA, Long M, Stunkard AJ, et al: Psychiatric diagnosis of morbidly obese gastric bypass patients. Am J Psychiatry 137:470–472, 1980.
28. Weissman M, Myers J: Affective disorders in a US urban community. Arch Gen Psychiatry 35:1304–1311, 1978.
29. Webb WW, Phares R, Abram HS, et al: Jejunoileal

bypass procedures in morbid obesity: Preoperative psychological findings. J Clin Psychol 32:82–85, 1976.

30. Lerner RM, Gellert E: Body build identification: Preference and aversion in children. Develop Psychol 1:456–462,1969.

31. Rand CS, Stunkard AJ: Psychoanalysis and obesity. J Am Acad Psychoanal 5:459–497, 1977.

32. Stunkard AJ: Eating patterns and obesity. Psychiatr Q 33:284–294, 1959.

33. Powers PS, Fernandez RC: Current Treatment of Anorexia Nervosa and Bulimia. Basel, S. Karger, 1984, pp 1–18.

34. Stunkard AJ, Grace WJ, Wolff HG: The night-eating syndrome: a pattern of food intake among certain obese patients. Am J Med 19:78–86, 1955.

35. Mayer A: Essai sur la Soif. Paris, Félix Alcan, 1901.

36. Stern J: Is obesity a disease of inactivity? In Stunkard AJ, Stellar E (eds): Eating and its Disorders. New York, Raven Press, 1984, pp 131–139.

37. Oscai LB: The role of exercise in weight control. Exerc Sports Med 1:103–123, 1973.

38. Bray GA: The myth of diet in the management of obesity. Am J Clin Nutr 23:1141–1148, 1970.

39. Bray GA: Effect of caloric restriction on energy expenditure in obese patients. Lancet 1:397–398, 1969.

40. Durrant ML, Garrow JS, Royston P, et al: Factors influencing the composition of the weight lost by obese patients on a reducing diet. Br J Nutr 44:275–284, 1980.

41. Mayer J, Roy P, Mitra KP: Relationship between calorie intake, body weight and physical work. Studies in an industrial male population in West Bengal. Am J Clin Nutr 4:169–175, 1956.

42. Edhalm OG, Fletcher JG, Widdowson EM, et al.: The food intake and individual expenditure of individual men. Br J Nutr 9:286–300, 1955.

43. Björntorp P, Berchtold P, Grimby G, et al: Effects of physical training on glucose tolerance, plasma insulin and lipids and on body composition in men after myocardial infarction. Acta Med Scand 192:439–443, 1972.

44. Stern JS, Schultz C, Mole P, et al: Effect of calorie restriction and exercise on basal metabolism and thyroid hormone. Proceedings of the Third International Congress of Obesity. Alim Nutr Metab 1:361, 1980.

45. Bray GA, Whipp BJ, Koyal SN: The acute effects of food intake on energy expenditure during cycle ergometry. Am J Clin Nutr 27:254–259, 1971.

46. Drenick EJ: Weight reduction by prolonged fasting. In Bray GA (ed): Obesity in Perspective. Fogarty International Center Series on Preventive Medicine, vol II, pt II. Washington, DC, US Govt Printing Office, 1976.

47. Björntorp P, de Jounge K, Krotkiewski M, et al: Physical training in human obesity. III. Effects of long-term physical training on body composition. Metabolism 22:1467–1475, 1973.

48. Pollock ML, Miller HS, Jr, Janeway R, et al: Effects of walking on body composition and cardiovascular function of middle-aged men. J Appl Physiol 30:126–130, 1971.

49. Skinner J, Holloszy JO, Cureton T: Effects of a program of endurance exercises on physical work: Capacity and anthropometric measurements of fifteen middle-aged men. Am J Cardiol 14:747–752, 1964.

50. Oscai LB, Williams BT: Effect of exercise on overweight middle-aged males. J Am Geriatr Soc 16:794–797, 1968.

51. Epstein LH, Wing RR: Aerobic exercise and weight. Addict Behav 5:371–388, 1980.

52. Sanne H: Exercise tolerance and physical training of non-selected patients after myocardial infarction. Acta Med Scand (Suppl 551), 1973.

53. Powers PS: Treatment of obesity: Drugs and surgery. In Powers PS: Obesity: The Regulation of Weight. Baltimore, Williams & Wilkins, 1980, pp 325–338.

54. Albrink MJ: Chorionic gonadotropin and obesity? (editorial). Am J Clin Nutr 22:681–685, 1969.

55. Birmingham CL, Smith KC: Human chorionic gonadotropin is of no value in the management of obesity. Can Med Assoc J 128:1156–1157, 1983.

56. Gwinup G, Poucher R: A controlled study of thyroid analogs in therapy of obesity. Am J Med Sci 254:416–420, 1967.

4

The Role of Gastrointestinal Peptides in the Regulation of Food Intake

STEPHEN M. COLLINS
HARVEY P. WEINGARTEN

Food intake and body weight are controlled by several mechanisms. This chapter addresses one of these mechanisms, namely the influence of gastrointestinal (GI) peptides on ingestion. Specifically, the review focuses on the ability of GI peptides to terminate feeding. We emphasize the role of cholecystokinin (CCK), since the analysis of CCK's role in satiety serves as a prototype for investigation of the involvement of other GI peptides in meal termination. This chapter does not address the role of GI peptides in the initiation of eating or their control of body weight through digestive, absorptive, or postabsorptive mechanisms. The reader will acknowledge that the gut, in general, and its peptides, in particular, make important contributions to body weight and adiposity through these mechanisms and that a comprehensive review of these areas is well beyond the scope of this chapter.

HISTORICAL OVERVIEW

The ingestion of nutrients is necessary for the homeostatic control of energy balance. In most mammals, including man, eating is a periodic event organized with meals as the basic unit. Regulatory physiology has viewed the mechanisms involved with meal initiation (i.e., "hunger") as distinct from those controlling meal termination (i.e., "satiety"). Mayer[1] proposed one of the earliest satiety mechanisms related to physiologic events emanating from the periphery. In his "glucostatic hypothesis," he suggested that the rate of glucose utilization provided the biologic signal for both hunger and satiety. He proposed that satiety was associated with a high rate of glucose utilization, measured by the difference of glucose concentration in arteries and veins (i.e., a high glucose arteriovenous gradient or a high Δ AV glucose). The major limitation of this proposal was that feeding terminates well before significant absorption of nutrient and, therefore, before meaningful changes in glucose utilization take place. The temporal incongruity between meal termination and postabsorptive glycemic changes led researchers to investigate preabsorptive satiety mechanisms. This search was focused by the demonstration that blood from a recently sated rat could inhibit feeding in food-deprived animals,[2,3] thus implicating a humoral signal. The origin of one such humoral factor was localized subsequently to the small intestine, when it was found that crude homogenates from this region induced satiety when injected into food-deprived rats.[4] Subsequent work, pioneered by G.P. Smith and J. Gibbs from the E. Bourne Laboratory of Cornell Medical Center, identified peptides secreted by the small intestine, most notably cholecystokinin (CCK), as the most likely candidates for this humoral intestinal preabsorptive satiety signal.[5]

It must be stressed that GI peptides are but one of a host of mechanisms involved in satiety. In fact, progress in the analysis of the biology of satiety permits the following general comments regarding meal termination:

1. The control of satiety is multifactorial. It is unlikely that any single physiologic signal is solely responsible for the termination of feeding. Rather, satiety is undoubtedly controlled by a host of physiologic responses, both peripheral and central, which act conjointly to determine the cessation of a meal. Thus, analysis of satiety must progress by first identifying each signal and then revealing how these signals interact with one another.

2. The controls of satiety are influenced by both short-term and long-term regulatory influences. Mechanisms must exist which, in the short term, are linked directly to meal termination. As discussed, these signals are likely to be preabsorptive. In the long term, factors such as the organism's weight, level of adiposity, recent eating history, and culture have an impact on meal size and frequency. These long-term factors may influence satiety by their modulatory role on short-term mechanisms.

CHOLECYSTOKININ (CCK) AS A MEDIATOR OF SATIETY

CCK is a peptide found in the gut and brain. Within the GI tract, high concentrations of this peptide are found in the duodenum and proximal jejunum, where it is synthesized, stored, and secreted by specialized endocrine cells.[6,7] CCK is released into the bloodstream after a meal;[8,9] fat and protein are potent secretagogues of the peptide.[10,11] Thus the anatomical location of CCK-containing cells, and their ability to respond to nutrient within the lumen of the proximal small intestine, provide structural and fuctional support for the role of CCK as a putative mediator of satiety.

Direct experimental evidence for the role of CCK in satiety was provided first by Gibbs and Smith in 1973 when they showed that intraperitoneal (ip) injections of CCK suppressed feeding in food-deprived rats eating normally[12,13] or sham feeding.[14] The finding that ip administration of exogenous CCK inhibits eating has been replicated in a variety of species and provides the basic support for CCK as a putative mediator of satiety. Other evidence implicating CCK as a physiologic satiety agent is:

1. The doses of CCK required to inhibit feeding (in the μg per kg range) are generally acknowledged not to be associated with overt signs of malaise,[15] although this issue is controversial.[16]

2. CCK, at doses which suppress eating, does not produce a general debilitation of behavior, as it does not suppress drinking in water-deprived rats[12] or apparent motivation for food.[17]

3. At appropriate doses, CCK inhibits eating by affecting the rate of eating in only the terminal part of the meal; rats injected with CCK simply terminate a meal sooner, thus resulting in a decreased meal size.[12,18]

4. The termination of eating in CCK-treated rats is accompanied by a behavioral sequence identical to that of spontaneous postprandial satiety.[19]

The major limitation of the CCK-satiety hypothesis is that all the evidence in its favor is based exclusively on experiments involving administration of the exogenous peptide. Thus, it cannot be determined whether the inhibition of eating produced by CCK represents a physiologic or pharmacologic effect of the peptide. As well, it is not clear whether sufficient quantities of the peptide can be, or are, released from the intestines to inhibit eating. The latter point is of practical importance in considering the therapeutic potential of CCK in the management of hyperphagic obesity and possible difficulties involved in the frequent administration of a peptide to suppress appetite. Thus, in order to evaluate the role of CCK in satiety and its possible therapeutic use, it is necessary to investigate the involvement of the endogenous peptide in the regulation of food intake.

Two procedures can be used to investigate the behavioral function of an endogenous peptide. The first involves measurement of CCK in plasma with radioimmunologic techniques and correlating levels of CCK with feeding behavior. This approach, however, is not definitive. Positive correlations do not imply causality. A lack of correlation does not

exclude a physiologic role for the peptide since its mode of action in inducing satiety may involve neurocrine or paracrine secretion, mechanisms not reflected in measurement of plasma levels. Thus, to evaluate the role of endogenous CCK, we chose a second strategy, the use of a selective antagonist.

The drug proglumide has been shown in vitro to be a competitive antagonist of the action of CCK on pancreatic acini,[20] gastric smooth muscle,[21,22] and gallbladder smooth muscle.[23] We demonstrated that proglumide also inhibited the satiety effect of exogenous CCK in the intact (normally feeding) rat.[24] This action was selective in that ip proglumide did not inhibit the satiety effect of the GI peptides glucagon or bombesin.[24] (The ability of the antagonist to attenuate the satiety produced by high-dose bombesin is interpreted that high-dose bombesin inhibits eating, in part, due to its ability to release CCK.) Proglumide also selectively inhibited the effect of CCK in the sham feeding rat, indicating that the effect of the antagonist on feeding was not due to its ability to influence gastric emptying, but, rather, on its ability to compete with CCK at the hitherto unidentified receptor responsible for the CCK satiety effect.[25]

If the endogenous peptide is important in the control of satiety, then administration of its antagonist should modulate eating in a predictable manner. Once we characterized the specificity of proglumide, we utilized it to investigate the role of endogenous CCK in eating. The original hypothesis of CCK as a mediator of intestinal satiety stated that the arrival of food in the proximal small intestine stimulated the release of CCK, which initiated a series of events culminating in satiety (Fig. 4.1). To test this experimentally, it was necessary to use an animal model which isolated this proposed intestinal satiety mechanism. Such a model, described first by Liebling et al.[26] consists of a rat with a chronically indwelling gastric fistula and duodenal catheter (Fig. 4.2). This arrangement permits the investigator to independently stimulate the intestinal satiety mechanism by infusing test solutions directly into the duodenum and to simultaneously observe the effects of this manipulation on food intake in the rat sham feeding through the open gastric fistula. Using this paradigm, Leibling et al.[26] demonstrated that intraduodenal infusion of nutrient, in volumes which approximated normal postprandial levels, suppressed sham feeding.

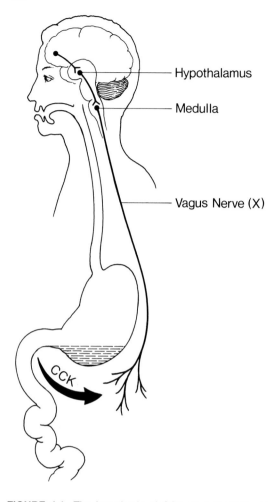

FIGURE 4.1. The hypothesis of CCK as a mediator of intestinal satiety. Food enters the proximal small intestine and releases CCK, which stimulates afferent vagal activity and induces a sequence of events culminating in satiety.

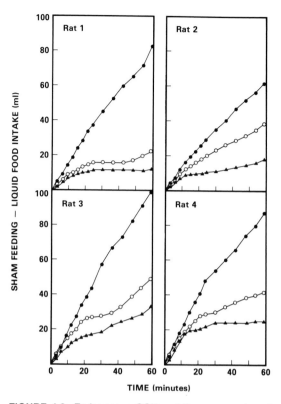

FIGURE 4.2. Endogenous CCK and the suppression of feeding: the effect of proglumide on the suppression of feeding induced by intraduodenal infusion of nutrient in the rat. The closed circles represent sham feeding during intraduodenal (id) infusion of saline and following an intraperitoneal (ip) injection of saline. The closed triangles represent sham feeding during an id infusion of nutrient and ip saline injection, and the open circles are data obtained following an ip injection of the CCK antagonist proglumide and an id infusion of nutrient. Note the partial reversal by proglumide of the id nutrient-induced suppression of feeding.

We tested whether the intestinal satiety mechanism demonstrated by Leibling et al. involved the action of CCK, as is implicit in the CCK-satiety hypothesis, by using the CCK antagonist proglumide. We found that intraduodenal infusion of nutrient suppressed sham feeding rapidly and profoundly. Administration of the CCK antagonist only partially reversed this suppression (Fig. 4.3). The partial reversal was not due to administration of insufficient proglumide since we used a dose, 150 mg/kg, which completely reversed the effects of a maximally effective dose of exogenous CCK in the normal and sham feeding rat.[24,25] Furthermore, we verified that this dose reversed a maximally effective dose of CCK in this particular preparation.[27] In addition, since a maximally effective dose of exogenous CCK suppressed sham feeding far less than that achieved by direct intraduodenal administration of nutrient,[27] these results indicate that factors in addition to CCK also mediated satiety induced by the presence of nutrient in the intestines. Regardless of the implication of these data to the physiologic role of CCK in postprandial satiety, the important finding from these experiments was that sufficient quantities of endogenous CCK could be released from the intestine to have an impact on eating. Since these studies were performed under experimental conditions in which the continuity of the alimentary tract was interrupted and large volumes of nutrient were infused, no statements may be made from these results regarding the physiologic role of CCK in satiety.

Experiments proposed to examine the *phys-*

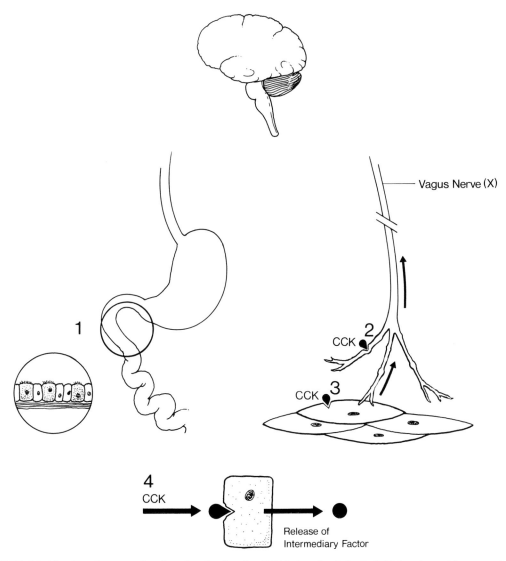

FIGURE 4.3. The theories regarding the site of action for CCK-induced satiety. 1. CCK is released from specialized endocrine cells in the duodenal mucosa. 2. CCK interacts with receptors on afferent vagal fibers, *or* 3. CCK interacts with receptors on smooth muscle to induce contraction, which is detected by mechanoreceptors and relayed to the brain via the vagus nerve, *or* 4. CCK interacts with an unidentified cell and releases a factor which stimulates afferent vagal nerve activity.

iologic role of CCK in feeding must incorporate several features:

1. Food and water must be available continuously to animals maintained under experimental conditions which approximate most closely those of the free-living animal.

2. The GI tract must be uninterrupted by surgical intervention, since the effectiveness of endogenous CCK may be influenced by interactions with signals emanating from other areas of the GI tract.

3. The route and dosage of CCK antagonists or other inhibitors (e.g., antibodies)

must be clearly shown to retain specificity under conditions used to assess the involvement of endogenous CCK in satiety.

MECHANISM UNDERLYING CCK-INDUCED SATIETY

It is believed that CCK induces a sequence of events culminating in satiety in the rat by interacting primarily with receptors located in the GI tract. This is based on the finding that subdiaphragmatic vagotomy abolishes satiety induced by ip administration of CCK in the intact rat.[28–31] In species other than rat, some have proposed a mechanism involving direct CCK effects on the central nervous system.[32,33] Although the site of action of CCK in the GI tract is not known, the following data suggest several likely hypotheses.

1. Since selective gastric vagotomy abolishes CCK-induced satiety, the site of action of that peptide must be within the area of distribution of that nerve, i.e., the stomach and proximal duodenum.

2. Autoradiographic studies have localized high concentrations of CCK receptors to the circular muscle layers of gastric antrum and pylorus.[34]

3. CCK stimulates contraction of smooth muscle by interacting directly with receptors on muscle cells[21] and also causes contractions of rat pyloric circular muscle by a direct effect on muscle (Collins et al., unpublished observations).

4. CCK slows gastric emptying in several species,[35] including rat (Weingarten et al., unpublished observations).

5. CCK receptors are located on the vagus nerve.[36,37]

From these data it is possible to generate a number of hypotheses regarding the site and mechanism of action of CCK. These hypotheses are not mutually exclusive. In fact, each may contribute to the sequence of events which originate in the GI tract and which culminate in meal cessation. Three hypotheses are best supported by the data:

Hypothesis 1: CCK produces satiety by interacting directly with receptors on the afferent vagal terminals (site 2 in Fig. 4.3).

Hypothesis 2: CCK produces satiety by interacting with receptors on pyloric smooth muscle with the net effect of inhibiting gastric emptying (site 3 in Fig. 4.3).

Hypothesis 3: CCK produces satiety by interacting with smooth muscle and/or enteric nerve receptors innervating smooth muscle, with the net effect of increasing tone within the gastric wall without necessarily affecting emptying. The change in gastric wall tension is detected by sensory nerve endings, and this signal is transmitted to the brain via the afferent vagus (sites 2 and 3 in Fig. 4.3).

It has recently been shown that the ability of CCK to suppress sham feeding in rats with chronic gastric fistulas is independent of vagal integrity.[38] This is in contrast to the vagal-dependent action of CCK in the normally-feeding animal. These findings indicate that more than one mechanism may exist for CCK-in-

duced satiety (although the sham feeding result is still consistent with Hypotheses 1 and 3). As a minimum, the demonstration that CCK can reduce intake in the sham feeding rat, albeit at higher doses, indicates that changes in gastric emptying are not the only mode of action of exogenous CCK. In the intact animal, the ability of CCK to suppress feeding is amplified by gastric distention.[35] Thus, while experimental evidence supports the existence of at least two distinct mechanisms whereby CCK may induce satiety, their relative contributions to meal termination are not known at this time.

OTHER PEPTIDES WITH SATIETY ACTION

Although CCK has been most widely investigated, it is not the only peptide which is associated with a reduction of eating. In fact, an extensive literature has been generated indicating that a host of peptides have the capacity to affect meal size.[39–42] In a consideration of this literature, it is important to keep in mind that several criteria must be met before any peptide can be reasonably considered as a satiety factor.[43] CCK has been the most widely investigated peptide in this regard and, at this time, it is unclear whether even it fulfills the defined criteria. Thus, claims of other peptides as physiologic satiety factors are, at present, speculative. However, the involvement of several other peptides as satiety agents is noteworthy.

Gibbs et al.[44,45] were the first to demonstrate that ip bombesin reduced meal size in normal and sham feeding rats. This effect is also obtained in man.[46] Bombesin-induced suppression of eating is accompanied by a behavioral sequence characteristic of satiety and is not accompanied by overt malaise.[44,45] However, in contrast to CCK, the action of bombesin is independent of vagal integrity.[28] Because bombesin is found in high concentrations in the stomach,[47,48] this peptide or its mammalian equivalent, gastrin-releasing peptide[49] may represent a gastric satiety factor.

Several pancreatic hormones are implicated in satiety, although their mechanism is not understood. Intraperitoneal injection of glucagon reduces eating, although high doses, relative to bombesin and CCK, are required.[24,50] In contrast to CCK and bombesin, glucagon is not effective in the sham feeding rat. A role for endogenous glucagon in the control of appetite is suggested by experiments demonstrating increased eating and body weight in rats treated with glucagon antibodies.[51] Pancreatic polypeptide (PP) has also been proposed as a satiety factor.[52] This hypothesis is based largely on the demonstrations that the hyperphagic ob/ob mouse fails to secrete PP in response to a meal.[53] However, whether PP is involved in postprandial satiety, and whether disturbances in its secretion are related to hyperphagia, is still controversial.[54,55]

THE ORIGIN OF OTHER SATIETY SIGNALS WITHIN THE GI TRACT

An understanding of the sites of origin of satiety signals within the GI tract is important in rationalizing new surgical techniques to reduce food intake. Evidence exists identifying various GI sites as contributing to the regulation of food intake. This review is focused specifically on the possible role of endogenous peptides released by these areas. For review of the role of GI mechanisms other than peptidergic ones in satiety, the reader is directed to references 56, 57 and 58.

The existence of a gastric humoral satiety factor is postulated by Koopmans.[59,60] In his experiments, the stomach of one rat is transplanted into the abdominal cavity of another. This supernumerary stomach is excluded from the GI tract of the recipient. Infusion of nutrient into the transplanted rat suppressed subsequent oral intake. The degree of inhibition of food intake produced by the infusion was equivalent (in terms of kcal) to the amount infused into the transplanted stomach. Since the transplant is denervated extrinsically and excluded from the gut of the recipient, the suppression of feeding must have been due to the release of a gastric humoral factor. The identification of the proposed gastic satiety factor is unknown. A leading candidate, however, is bombesin (mammalian GRP), since it is found in high concentrations in the stomach[47,48] and exogenous administration of this peptide produces satiety.[44,45]

The leading candidate for the intestinal satiety factor is CCK. However, the results of recent experiments from our laboratory indicate that the contribution of CCK to satiety produced by nutrient in the intestines may not be large.[27] Other factors, in addition to CCK, also mediate intestinal satiety.[27] The identity of these factors is not currently known. Although secretin and gastrin are both released from the proximal intestine, neither of these substances appears able to inhibit eating when administered exogenously.[61] Aside from possible osmotic or distension mechanisms,[56] other putative peptide mediators of intestinal satiety are somatostatin[42] and enteroglucagon.

Finally, there is evidence to suggest that the lower intestine may also be the origin of satiety signals. While not situated strategically to function as early postprandial signals, they may play a back-up role if and when sufficient nutrient remains after digestion and absorption. Or, such signals may be involved primarily in the control of daily food intake (i.e., a long-term regulatory mechanism), and not concerned directly with the regulation of individual meal size. Evidence for an ileal signal is derived from experiments by Koopmans demonstrating that preparations which provide greater nutrient stimulation of the ileum, either through jejunoileal bypass or ileal transposition, result in reductions of eating and body weight.[62–64]

USE OF CCK FOR THE MANAGEMENT OF OVEREATING IN OBESITY: THERAPEUTIC POTENTIAL

Obesity represents a disorder of energy balance in which energy intake exceeds output. Obesity directly causes, or indirectly exacerbates, a number of medical conditions including diabetes and cardovascular disorders. The incidence of obesity within North America renders it a major health risk. It is recognized that at least some obesities may be determined by a primary metabolic disorder and, thus, would be relatively resistant to a therapeutic intervention which focused on manipulation of eating. However, it is also clear that many obesities are characterized by an excessive level of caloric intake and that this disturbance in the control of eating directly causes, or at least amplifies, the obese condition. In such cases, interventions aimed to decrease the level of ingestion would provide some therapeutic value in the control of the obesity and the accompanying clinical conditions.

The possibility that CCK can be used in a therapeutic way in the control of appetite is left open by the demonstrations that CCK can reduce meal size in humans and that the inhibition of eating is not accompanied by dramatic negative side-effects or overt malaise.[65–67] The fundamental question, however, is whether CCK could be effective in reducing the excessive food intake characteristic of obesity. Several animal studies address this issue. Although they are less responsive to exogenous CCK than their lean littermates, the genetically obese Zucker rats do decrease food intake in response to ip administration of CCK-8,[55,68,69] as do obese ventromedial hypothalamic-lesioned rats.[70] In fact, the food intake changes of the obese Zucker rat may be more responsive than its lean littermate to experimental manipulations believed to modulate endogenous CCK secretion[71] (although see reference 72). In the most direct test of the ability of CCK to promote a reduction of eating and weight in obesity, Campbell and Smith[73] allowed fat Zucker rats to eat three meals per day. For one group, each meal was preceded by an ip injection of CCK-8; for a second group it was not. Over a 3-week period, the obese rats which were injected with CCK before meals lost more weight than obese animals on the same diet without CCK. The differential weight loss appeared to be a direct result of decreased meal size in fat rats injected with CCK before eating.

It may be possible to exploit our understanding of GI satiety signals to therapeutic advantage in the management of eating disorders, especially in the manipulation of the hyperphagia associated with obesity. The data described above appear promising. However, several considerations mitigate the successful therapeutic use of CCK in the treatment of overeating. First, the effects of long-term administration of CCK on food intake and body weight in man are unknown. In rats, the results of chronic administration of CCK have been disappointing in that animals, when permitted free access to food after CCK injection, compensate for the CCK-induced suppression of eating by increasing the size of the subsequent meals or reducing intermeal interval.[74,75] Three factors may explain this result. 1) The short half-life of CCK (about 15 minutes)[76] results in rapid reduction in the effective concentration of CCK. 2) CCK-induced desensitization of many target tissues results in the rapid loss of biologic effect on repeated or prolonged exposure to the peptide.[77] 3) It is possible that the body adapts to CCK-induced suppression of eating by activating one or several compensatory factors.

In an attempt to overcome the problem related to the short half-life of the peptide, we have recently investigated the effect of an acetylated derivative of CCK, which is relatively resistant to degradation and has a prolonged half-life,[78] on food intake in the rat. We found that although we could increase the efficacy of the peptide with respect to the suppression of eating, the animal was able to compensate for this by decreasing subsequent intermeal interval and increasing meal size. In other studies, we investigated the possibility that the timing of CCK administration with respect to feeding may alter its satiety action. We found,[79] similar to a previous report,[80] that the efficacy of exogenous CCK was enhanced by administering the peptide after the animal had tasted food for some brief period. Thus, although oropharyngeal stimulation is synergistic with CCK-induced satiety, it would appear inconvenient to apply this finding to the management of feeding disorders in man. These problems, including the necessity of injecting the peptide, suggest that the therapeutic use of CCK is confounded by too many problems to be of practical use in the management of hyperphagia in man.

A reasonable alternative to the administration of exogenous CCK to control feeding might be the use of CCK secretagogues. Such substances could be incorporated into food and result in the exaggerated release of endogenous CCK, thus inducing early satiety. Our recent demonstration of the capacity of endogenous intestinal CCK to suppress feeding in animals[27] supports such an approach. However, it should be remembered that while this approach overcomes some of the technical difficulties associated with the administration of exogenous CCK, it is still subject to the constraints imposed by CCK-induced desensitization and the organism's adaptive responses to CCK.

REFERENCES

1. Mayer J: Regulation of energy intake and the body weight: The glucostatic theory and the lipostatic hypothesis. Ann NY Acad Sci 63:15–43, 1955.
2. Fleming DG: V. Humoral and metabolic factors in the regulation of food and water intake. Food intake studies in parabiotic rats. Ann NY Acad Sci 157:985–1003, 1969.
3. David JD, Gallagher RJ, Ladove RF, et al: Inhibition of food intake by a humoral factor. J Comp Physiol Psychol 67:407–414, 1969.
4. Glick Z, Mayer J: Preliminary observations on the effect of intestinal mucosa extract on food intake of rats. Fed Proc 27:485, 1968.
5. Smith GP, Gibbs J: Brain-gut peptides and the control of food intake. In Martin JB, Reichlin S, Bick KL (eds):

Neurosecretion and Brain Peptides. New York, Raven Press, 1981, pp 389–395.

6. Polak JM, Bloom SR, Rayford PL, et al: Identification of cholecystokinin-secreting cells. Lancet 2:1016–1018, 1975.

7. Rehfeld JF: Immunochemical studies on cholecystokinin. II. Distribution and molecular heterogeneity in the central nervous system and small intestine of man and hog. J Biol Chem 253:4022–4030, 1978.

8. Chang TM, Chey WY: Radioimmunoassay of cholecystokinin. Dig Dis Sci 28:456–468, 1983.

9. Rayford PL, Schafmayer A, Teichman RK, et al: Cholecystokinin radioimmunoassay. In Bloom SR (ed): Gut Hormones. Edinburgh, London and New York, Churchill Livingstone, 1978, pp 208–212.

10. Himeno S, Tarui S, Kanayama S, et al: Plasma cholecystokinin responses after ingestion of liquid meal and intraduodenal infusion of fat, amino acids, or hydrochloric acid in man: Analysis with region specific radioimmunoassay. Am J Gastroenterol 78:703–707, 1983.

11. Makhlouf GM: The neuroendocrine design of the gut: The play of chemicals in a chemical playground. Gastroenterology 67:159–184, 1974.

12. Smith GP, Gibbs J, Young RC: Cholecystokinin and intestinal satiety in the rat. Fed Proc 33:1146–1149, 1974.

13. Gibbs J, Young RC, Smith GP: Cholecystokinin decreases food intake in rats. J Comp Physiol Psychol 84:488–495, 1973.

14. Gibbs J, Young RC, Smith GP: Cholecystokinin elicits satiety in rats with open gastric fistulas. Nature 245:323–325, 1973.

15. Holt J, Antin J, Gibbs J, et al: Cholecystokinin does not produce bait shyness in rats. Physiol Behav 12:497–498, 1974.

16. Deutsch JA, Hardy WT: Cholecystokinin produces bait shyness in rats. Nature 266:196, 1977.

17. Cox JE, Toney RJ, Wiebe DJ: Effects of cholecystokinin on runway performance. Neurosci Abstr 9:901, 1983.

18. Weingarten HP: Meal initiation controlled by learned cues: Effects of peripheral cholinergic blockade and cholecystokinin. Physiol Behav 32:403–408, 1984.

19. Antin J, Gibbs J, Holt J, et al: Cholecystokinin elicits the complete behavioral sequence of satiety in rats. J Comp Physiol Psychol 89:784–790, 1975.

20. Hahne WF, Jensen RT, Lemp GF, et al: Proglumide and benzotript: members of a different class of cholecystokinin receptor antagonists. Proc Natl Acad Sci USA 78:6304–6308, 1981.

21. Collins SM, Gardner JD: Cholecystokinin-induced contraction of dispersed smooth muscle cells. Am J Pysiol 243:G497–504, 1982.

22. Bitar KN, Makhlouf GM: Receptors on smooth muscle cells: characterization by contraction and specific antagonists. Am J Physiol 242:G400–407, 1982.

23. Davison JS, Najafi-Farashah SA: Proglumide: a specific antagonist to the actions of cholecystokinin-like pepides in guinea-pig gallbladder and ileum. IRCS Medical Sci 10:409–410, 1982.

24. Collins SM, Walker D, Forsyth P, et al: The effects of proglumide on cholecystokinin-, bombesin-, and glucagon-induced satiety in the rat. Life Sci 32:2223–2229, 1983.

25. Collins SM, Weingarten HP: Inhibition of satiety by a cholecystokinin antagonist is independent of gastric emptying. Peptides 5:481–484, 1984.

26. Liebling DS, Eisner JD, Gibbs J, et al: Intestinal satiety in rats. J Comp Physiol Psychol 89:955–965, 1975.

27. Collins SM, Conover KL, Forsyth PA, et al: Endogenous cholecystokinin and intestinal satiety. Am J Physiol 249:R667–671, 1985.

28. Smith GP, Jerome C, Cushin BJ, et al.: Abdominal vagotomy blocks the satiety effect of cholecystokinin in the rat. Science 213:1036–1037, 1981.

29. Smith GP, Jerome C, Norgren R: Vagal afferent axons mediate the satiety effect of CCK-8, Neurosci Abstr 9:902, 1983.

30. Morley JE, Levine AS, Kneip J, et al: The effect of vagotomy on the satiety effects of neuropeptides and naloxone. Life Sci 30:1943–1947, 1982.

31. Lorenz DN, Goldmn SA: Vagal mediation of the cholecystokinin satiety effect in rats. Physiol Behav 20:599–604, 1982.

32. Della-Fera MA, Baile CA, Schneider BS, et al: Cholecystokinin antibody injected in cerebral ventricles stimulates feeding in sheep. Science 212:687–689, 1981.

33. Della-Fera MA, Baile CA: Cholecystokinin octapeptide: continuous picomole injections into the cerebral ventricles of sheep suppress feeding. Science 206:471–473, 1979.

34. Smith GT, Moran TH, Coyle JT, et al: Anatomic localization of cholecystokinin receptors to the pyloric sphincter. Am J Physiol 246:R127–130 1984.

35. Moran TH, McHugh PR: Cholecystokinin suppresses food intake by inhibiting gastric emptying. Am J Physiol 242:R491–497, 1982.

36. Zarbin MA, Wamsley JK, Innis RB, et al.: Cholecystokinin receptors: presence and axonal flow in the rat vagus nerve. Life Sci 29:697–705, 1981.

37. Rehfeld, JF, Lundberg JM: Cholecystokinin in feline vagal and sciatic nerves: concentration, molecular form and transport velocity. Brain Res 275:341–347, 1983.

38. Kraly FS: Vagotomy does not alter cholecystokinin's inhibition of sham feeding. Am J Physiol 246:R829–831, 1984.

39. Woods SC, West DB, Stein LJ, et al: Peptides and the control of meal size. Diabetologia 20 (Suppl):305–313, 1981.

40. Morley JE, Levine AS, Yim GK, et al: Opioid modulation of appetite. Neurosci Biobehav Rev 7:281–305, 1983.

41. Morley JE: The neuroendocrine control of appetite: the role of the endogenous opiates, cholecystokinin, TRH, gamma-amino-butyric-acid and the diazepam receptor. Life Sci 25:355–368, 1980.

42. Lotter EC, Krinsky R, McKay JM, et al: Somatostatin decreases food intake of rats and baboons. J Comp Physiol Psychol 95:278–287, 1981.

43. Smith GP: Gut hormone hypothesis of postprandial satiety. In Stunkard AJ, Stellar E (eds): Eating and Its

Disorders. Association for Research in Nervous & Mental Disease (ARNMD) Research Publications Service. New York, Raven Press, 1984, vol 62, pp 67–75.

44. Gibbs J, Kulkosky PJ, Smith GP: Effects of peripheral and central bombesin on feeding behavior of rats. Peptides 2 (Suppl):179–183, 1981.

45. Gibbs J, Fauser DJ, Rowe EA, et al: Bombesin suppresses feeding in rats. Nature 282:208–210, 1979.

46. Muurahainen WE, Kissileff H, Smith GP: Bombesin: another peptide that inhibits feeding in man. Neurosci Abstr 9:156, 1983.

47. Brown M, Allen R, Villareal J, et al.: Bombesin-like activity: radioimmunologic assessment in biological tissues. Life Sci 23:2721–2728, 1978.

48. Walsh JH, Wong HC, Dockray GJ: Bombesin-like peptides in mammals. Fed Proc 38:2315–2319, 1979.

49. Brown M, Märki W, Rivier J: Is gastrin releasing peptide mammalian bombesin? Life Sci 27:125–128, 1980.

50. Geary N, Smith GP: Pancreatic glucagon and postprandial satiety in the rat. Physiol Behav 28:313–322, 1982.

51. Langhans W, Zeiger U, Scharrer E, et al: Stimulation of feeding in rats by intraperitoneal injection of antibodies in glucagon. Science 218:894–896, 1982.

52. Malaisse-Lagae F, Carpentier JL, Patel YC, et al.: Pancreatic polypeptide: a possible role in the regulation of food intake in the mouse. Hypothesis. Experientia 33:915–917, 1977.

53. Jia BQ, Taylor IL: Failure of pancreatic polypeptide release in congenitally obese mice. Gastroenterology 87:338–343, 1984.

54. Taylor IL, Garcia R: Effects of pancreatic polypeptide, caerulein, and bombesin on satiety in obese mice. Am J Physiol 248:G277–280, 1985.

55. McLaughlin CL, Baile CA: Obese mice and the satiety effects of cholecystokinin, bombesin and pancreatic polypeptides. Physiol Behav 26:433–437, 1981.

56. David JD, Collins BJ: Distension of the small intestine, satiety, and the control of food intake. Am J Clin Nutr 3:S255–S258, 1978.

57. Deutsch JA: The stomach in food satiation and the regulation of appetite. Prog Neurobiol 10:135–153 1978.

58. Smith GP, Gibbs J: Postprandial satiety. In Sprague JM, Epstein AN (eds): Progress in Psychobiology and Physiological Psychology. New York, Academic Press, 1979, vol 8, pp 179–242.

59. Koopmans HS: The role of the gastrointestinal tract in the satiation of hunger. In Cioffi LA, James WPT, Van Itallie TB (eds): The Body Weight Regulatory System: Normal and Disturbed Mechanisms. New York, Raven Press, 1981, pp 45–55.

60. Koopmans HS: A stomach hormone that inhibits food intake. J Auton Nerv Syst 9:157–171, 1983.

61. Lorenz DN, Krielsheimer G, Smith GP: Effect of cholecystokinin, gastrin, secretion and GIP on sham feeding in the rat. Physiol Behav 23:1065–1072, 1979.

62. Sclafani A, Koopmans HS, Appelbaum KA: Hypothalamic hyperphagia and obesity in rats with jejunoileal bypass. Am J Physiol 239:G387–394, 1980.

63. Koopmans HS, Sclafani A, Fichtner C, et al: The effects of ileal transposition on food intake and body weight loss in VMH-obese rats. Am J Clin Nutr 35:284–293, 1982.

64. Canbeyli RS, Koopmans HS: Comparison of gastric, duodenal and jujunal contributions to the inhibition of food intake in the rat. Physiol Behav 33:951–957, 1984.

65. Kissileff HR, Pi-Sunyer FX, Thornton J, et al: C-terminal octapeptide of cholecystokinin decreases food intake in man. Am J Clin Nutr 34:154–160, 1981.

66. Stacher G, Steinringer H, Schmierer G, et al: Cholecystokinin octapeptide decreases intake of solid food in man. Peptides 3:133–136, 1982.

67. Sturdevant RA, Goetz H: Cholecystokinin both stimulates and inhibits human food intake. Nature 261:713–715, 1976.

68. McLaughlin CL, Baile CA: Feeding and drinking behavior responses of adult Zucker obese rats to cholecystokinin. Physiol Behav 25:535–541, 1980.

69. McLaughlin CL, Baile CA: Decreased sensitivity of Zucker obese rats to the putative satiety agent cholecystokinin. Physiol Behav 25:543–548, 1980.

70. Kulkosky PJ, Breckenridge C, Krinsky R, et al: Satiety elicited by the C-terminal octapeptide of cholecystokinin-pancreozymin in normal and VMH-lesioned rats. Behav Biol 18:227–234, 1976.

71. McLaughlin CL, Peikin SR, Baile CA: Food intake response to modulation of secretion of cholecystokinin in Zucker rats. Am J Physiol 244:R676–685, 1983.

72. McLaughlin CL, Baile CA, Buonomo FC: Effect of CCK antibodies on food intake and weight gain in Zucker rats. Physiol Behav 34:277–282, 1985.

73. Campbell RG, Smith GP: CCK-8 decreases body weight in Zucker rats. Neurosci Abstr 9:902, 1983.

74. West DB, Fey D, Woods SC: Cholecystokinin persistently suppresses meal size but not food intake in free-feeding rats. Am J Physiol 246:R776–787, 1984.

75. Weingarten HP, Collins SM: Unpublished data.

76. Bennett HPJ, McMartin C: Peptide hormones and their analogues: distribution, clearance from the circulation, and inactivation in vivo. Pharmacol Rev 30:247–292, 1978.

77. Crawley JN, Beinfeld MC: Rapid development of tolerance to the behavioral actions of cholecystokinin. Nature 302:703–706, 1983.

78. Praissman M, Fara JW, Praissman LA, et al.: Preparation of an N-acetyl-octapeptide of cholecystokinin. Biochim Biophys Acta 716:240–248, 1982.

79. Forsyth PA, Weingarten HP, Collins SM: Role of oropharyngeal stimulation in cholecystokinin-induced satiety in the sham feeding rat. Physiol Behav 35:539–543, 1985.

80. Antin J, Gibbs J, Smith GP: Cholecystokinin interacts with pregastric food stimulation to elicit satiety in the rat. Physiol Behav 20:67–70, 1978.

5

Other Eating Disorders— Anorexia Nervosa and Bulimia Nervosa

DAVID S. GOLDBLOOM
PAUL E. GARFINKEL

**ANOREXIA NERVOSA
    AND BULIMIA NERVOSA
TREATMENT
RELATIONSHIP TO OBESITY**

At first glance, it may seem surprising that a chapter on anorexia nervosa and bulimia nervosa appears in a text on surgical approaches to morbid obesity. However, important connections exist between these eating disorders and obesity and may color both the clinical characteristics of obese patients and the sequelae of treatment for their obesity.

A significant minority of obese patients engage in bulimic behavior that may have multiple medical and psychologic consequences. Weight loss in the obese can precipitate a partial or full-blown syndrome of anorexia nervosa. Finally, evidence indicates that the emergence following gastroplasty of symptoms associated with anorexia nervosa and bulimia nervosa may be confused with more purely surgical postoperative complications. In order to emphasize the meaning and importance of these associations, it is necessary to provide an overview of these eating disorders.

ANOREXIA NERVOSA AND BULIMIA NERVOSA

Anorexia nervosa is characterized by self-imposed starvation due to a relentless pursuit of thinness and fear of fatness; this leads to varying degrees of emaciation. While theories of etiology continue to evolve, including contributions from biology, psychology, and culture, the clinical features of the disorder have been well described since the late 17th century. Current standard diagnostic criteria are presented in Table 5.1. Anorexia nervosa in a serious form occurs in about 1% of adolescent and young adult women, with more mild variants found in approximately 5% of the female population. It is a disorder largely but not exclusively of women, with up to 5% of cases reported among men. It continues to carry a significant mortality of about 5%, despite increased diagnostic awareness and improved treatment. Its morbidity emanates from the starvation and the variety of means to pursue and maintain thinness, and the sequelae are both medical and psychiatric.

Bulimia nervosa exists as a symptom of a variety of medical disorders, including obesity, as a subtype of anorexia nervosa, and as an autonomous syndrome (bulimia nervosa) in women at relatively normal weight. As a symptom, it describes a pattern of binge-eating involving the ingestion of huge quantities of food with a feeling of being out of control. Typically, this is associated with a desire to

TABLE 5.1. DIAGNOSTIC CRITERIA*

ANOREXIA NERVOSA
A. Refusal to maintain body weight over a minimal normal weight for age and height: e.g., weight loss leading to maintenance of body weight 15% below expected; failure to make expected weight gain during period of growth, leading to body weight 15% below expected.
B. Intense fear of becoming obese, even though underweight.
C. Disturbance in the way in which one's body weight, size or shape is experienced: e.g., claiming to "feel fat" even when emaciated; belief that one area of the body is "too fat" even when obviously underweight.
D. In females, absence of at least three consecutive menstrual cycles when otherwise expected to occur (primary or secondary amenorrhea).

BULIMIA NERVOSA
A. Recurrent episodes of binge-eating (rapid consumption of a large amount of food in a discrete period of time, usually less than 2 hours).
B. During the eating binges, there is a feeling of lack of control over the eating behavior.
C. The individual regularly engaged in either self-induced vomiting, use of laxatives or diuretics, rigorous dieting or fasting, or vigorous exercise in order to counteract the effects of the binge-eating.
D. A minimum average of two binge-eating episodes per week for at least 3 months.
E. Persistent overconcern with body weight and shape.

*Diagnostic and Statistical Manual, 3rd Edition. Revised. American Psychiatric Association, 1987.

be thinner and depressive moods. This is often complicated and perpetuated by purging behavior, including self-induced vomiting and diuretic and laxative abuse. Current standard diagnostic criteria for the syndrome of bulimia nervosa are presented in Table 5.1.

Estimates of the incidence of bulimia nervosa vary depending on the stringency of diagnosis and population studied; an incidence of 2 to 5% of adolescent and young adult women reflects a form of the disorder associated with chronicity and significant medical and psychiatric severity. As in the related disorder of anorexia nervosa, individuals with bulimia nervosa are overwhelmingly female. The incidence of anorexia nervosa has increased at a much less dramatic rate than the incidence of bulimia nervosa in the last decade; doubtless this reflects a confluence of factors from heightened diagnostic awareness to mounting sociocultural pressures.

The etiology of these disorders is unknown. Most clinicians and researchers embrace a multidetermined model of etiology that acknowledges risk factors at several levels.[1] In terms of culture, readers of this text will know that prejudice against obesity in Western society is strong; the corollary is that exaltation of thinness has reached unparalleled heights.

Professions such as ballet and modeling further intensify this pressure to be thin. In terms of family, a familial history of depression, alcoholism, or anorexia nervosa increases risk for development of anorexia nervosa. In the development of bulimia nervosa, a family history of obesity may also augment risk. At the level of the individual, a sense of personal helplessness and fear of losing control may predispose to the development of these disorders. Certain personality characteristics (in which the person's self-worth is highly tied to performing or pleasing others) and thinking styles (in which the person sees only the extremes in a situation) may provide added risk. The onset of puberty for such a person may result in overwhelming fear in terms of expectations for maturity and independence. The individual responds by dieting, and achieving an illusory sense of mastery through weight control. Other precipitants include separations and losses—these include the individual going away to college or a new summer camp, where there may be a feeling of being threatened by the competition of another person. Family disruption such as divorce and separation may also provoke the individual into dieting to feel a sense of personal control. Infrequently, sudden weight loss for any reason, such as an intercurrent physical illness, may be the event that triggers relentless dieting. A variety of circumstances may coalesce to provide the individual with a maladaptive sense of personal meaning through pursuit of thinness and avoidance of weight gain. Physiologic factors may then intercede to perpetuate the disorder.

Typically, these individuals demonstrate an "all-or-nothing" thinking style that permeates their perceptions of life in general and food in particular; this and the biology of starvation itself often compel them into a cyclical pattern of severe dietary restriction and bingeing, often followed by purging behavior. Self-esteem is chronically low and highly dependent on the opinion of others; these individuals often do not know or trust their perceptions of themselves in terms of self-worth, mood, hunger, satiety, and body weight and shape. Those who suffer from bulimia nervosa as either a component of anorexia nervosa or as an autonomous disorder have some distinctive individual features, including a history of premorbid obesity, general impulsivity, which may manifest as drug and alcohol abuse, stealing, or suicidal behavior, and prominent depressive symptoms.[2]

Many of the symptoms attributed to anorexia nervosa and bulimia nervosa reflect the pathology of starvation due to any cause. Food preoccupation in the context of non-ingestion, sleep and mood disturbances, alterations in perceptions of hunger and satiety, and decreased libido can occur in any starved individual. Similarly, bulimic behavior may emerge from food abstinence. However, because of the drive for thinness, a bulimic episode often if not always is followed by some kind of purging behavior—self-induced vomiting, diuretic or laxative abuse, as well as rigorous exercise and food restriction. A small group of people are unable to induce vomiting and resort to using syrup of ipecac. This contains emetine, a potent muscle toxin, which can result in a serious peripheral or cardiac myopathy.

Because of secrecy and shame in the patient and lack of awareness of these disorders among physicians, diagnosis may be delayed until medical complications emerge. These complications are summarized in Table 5.2. Of particular interest to readers of this text may be gastrointestinal complications of these disorders. Painless parotitis and hyperamylasemia of both salivary and pancreatic origin may betray covert self-induced vomiting. In emaciated anorexics, radiographically confirmed delay in gastric emptying may present as bloating and early satiety. Less commonly, gastric dilatation, infarction, and even rupture have been documented in these patients for the past 20 years. Constipation is a common sequela of food abstinence or laxative abuse and may perpetuate the latter.

TREATMENT

Anorexia nervosa and bulimia nervosa are disorders of ingestive behavior that reflect significant disturbances in intrapsychic functioning. The first step—and often the longest delay—in treatment is adequate diagnosis. For a variety of reasons, these patients often do not initially seek out psychiatric help. As a result, they may only present to non-psychiatric physicians with complications of their eating disorder.

Referral to a psychiatrist familiar with eating disorders is recommended. Treatment will not be described in detail here, except to note that it includes the following components:

TABLE 5.2. COMPLICATIONS

	Frequency	Cause	Treatment
Cardiovascular System			
Bradycardia	Common	Starvation	Responds to weight restoration
Hypotension	Common	Starvation; fluid depletion	Responds to weight restoration
Arrhythmias	Infrequent	Usually provoked by exercise in starvation; may be due to hypokalemia	Responds to weight restoration or potassium supplements
Cardiomyopathy	Rare	Emetine toxicity from ipecac	Stop the ipecac
Central Nervous System			
Nonspecific EEG changes	Common	Starvation	Weight restoration
Reversible cortical atrophy	Uncommon	Starvation	Weight restoration
Renal/Electrolytes			
Hypokalemia	Common	Loss of potassium from multiple routes (vomiting, diarrhea and diuretics); Salt restriction and water intoxication (to meet weight goals)	Prevent purging; may need a potassium supplement Well-balanced diet with appropriate amount of fluids
Increased BUN	Uncommon	Dehydration	Rehydration
Metabolic alkalosis	Common	Purging	Prevent purging
Edema	Common	Not clearly understood	Elevate feet for 1 hour t.i.d.; avoid salt; do not use diuretics
Gastrointestinal System			
Parotitis	Common	Mechanical trauma; starvation	No specific treatments; stop binges and vomiting
Early satiety	Common	Delayed gastric emptying	Domperidone 20 mg t.i.d.
Gastric dilatation	Rare	Rapid refeeding	Avoid oral feeding; use I.V. feeding
Constipation	Common	Starvation; reliance on laxative	Use diet—emphasis on dietary bulk, fruits, vegetables, and try to avoid laxatives
Dental caries	Common	Acidic nature of vomitus	Dental consult
Hyperamylasemia	Common in bulimia nervosa	Unknown	Prevent purging
Gastric rupture	Rare	Bingeing	Surgery
Superior mesenteric artery syndrome	Rare	Weight loss	Weight restoration
Musculoskeletal System			
Myopathy	Uncommon	Starvation; hypokalemia; emetine myotoxicity of ipecac	Weight restoration; stop ipecac abuse
Osteoporosis	Rare	Starvation	Weight restoration
Endocrine System			
Decreased serum T3 and increased reverse T3	Common	Starvation	Weight restoration
Altered insulin sensitivity	Common	Starvation	Weight restoration
Persistent amenorrhea	Infrequent	Low weight; emotional stress	Restore weight to 90% of average
Hematological Changes			
Anemia	Infrequent	Bone marrow hypoplasia; due to starvation	Weight restoration; may need iron
Thrombocytopenia	Rare	Starvation	Weight restoration
Hypercholesterolemia	Common	Unknown	Balanced diet
Hypercarotenemia	Infrequent	Ingestion of high carotene foods	Balanced diet

a) Restoration and maintenance of body weight to a level appropriate for biologic and psychologic health of the patient.

b) Education about the illness and resumption of normal eating patterns.

c) Psychotherapy directed toward those particular psychologic issues which are prominent in the meaning of the eating disorder for the patient. Family therapy may also be indicated.

d) Pharmacotherapy may play a role in the larger treatment of these patients. In particular, a variety of antidepressant medications have demonstrated efficacy in the treatment of bulimia nervosa.

e) Hospitalization may be required for severe emaciation, complications such as hypokalemia and arrhythmia, or suicidality.

RELATIONSHIP TO OBESITY

Stunkard[3] has estimated that roughly 5% of obese persons experience the symptom of bulimia, but unlike their emaciated or normal-weight counterparts, they usually do not vomit after binges. However, it is possible that vomiting, which is a known complication of gastroplasty, may become incorporated into the behavioral repertoire of a bulimic individual. Indeed, such a case has recently been described in one gastroplasty patient coupled with an informal survey of gastroplasty patients, revealing a 40% incidence of self-induced vomiting.[4] Such reports demand further research evaluation as well as clinical concern. Otherwise, eating disorders and their sequelae may masquerade as postoperative complications.

Research on the long-term outcome of anorexia nervosa, bulimia nervosa, and surgery for morbid obesity is in its infancy. Affected individuals share a preoccupation with weight and shape that demands of clinicians a familiarity with areas of common ground.

REFERENCES

1. Garfinkel PE, Garner DM: Anorexia Nervosa: a Multidimensional Perspective. New York, Brunner/Mazel, 1982.
2. Garfinkel PE, Maldofsky H, Garner DM: The heterogeneity of anorexia nervosa: Bulimia as a distinct subgroup. Arch Gen Psychiatry 37:1036–1040, 1980.
3. Stunkard AJ: Obesity. In Hales RE, Frances AJ (eds): American Psychiatric Association Annual Review 4:419–437, 1985.
4. Thompson JK, Weinsier RL, Jacobs B: Self-induced vomiting and subclinical bulimia following gastroplasty surgery for morbid obesity. Int J Eating Disorders 4:609–615, 1985.

6

Perioperative Risk Management in Obese Patients

JOHN G. KRAL
RICHARD J. STRAUSS
LESLIE WISE

The challenge of surgery in the overweight patient lies in the special care and knowledge that are required for successful preoperative, intraoperative and postoperative management. From the outset, the obese patient is at a surgical disadvantage because differential diagnosis is more difficult, anesthesia is more troublesome and technical procedures are more complicated.

The obese have an increased prevalence of serious systemic diseases such as diabetes, hypertension and dyslipoproteinemia and of various medical conditions that impair their general level of health.[1] Several surgical diseases are also more prevalent in obesity (Table 6.1), although many surgeons defer operating on the obese for fear of the increased risk of complications. It is true that obesity is associated with an increase in complications (Table 6.2), but significant advances have been made in recent years from the experience gained through the development and use of surgical procedures specifically for the treatment of morbid obesity. The reader is referred to excellent summaries which review anesthetic and surgical management of the morbidly obese.[2–4]

Obesity is a prevalent disease in those parts of the world where such statistics are available. Taking into account different criteria for obesity and differences in age and sex distribution and sampling methods, a recent compilation of European statistics demonstrates a prevalence of obesity in males of 5–44% and in females of 6–49%.[5] In the United States the Health and Nutrition Survey 1976–1980 (NHANES II) demonstrated that 26% of

TABLE 6.1. SURGICAL DISEASES PREVALENT IN OBESITY

A. Metabolic etiology
  1) Cholelithiasis
  2) Thromboembolism
  3) Peripheral vascular
  4) Urolithiasis
  5) Neoplasia
    a) Malignant
      1. Endocrine: endometrial, breast, prostate cancer
      2. Colon cancer
      3. Renal cancer
    b) Benign
      1. Uterine fibroma
      2. Ovarian cysts
      3. Fibroadenoma of the breast
B. Physical etiology
  1) Osteoarthritis
  2) Esophagitis
  3) Cesarean section
  4) Hernia (primary)

TABLE 6.2. SURGICAL COMPLICATIONS IN OBESE PATIENTS

A. Anesthesia-related
  1) Respiratory—hypoventilation
  2) Pulmonary—atelectasis, pneumonia
  3) Circulatory—thromboembolism
B. Wound healing
  1) Infection
  2) Hernia (secondary)
C. Technical
  1) Hemorrhage
  2) Leaks

adults aged 20–75 years are overweight[6] with significantly higher prevalence in specific groups based on age and sex.

Apart from the increased morbidity associated with obesity, the excess mortality is substantial.[7] It is principally caused by death from coronary heart disease, stroke and diabetes mellitus, although sudden unexplained death,[8] malignancies and fatal accidents are also more prevalent in the obese. Drenick et al.[9] have shown that there is a twelve-fold excess mortality in men in the age group 25–34 years and a six-fold excess in those aged 35–44 years.

Obesity is a risk factor for development of postoperative complications as outlined in Table 6.2. The following review will present systemic complications of obesity that influence perioperative management as well as specific surgical and anesthesiologic risks and will provide recommendations for managing obese patients undergoing surgery.

SYSTEMIC COMPLICATIONS OF OBESITY

CARDIOVASCULAR PROBLEMS

Obesity has an adverse effect on the cardiovascular system. The heart often enlarges, and the cardiac output, stroke volume, and blood volume[10] as well as extracellular fluid volume[11] all may increase. As reported in several studies[12,13] the hemodynamic status in the resting state becomes adapted to the increased metabolic need of the obese patient as evidenced by increased cardiac output, stroke volume, cardiac index, left ventricular stroke work, right ventricular stroke work, higher filling pressures of the right and left side of the heart and increased mean pulmonary artery pressure.

In a study by Agarwal et al.[12] hemodynamic changes in the morbidly obese were studied in the preoperative, intraoperative and postoperative period and these results were compared with those of non-obese patients. Obese patients demonstrated significantly elevated preoperative, intraoperative and postoperative right atrial, mean pulmonary artery and pulmonary artery wedge pressures. Preoperatively, hemodynamic variables were in the high range of normal in obese patients, but in the intraoperative period, significantly greater decreases in cardiac index, right ventricular stroke work and left ventricular stroke work were noted. According to Agarwal et al.,[12] the cardiac index and left ventricular stroke work remained depressed in the postoperative period. Obese patients, therefore, reacted to the stress of surgery and anesthesia by a left ventricular dysfuction represented by a low cardiac index and reduced left ventricular contractility in the early postoperative period.

In a study by Clowes, Del Guercio and Barwinsky,[14] it was demonstrated that in the event that the intraoperative phase, characterized by depression of cardiac output and cardiac index, was not followed by the normal elevation of cardiac output and cardiac index in the immediate postoperative period, the patients did poorly. Thus, we may conclude that the abnormal response of obese patients in the immediate postoperative period may be an important contributory factor for the increased operative mortality in the morbidly obese.[12]

Systemic hypertension is common among obese surgical patients, and prospective studies show a correlation between obesity and systemic hypertension.[15,16] A large Scandinavian study of more than 67,000 adults found an increase in systolic pressure of 3 mm Hg and a rise in diastolic pressure of 2 mm Hg for every 10-kg increase in body weight.[17] Clinical studies have also shown that weight reduction produces a significant drop in blood pressure, heart rate, stroke volume, cardiac output and oxygen uptake.[16,18]

The mechanism for hypertension is not known although several have been implicated. The increase in extracellular fluid volume in obesity, which is an important independent factor in obesity—hypertension,[19] can be attributed to hyperinsulinemia with sodium retention[20] as well as other hormonal effects.[21,22]

RENAL FAILURE

Hypertension produces vascular changes throughout the body, particularly in the kidneys, and induces nephrotic changes. This causes the small arteries to thicken, and in time they undergo collagenous fibrosis with marked luminal narrowing. The kidneys gradually undergo a slow, progressive atrophy and fibrosis. Since obese patients have a higher incidence of hypertension than the general population, they suffer more often from the renal consequences of hypertension.

Hypertension reduces renal blood flow and tubular function, and because of the vascular changes noted above, the obese may exhibit mild proteinuria and, occasionally, uremia. Nephrosis has been described in morbidly obese patients[23,24] and renal vein thrombosis is also a cause of renal failure according to one study.[25]

DIABETES

There is a complex relationship between diabetes mellitus and obesity. Increased body weight and age are both correlated with an increased incidence of diabetes. In one study[26] less than 1% of women of normal weight between the ages of 25 and 44 had diabetes, but 7% of those in the same age group who were 100% overweight had diabetes. Ogilvie[27] has shown that the beta-cells in the islets of Langerhans are enlarged in obese patients and glucose tolerance is frequently impaired.[28] Obese subjects have reduced numbers of insulin receptors, which have been shown to increase after weight loss induced by gastric bypass.[29]

One of us (LW) studied intraoperative glucose metabolism in seven grossly obese patients.[30] Preoperative fasting plasma glucose levels were all in the low normal range, and in three of the seven, intravenous glucose tolerance studies during the preoperative period suggested impaired glucose utilization. During surgery, glucose utilization was found to be impaired in all patients. Although this study did not demonstrate a marked osmotic diuresis leading to hypovolemia, the decreased glucose utilization suggests that the obese patient may require cautious administration of glucose during the procedure. Impaired glucose tolerance has been implicated in the poor immune response of obese patients[31] which will be discussed below.

HYPOVENTILATION

Markedly obese patients are particularly susceptible to hypoventilation, although many other characteristics have also been described in patients with only moderate obesity.[32] Pulmonary function studies in obese patients demonstrate large anatomic shunts and increased ventilation/perfusion inequalities both at rest and during exercise.[33] It also appears that some element of venous admixture leads fairly consistently to modest degrees of decreased arterial oxygenation without increase in arterial CO_2 content.[34] It is unclear whether this has any clinical significance. The numerous pulmonary abnormalities contributing to the decreased arterial oxygenation in obesity are summarized in Figure 6.1, which will serve as a baseline for the discussion of perioperative changes.

PREOPERATIVE EVALUATION AND TREATMENT

The systemic complications discussed above have to be evaluated and treated if present prior to surgery. It is often necessary to postpone elective surgery on obese patients, simply to improve their preoperative status. Routine physical examination with special attention to peripheral edema, repeated blood pressure measurement with a wide cuff, and routine EKG and chest X-ray should be supplemented with rhythm strip EKG to detect arrhythmia, exercise testing (if physically possible), and radionuclide cardiography if the patient's history discloses risk factors or manifest symptoms or episodes of cardiovascular compromise. Smoking is the most serious risk factor complicating obesity and might even be considered a contraindication to elective surgery. It is impossible to design stringent controlled studies to determine a minimum preoperative smoking-free interval but a 6-week period is rec-

ommended[35,36] and should preferably be complemented with vigorous chest physical therapy. Obesity is associated with elevated extracellular water as pointed out above, and it is often appropriate to pretreat the patient with a course of diuretics (with K supplements!).

Pulmonary function tests are essential in view of the high prevalence of abnormalities outlined above. Arterial blood gas determination is most important. Chest physical therapy with breathing exercises and instruction in the use of the incentive spirometer should be routine in obese patients. Taking of the patient's history should specifically be directed toward present or past history of smoking and symptoms of hypoventilation or obstructive sleep apnea, inquiring about snoring, orthopnea, daytime somnolence, depression and nocturnal shortness of breath, since routine pulmonary fuction tests might not disclose any abnormalities. If sleep apnea is suspected, an ENT consult should be obtained and sleep provocation tests be performed. Preoperative weight loss and possibly surgical correction of airway obstruction will significantly reduce the likelihood of the patient remaining intubated postoperatively, and thus reduce the frequency of postoperative complications. A course of continuous positive airway pressure (CPAP) can dramatically improve the pulmonary function of an obese patient.

Obese patients are susceptible to wound infections, partly because of their diabetic tendency and partly because of difficulties in managing their personal hygiene, particularly if they have a pendulous abdomen. Preoperative skin care with bactericidal showers twice daily and perioperative antibiotic cov-

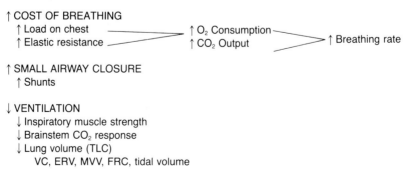

$\downarrow$ **Pao$_2$**

$\uparrow$ COST OF BREATHING
  $\uparrow$ Load on chest ———————→ $\uparrow$ O$_2$ Consumption
  $\uparrow$ Elastic resistance ———————→ $\uparrow$ CO$_2$ Output ————————→ $\uparrow$ Breathing rate

$\uparrow$ SMALL AIRWAY CLOSURE
  $\uparrow$ Shunts

$\downarrow$ VENTILATION
  $\downarrow$ Inspiratory muscle strength
  $\downarrow$ Brainstem CO$_2$ response
  $\downarrow$ Lung volume (TLC)
     VC, ERV, MVV, FRC, tidal volume

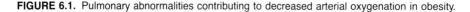

FIGURE 6.1. Pulmonary abnormalities contributing to decreased arterial oxygenation in obesity.

erage have dramatically reduced the wound infection rate in these patients.

ANESTHESIA AND OPERATION

ACCESS

The obese patient poses special problems for the anesthetist. These arise from difficulties in intravenous access, difficulties in intubation and airway maintenance, ventilatory problems both before and after operation, factors influencing the uptake and distribution of anesthetic agents, and anatomic problems encountered with regional anesthesia. An intravenous infusion (I.V.) may be difficult to start and may be time-consuming because of the paucity of visible and palpable veins. A large-bore I.V. or preferably a central line should be started the day before surgery, allowing infusion of potassium and glucose (to be discussed below).

Both subclavian and internal jugular catheters are difficult to place in the obese. Preference should be given to an internal jugular since the complications are fewer and less serious. If preoperative placement is not feasible, a central line should be inserted after induction of anesthesia in severely obese patients having major surgery, particularly where prolonged postoperative parenteral nutrition is expected, but also to monitor central venous pressure.

It is often difficult to obtain and maintain an airway in obese patients. The mask does not fit well, and reduced mobility of the cervical spine in patients with obese necks makes intubation difficult. Furthermore, it is not uncommon to encounter airway obstruction from a large tongue, swollen tonsils or frank narrowing of the glottis.

ASPIRATION

Obese patients have a higher risk of aspiration pneumonia than controls. Teabeaut[37] pointed out that the predominant insult from the aspiration of liquid gastric contents was a result of the acidity and the volume. He also showed that as the pH of the aspirate decreased to 1.5, pulmonary parenchymal damage increased to a maximum. In a study of 106 patients, one of us showed that obese patients had a significantly higher residual gastric volume (42 mL vs 14 mL; $p < 0.01$) and a lower pH (1.7 vs 3.7; $p < 0.01$) than nonobese controls.[38] These findings can be explained by delayed gastric emptying[39] (although data are conflicting) and an elevated acid secretory capacity,[40] which are found in the obese. For these reasons, particular care should be exercised in the induction of anesthesia in obese patients, and even in elective operations they should be treated as if they had a full stomach. As suggested by Vaughan et al.,[38] one should consider either tracheal intubation under topical anesthesia with the patient awake or a rapid intravenous induction-intubation sequence. Wilson et al.[41] reported that in morbidly obese patients, cimetidine 300 mg, administered orally at midnight and repeated with a sip of water 2 to 4 hours before surgery, is highly effective in increasing gastric pH values, and therefore may be effective in reducing the risk of aspiration pneumonia in this high-risk group during intubation. However, studies culturing gastric mucosa obtained during gastroplasty have revealed elevated bacterial counts that might be due to overgrowth after suppression of acid.[42]

INDUCTION AND EXTUBATION

Induction of anesthesia may be greatly prolonged in obese patients,[43] probably because their more difficult ventilation makes it harder to raise the alveolar concentration of the anesthetic gas.[44] Anesthetic agents are highly soluble in fat[45,46] and there is a decreased clearance of various drugs in obesity,[47] particularly halothane.[48] Thus, it is important to begin anesthetic washout earlier in these cases to enable expeditious extubation. During the anesthesia it is possible to misjudge the level of relaxation if the anesthesiologist relies solely on bag pressure. In view of the reduced compliance of the chest wall in obese patients a false impression of increased needs for relaxants might lead to unnecessary administration of anesthetic gas or muscle relaxants. Routine use of a nerve stimulator to evaluate degree of relaxation is appropriate in severely obese patients.

REGIONAL ANESTHESIA

To try to avoid some of the problems of general endotracheal anesthesia, regional anesthesia has been suggested,[49] although it is understood that anatomic landmarks are obscured in obese patients. It is also dangerous to estimate the proper dose of local anesthetic on the basis of body weight alone; the obese patient often needs 30 to 40% less epidural anesthesia than does the individual of average weight.[50] Spinal anesthesia in the obese also carries with it the threat of unintentional overdose, which is primarily due to a decrease in the effective volume of the subarachnoid space secondary to the accumulation of excessive amounts of adipose tissue in the peridural space[51] or to increased epidural venous blood volume reducing the volume of the epidural space. If this need for lower doses is not recognized, the anesthesiologist may be faced with an apneic patient who can be intubated only with extreme difficulty. In the event that intubation proves impossible, tracheostomy will have to be performed, and this may be extremely difficult in a patient with an obese immobile neck.

INTRAOPERATIVE OXYGENATION

Vaughan and Wise studied the intraoperative arterial oxygenation pattern of obese patients and the effect on arterial oxygenation of changes in operative position or the placement of a subdiaphragmatic laparotomy pack.[52] This study demonstrated that 40% oxygen concentrations did not uniformly produce adequate arterial oxygenation during intra-abdominal surgery in otherwise healthy obese patients. The placement of a subdiaphragmatic abdominal laparotomy pack with no change in operative position produced a consistent fall in Pa_{O_2} to less than 65 torr even though 40% oxygen was being administered. They also found that a change from a supine to a 15° head-down operative position resulted in a significant ($p < 0.001$) reduction in mean Pa_{O_2} (73.0 ± 26.3 torr). On 40% oxygen, 77% of these patients had Pa_{O_2} values of less than 80 torr.

These findings suggest that the Trendelenburg position and the use of subdiaphragmatic laparotomy packs should be avoided in obese patients. In fact, most upper abdominal procedures in morbidly obese patients are routinely performed with the patient in a 30–45° head-up position, ameliorating oxygenation and improving operative exposure.[53] This requires a foot-rest on the operating-table and the use of intermittent compression leggings to improve venous return.

POSTOPERATIVE OXYGENATION

The reduced arterial oxygen tension in obese patients preoperatively is further re-duced postoperatively as demonstrated by Vaughan et al. in 1974.[54] In a group of 20 morbidly obese patients the decrease in mean Pa_{O_2} averaged −9.2 2 hours postoperatively, −15.0 on day 1, −15.5 on day 2 and −11.7 on day 3 (all $p < 0.001$ compared to preoperatively). Similar results were obtained in 56 patients having gastric bypass.[55] Full recovery was not evident until the fifth day, which is in agreement with pulmonary function studies performed postoperatively by Catenacci et al.[56]

Postoperatively, Pa_{O_2} may reach dangerously low levels due to multiple factors which are enumerated in Table 6.3. One of us (LW) has addressed the importance of the effects of the operative incision (midline vs transverse)[57] and of the position of the patient (supine vs semi-recumbent)[58] on postoperative oxygenation. Patients with midline incisions had significantly increased alveolar-arterial oxygen tension differences compared to those with transverse incisions without return to preoperative values throughout the first 5 days postoperatively.[57] Often upper midline incisions are necessary for reasons of exposure in these patients, but wherever possible, transverse incisions should be chosen. The other study[58] revealed that the supine position during the first 48 hours postoperatively reduced arterial oxygenation. Thus, the semi-recumbent position recommended above for use intraoperatively should be maintained at all times also after extubation, as an aid to improving arterial oxygenation. Furthermore, most surgeons performing obesity surgery routinely administer oxygen via nasal prongs or face mask for at least 12 hours following extubation, and one paper suggests maintaining supplemental oxygen for 3 days.[55] An indwelling arterial line placed intraoperatively is invaluable for postoperative monitoring of blood gases and true blood pressure during the first 12 hours after surgery.

POSTOPERATIVE COMPLICATIONS AND THEIR PREVENTION

PULMONARY

Although respiratory parameters have been amply studied as outlined above, there are relatively few studies on the importance of obesity for development of pulmonary complications postoperatively. Atelectasis has been shown to be more prevalent in obese patients,[59-61] which emphasizes the impor-

TABLE 6.3. FACTORS CONTRIBUTING TO POSTOPERATIVE DECREASED Pa$_{O_2}$ IN MORBIDLY OBESE PATIENTS

Sedation	Atelectasis	Position
Immobilization	Pneumonia	Incision
Pain	Retained secretions	

tance of the reverse-Trendelenburg position, intermittent hyperinflation ("sighs") during intubation anesthesia, and postoperative breathing exercises with chest physical therapy. Although two studies were unable to document a statistically significant difference in incidence of pneumonia in obese patients,[59,60] obesity is considered a risk factor for the development of pneumonia and vigorous steps should be taken to prevent it. Particularly important measures are early postoperative ambulation, usually within four hours of extubation, and chest physical therapy.

Since pain medication, especially parenteral narcotics, causes respiratory depression as well as sedation, great care must be taken in the administration of such medication. Two strategies have been developed that drastically reduce the total need for narcotics. Patient-controlled analgesia (PCA), allowing the patient to self-administer I.V. narcotics with maximized single and cumulative dosage, reduces the total narcotic dose by 50%. Furthermore, epidural morphine seems to be highly effective in promoting ambulation and reducing hospital stay in morbidly obese patients.[62,63]

THROMBOSIS AND EMBOLISM

Obesity is a risk factor predisposing to thromboembolism.[64] In a study of 4600 autopsies, 12.3% has pulmonary embolism. The prevalence of embolism in the study was 21.9% in 544 obese (>20% overweight) adults compared with 14.4% in the non-obese (p <0.005) irrespective of sex.[65] In the Framingham study overweight was the only independent factor associated with death from pulmonary embolism, and only among women (p <0.001) although there was a trend in men.[64] Pulmonary embolism was the most common pulmonary complication in a study of postsurgical morbidly obese patients having various types of procedures including orthopedic, thoracic, pelvic, abdominal and "superficial" surgery.[66] Excessive weight was a significant predictor of the development of deep vein thrombosis after gynecologic surgery in several studies.[67,68]

Several mechanisms may be involved in the pathogenesis of thromboembolism in obesity. Low vascular fibrinolytic activity,[69] increased blood viscosity associated with dyslipoproteinemia[70] and low antithrombin III[71] increase the likelihood of thrombus formation. The characteristically elevated blood levels of free fatty acids in the obese increase still more during the routine fast preceding surgery and are augmented by catecholamine release during surgery, as has been pointed out by Mason and coworkers.[72] Infusion of glucose (evoking an endogenous insulin response) inhibits lipolysis and reduces hemoconcentration, both of which should be beneficial in preventing thrombosis.

A recent NIH Consensus Conference on prevention of venous thrombosis and pulmonary embolism,[73] affirming the role of obesity as a risk factor, recommended external pneumatic compression as a safe antithrombotic measure, virtually without contraindications in any field of surgery. This technique is particularly suitable in obese patients for several reasons. The obese have an increased incidence of varicose veins with peripheral pooling of blood which is counteracted by intermittent compression of the legs. Furthermore, compression stimulates the release of venous fibrinolytic factors, which are known to be reduced in obesity.[71] As pointed out above, leg compression is an important adjunct to the semi-recumbent position required to improve respiratory function in these patients.

WOUND INFECTION, DEHISCENCE AND HERNIA

Several series have demonstrated increased prevalence of wound infections in obese patients after ulcer surgery,[60] cholecystectomy,[59] colo-rectal surgery,[74] and gynecologic-obstetric procedures.[75,76] However, 23 obese patients with frankly contaminated wounds where drains had been placed had a lower infection rate in a prospective randomized study undertaken to determine the effect of wound drains.[77] The study did show that the infection rate was greater in both clean and potentially contaminated wounds in the presence of a drain in the overall surgical population, implying that drains in fact contaminated the wounds.[77] Most surgeons performing obesity surgery will avoid placing subcutaneous drains, and intraabdominal drains are contraindicated if foreign material is being used as in banded gastroplasty. The principle of delayed primary wound closure is particularly appropriate in obese and diabetic patients with obvious contamination at operation.[78]

There are several explanations for the increased susceptibility of obese patients to wound infections. Technical difficulties lead to longer operating times and more trauma to the abdominal wall and subcutaneous tissue during retraction. Apposition of the wound is difficult and the subcutaneous adipose tissue provides substrate for bacteria. There is also evidence in obesity of impaired immunocompetence,[79,80] of unknown etiology, although the diabetic or at least pre-diabetic glucose disposal in obesity is known to interfere with leukocyte function.[81]

The increased frequency of wound infection, stress on the incision and encumbered apposition increase the risk of wound dehiscence in obesity. There are no controlled prospective studies comparing dehiscence in obese versus non-obese patients, although one retrospective study found 4 cases among 225 obese patients and none among 225 of normal weight. In another retrospective analysis of 18,000 abdominal procedures the predominant factor in the 70 patients with dehiscence was obesity.[82] In this context, it is probable that a vertical incision is subjected to less tension than a horizontal incision, which has to be taken into account in the choice of method of closure.

Dehiscence, wound infection, and development of seroma predispose to incisional hernia. Indeed, obese patients have an increased incidence of incisional hernia as well as primary hernias. Branch reported that 48 of his 100 patients with incisional hernias were obese.[83] In 13 he found no other factor than obesity to explain the hernia. Several studies have documented the increased incidence of dehiscence and hernia in obstetric and gynecologic populations.[84,85]

Incison and Retraction

The extensive performance of surgery for obesity has led to the development of techniques and routines for reducing wound complications in obese patients having other types of surgery. It is a truism to stress atraumatic technique, but some details deserve mentioning. Once the skin has been opened, tearing the adipose tissue by forceful traction with rake retractors reduces the amount of bleeding. It can usually be stopped by compression with dry laparotomy pads, obviating the need for electrocautery and ligatures. Sutures and ligatures should be avoided in adipose tissue. If they are needed, the choice should be synthetic absorbables (e.g. polyglycolic acid). Rake retractors cause less compression and crushing of tissue, and throughout the operation retractors should be relaxed periodically and saline applied to wound edges. Exposure is significantly enhanced by adjustable mounted retraction systems, but these should be released intermittently.

Infection Control

Vigorous irrigation of the abdomen, with or without antibiotics (no prospective randomized trial to prove the benefit of antibiotics), and of the subcutaneous tissue is recommended. Many surgeons routinely use preoperative systemic antibiotics, continued postoperatively, and antibacterial showers 2–3 times preoperatively are probably beneficial. Paper drapes and gowns in the operating-room have been proven to cut infection rates in orthopedic and vascular surgery and it is reasonable to use them for obese patients.

Closure

Fascia closure with running #2 polyglycolic acid is sufficient for most purposes. However, morbidly obese patients with well-developed muscles (particularly all men) should probably have retention sutures to relax the fascial closure. As mentioned above, sutures and ligatures should be avoided in the subcutaneous tissues. Apposition of the thick layer of adipose tissue can best be achieved by #1 monofilament semi-retention mattress sutures through the skin down to the level of the fascia, taking care to eliminate dead space. These sutures should be removed on the 3rd–4th postoperative day to avoid skin necrosis. Drains should only be used under special circumstances, as pointed out earlier. Preoperative physical therapy to teach the patient how to roll in and out of bed avoiding stress on the abdominal muscles and Valsalva maneuvers, might be helpful for the first 7–10 days after surgery as a measure to prevent dehiscence.

NUTRITIONAL STATE

It is important to recognize patients with nutritional compromise in the face of their obesity. A subgroup of obese patients have reduced body cell mass with concomitant elevated extracellular water, making them less able to withstand operative stress and postoperative catabolism. In one study, 8 of 44 morbidly obese patients demonstrated significant reduction in body cell mass prior to surgery.[86] On the other hand the majority of extremely obese patients have a greater absolute cell mass than the normal-weight population. A particularly compromised group is patients who have had prior surgery for obesity. They must always be considered to have latent malnutrition and thus present a greater risk for the development of postoperative complications. This is especially true of patients who have had malabsorptive operations. They may require preoperative total parenteral nutrition to improve their nitrogen balance.

Weight loss prior to surgery is obviously beneficial to ameliorate many of the complicating conditions afflicting the obese. However, it is important that the loss not occur at the expense of lean body mass and that sufficient protein (1.5 g/kg of ideal body weight per day) be provided.[87] Reduction in simple carbohydrates reduces glycemia and lipogenesis, and should be recommended routinely. An important adjunct to dietary management is implementation of an exercise program whenever feasible, since the majority of obese patients are sedentary and exercise improves

glucose tolerance and respiratory capacity, and helps maintain lean body mass. Even though the modalities of diet and exercise are generally unsuccessful in treating obesity per se, they are invaluable adjuncts in preparing the obese patient for surgery.

SUMMARY

Numerous preoperative, intraoperative and postoperative problems, including those of diagnosis, anesthesia, technical difficulties, postoperative respiratory insufficiency, wound complications and thromboembolism, are associated with obesity. Lessons learned from 30 years of risk-reduction in obesity operations are pertinent to general surgical practice. Table 6.4 lists pre-, peri- and postoperative measures to prevent surgical complications in obese patients. Improved management should ultimately influence the negative selection bias that has excluded obese patients from elective surgery for fear of complications, potentially resulting in emergency procedures in those already compromised patients.[88] Over the long term, surgical morbidity and mortality statistics for obese patients are expected to improve.

TABLE 6.4. MEASURES TO PREVENT SURGICAL COMPLICATIONS IN OBESE PATIENTS

A. Preoperative
  1) Patient selection
  2) D/C smoking, oral contraceptives
  3) Diet
  4) Physical therapy, CPAP, incentive spirometer
  5) Antibacterial showers
  6) Antibiotic prophylaxis
B. Perioperative
  1) Antibiotics, paper drapes, irrigation
  2) Antithrombotic measures—low-dose heparin, stockings/wraps, intermittent compression, hemodilution
  3) Pulmonary precautions—reverse Trendelenburg, empty stomach, sigh, immediate extubation
  4) Surgical technique—access with adjustable retractors, avoid subcutaneous sutures
C. Postoperative
  1) Early ambulation
  2) Oxygen support
  3) Close monitoring—central venous pressure, ABG, glycemia
  4) Semi-recumbent position

REFERENCES

1. Kral JG: Morbid obesity and related health risks. Ann Intern Med 103:1043–1047, 1985.
2. Gayes JM: Anesthesia for the morbidly obese patient. In Linner JH (ed): Surgery for Morbid Obesity. New York, Springer-Verlag, 1984, pp 133–144.
3. Mason EE: Surgical Treatment of Obesity. Philadelphia, WB Saunders, 1981.
4. Brown BR: Anesthesia and the Obese Patient. Philadelphia, WB Saunders, 1982.
5. Kluthe R, Schubert A: Obesity in Europe. Ann Intern Med 103:1037–1042, 1985.
6. Van Itallie TB: Health implications of overweight and obesity in the United States. Ann Intern Med 103:983–988, 1985.
7. Simopoulos AP, Van Itallie TB: Body weight, health and longevity. Ann Intern Med 100:285–295, 1984.
8. Drenick EJ: Incidence of sudden unexplained death in morbidly obese patients. Clin Nutr 5 (suppl):iii, 1986.
9. Drenick EJ, Bale GS, Saltzer F, et al: Excessive mortality and causes of death in morbidly obese men. JAMA 243:443–445, 1980.
10. Alexander JK, Amad KH, Cole VW: Observations on some clinical features of extreme obesity with particular reference to the cardiorespiratory effects. Am J Med 32:512–524, 1962.
11. Pierson RN Jr, Wang J, Yang MU, et al: The assessment of human body composition during weight re-

duction: evaluation of a new model for clinical studies. J Nutr 106:1694–1701, 1976.

12. Agarwal N, Shibutani K, SanFillipo J, et al: Hemodynamic and respiratory changes in surgery of the morbidly obese. Surgery 92:226–234, 1982.

13. Divitiis OD, Fazio S, Petitto M, et al: Obesity and cardiac function. Circulation 64:477–482, 1981.

14. Clowes GHA Jr, Del Guercio LRM, Barwinsky J: The cardiac output in response to surgical trauma. Arch Surg 81:212–222, 1960.

15. Keys A, Aravanis C, Blackburn H, et al: Coronary heart disease, overweight and obesity as risk factors. Ann Intern Med 77:15–27, 1972.

16. Chang BN, Periman LV, Epstein FH: Overweight and hypertension: a review. Circulation 39:403–421, 1969.

17. Bjerkedal T: Overweight and hypertension. Acta Med Scand 159:13–26, 1957.

18. Alexander JK, Peterson KL: Cardiovascular effects of weight reduction. Circulation 45:310–318, 1972.

19. Raison J, Achimastos A, Asmar R, et al: Extracellular and interstitial fluid volume in obesity with and without associated systemic hypertension. Am J Cardiol 57:223–226, 1986.

20. De Fronzo RA, Cooke RE, Andres R: The effects of insulin on renal handling of sodium, potassium, calcium, and phosphate in man. J Clin Invest 55:845–855, 1975.

21. Evans DJ, Hoffmann RG, Kalkhoff RK, et al: Relationship of androgenic activity to body fat topography, fat cell morphology and metabolic aberrations in premenopausal women. J Clin Endocrinol Metab 57:304–310, 1983.

22. Hiramatsu K, Yamada T, Schikawa K, et al: Changes in endocrine activities relative to obesity in patients with essential hypertension. J Am Geriatr Soc 29:25–30, 1981.

23. Warnke RA, Kempson RL: The nephrotic syndrome in massive obesity: a study by light, immunofluorescence, and electron microscopy. Arch Pathol Lab Med 102:431–438, 1978.

24. Weisinger JR, Kempson RL, Eldridge FL, et al: The nephrotic syndrome: a complication of massive obesity. Ann Intern Med 81:440–447, 1974.

25. Luft FC, Walker PD, Hamburger RJ, et al: Thrombosis of the renal veins and vena cava: occurrence in morbid obesity. JAMA 234:1158–1160, 1975.

26. Rimm AA, Werner LH, Bernstein R, et al: Disease and obesity in 73,532 women. Obesity Bariatric Med 1:77–84, 1972.

27. Ogilvie RF: The islands of Langerhans in 19 cases of obesity. J Pathol Bacteriol 37:473–481, 1933.

28. Sanderson I, Deitel M, Bojm M: The handling of glucose and insulin response before and after weight loss with jejuno-ileal bypass. JPEN 7:274–276, 1983.

29. Kramer JL, Halverson JD, Thomas L, et al: Increased binding of insulin to mononuclear blood cells following gastric bypass for morbid obesity. J Surg Res 32:343–346, 1982.

30. Stein T, Vaughan R, Wise L: Glucose tolerance in the obese surgical patient. Surg Gynecol Obstet 148:380–384, 1979.

31. Kolterman, OG, Olefsky JM, Kurahara C, et al: A defect in cell-mediated immune function in insulin-resistant diabetic and obese subjects. J Lab Clin Med 96:535–543, 1980.

32. Bray GA: Complications of obesity. Ann Intern Med 103:1052–1062, 1985.

33. Barrera F, Hillyer P, Ascanio G, et al: The distribution of ventilation, diffusion, and blood flow in obese patients with normal and abnormal blood gases. Am Rev Respir Dis 108:819–830, 1973.

34. Douglas FG, Chang PY: Influence of obesity on peripheral airways patency. J Appl Physiol 33:559–563, 1972.

35. Jones RM: Smoking before surgery: the case for stopping (editorial). Br Med J 290:1763–1764, 1985.

36. Wilhelmsen L: Effects on bronchopulmonary symptoms, ventilation, and lung mechanics of abstinence from tobacco smoking. Scand J Respir Dis 48:407–410, 1967.

37. Teabeaut JR II: Aspiration of gastric contents: an experimental study. Am J Pathol 28:51–67, 1952.

38. Vaughan RW, Bauer S, Wise L: Volume and pH of gastric juice in obese patients. Anesthesiology 43:686–689, 1975.

39. Horowitz M, Collins PJ, Cook DJ, et al: Abnormalities of gastric emptying in obese patients. Int J Obes 7:415–421, 1983.

40. Kral JG, Granerus G: Gastric acid secretion in morbid obesity (abstract). Gastroenterology 80:1199, 1981.

41. Wilson S, Mantena NR, Halverson JD: Effect of atropine, glycopyrrolate, and cimetidine on gastric secretions in morbidly obese patients. Anesth Analg 60:37–40, 1981.

42. Cowan GSM Jr: Presence of intra-gastric organisms in the bariatric surgical field. Proceedings, 3rd annual meeting, American Society for Bariatric Surgery, Iowa City, June 18–20, 1986, p 93.

43. Warner WA, Garrett LP: The obese patient and anesthesia. JAMA 205:102–106, 1968.

44. Eger EI: Uptake, distribution, and elimination of inhaled anaesthetics. In Scurr C, Feldman S (eds): Scientific Foundations of Anaesthesia. Chicago, Year Book Medical Publishers, 1974, p 444.

45. Young SR, Stoelting RK, Peterson C, et al: Anesthetic biotransformation and renal function in obese patients during and after methoxyflurane or halothane anesthesia. Anesthesiology 42:451–457, 1975.

46. Vaughan WR, Sipes IG, Brown BR: Role of biotransformation in the toxicity of inhalation anesthetics. Life Sci 23:2447–2462, 1978.

47. Abernethy DR, Greenblatt DJ, Divoll M, et al: Alterations in drug distribution and clearance due to obesity. J Pharmacol Exp Ther 217:681–685, 1981.

48. Saraiva RA, Lunn JN, Mapleson WW, et al: Adiposity and the pharmacokinetics of halothane: the effect of adiposity on the maintenance of and recovery from halothane anaesthesia. Anaesthesia 32:240–246, 1977.

49. Brodsky JB: Anesthetic management of the morbidly obese patient. Int Anesthesiol Clin 24:93–103, 1986.

50. Bromage PR: Physiology and pharmacology of epidural analgesia. Anesthesiology 28:592–622, 1967.

51. Lund PC: Principles and Practice of Spinal Anesthesia. Springfield, Ill., Charles C Thomas, 1971, p. 481.
52. Vaughan RW, Wise L: Intraoperative arterial oxygenation in obese patients. Ann Surg 184:35–42, 1976.
53. Linner JH: Gastric operations: specific tecniques. In Linner JH (ed): Surgery for Morbid Obesity. New York, Springer-Verlag, 1984, pp 65–92.
54. Vaughan RW, Engelhardt RC, Wise L: Postoperative hypoxemia in obese patients. Ann Surg 180:877–882, 1974.
55. Taylor RR, Kelly TM, Elliott CG, et al: Hypoxemia after gastric bypass surgery for morbid obesity. Arch Surg 120:1298–1302, 1985.
56. Catenacci AJ, Anderson JD, Boersma D: Anesthetic hazards of obesity. JAMA 175:657–661, 1961.
57. Vaughan RW, Engelhardt RC, Wise L: Postoperative alveolar-arterial oxygen tension difference: its relation to the operative incision in obese patients. Anesth Analg 54:433–437, 1975.
58. Vaughan RW, Bauer S, Wise L: Effects of position (semi-recumbent vs. supine) on postoperative oxygenation in markedly obese subjects. Anesth Analg 55:37–41,1976.
59. Pemberton LB, Manax WG: Relationship of obesity to postoperative complications after cholecystectomy. Am J Surg 121:87–90, 1971.
60. Postlethwait RW, Johnson WD: Complications following surgery for duodenal ulcer in obese patients. Arch Surg 105:438–440, 1972.
61. Hansen G, Drablos PP, Steinert R: Pulmonary complications, ventilation and blood gases after upper abdominal surgery. Acta Anaesthesiol Scand 21:211–215, 1977.
62. Brodsky JB, Merrell RC: Epidural administration of morphine postoperatively for morbidly obese patients. West J Med 140:750–753, 1984.
63. Rawal N, Sjöstrand U, Christoffersson E, et al: Comparison of intramuscular and epidural morphine for postoperative analgesia in the grossly obese: influence on postoperative ambulation and pulmonary function. Anesth Analg 63:583–592, 1984.
64. Goldhaber SZ, Savage DD, Garrison RJ, et al: Risk factors for pulmonary embolism: The Framingham study. Am J Med 74:1023–1028, 1983.
65. Coon WW: Risk factors in pulmonary embolism. Surg Gynecol Obstet 143:385–390, 1976.
66. Putnam L, Jenicek JA, Allen R, et al: Anesthesia in the morbidly obese patient. South Med J 67:1411–1417, 1974.
67. Clayton JK, Anderson JR, McNicol GP: Preoperative prediction of postoperative deep vein thrombosis. Br Med J 2:910–912, 1976.
68. Rakoczi I, Chamone D, Collen D, et al: Prediction of postoperative leg-vein thrombosis in gynaecological patients (letter). Lancet 1:509–510, 1978.
69. Almer L, Janzon L: Low vascular fibrinolytic activity in obesity. Thromb Res 6:171–175, 1975.
70. Elkeles RS, Chakrabarti R, Vickers M, et al: Effect of treatment on hyperlipidaemia on haemostatic variables. Br Med J 28:973–974, 1980.
71. Batist G, Bothe A Jr, Bern M, et al: Low antithrombin III in morbid obesity: return to normal with weight reduction. JPEN 7:447–449, 1983.
72. Mason EE, Gordy DD, Chernigoy FA, et al: Fatty acid toxicity. Surg Gynecol Obstet 133:992–998, 1971.
73. NIH Consensus Conference: Prevention of venous thrombosis and pulmonary embolism. JAMA 256:474–479, 1976.
74. Pollock AV, Arnot RS, Leaper DJ, et al: The role of antibacterial preparation of the intestine in the reduction of primary wound sepsis after operations on the colon and rectum. Surg Gynecol Obstet 147:909–912, 1978.
75. Pitkin RM: Abdominal hysterectomy in obese women. Surg Gynecol Obstet 142:532–536, 1976.
76. Shapiro M, Munoz A, Tager IB, et al: Risk factors for infection at the operative site after abdominal or vaginal hysterectomy. N Engl J Med 307:1661–1666, 1982.
77. Higson RH, Kettlewell MG: Parietal wound drainage in abdominal surgery. Br J Surg 65:326–329, 1978.
78. Brown SE, Allen HH, Robins RN: The use of delayed primary wound closure in preventing wound infections. Am J Obstet Gynecol 127:713–717, 1977.
79. Weber DJ, Rutala WA, Samsa GP, et al: Impaired immunogenicity of hepatitis B vaccine in obese persons (letter). N Engl J Med 314:1393, 1986.
80. Krishnan EC, Trost L, Aarons S, et al: Study of function and maturation of monocytes in morbidly obese individuals. J Surg Res 33:89–97, 1982.
81. Kolterman OG, Olefsky JM, Kurakara C, et al: A defect in cell-mediated immune function in insulin-resistant diabetic and obese subjects. J Lab Clin Med 96:535–543, 1980.
82. Haddad V, Macon WL: Abdominal wound dehiscence and evisceration: Contributory factors and improved mortality. Am Surg 46:508–518, 1980.
83. Branch CD: Incisional hernia: analysis of 300 cases. N Engl J Med 211:949–952, 1934.
84. Helmkamp BF: Abdominal wound dehiscence. Am J Obstet Gynecol 128:803–807, 1977.
85. Tracy TA, Miller GL: Obstetric problems of the massively obese. Obstet Gynecol 33:204–208, 1969.
86. Shizgal HM, Forse RA, Spanier AH, et al: Protein malnutrition following intestinal bypass for morbid obesity. Surgery 86:60–69, 1979.
87. Hoffer LJ, Bistrian BR, Young VR, et al: Metabolic effects of very low calorie weight reduction diets. J Clin Invest 73:750–758, 1984.
88. Kral JG: Surgical risks in obese patients. In Schettler G, Gotto AM, Middelhoff G, Habenicht AJR, Jurutka KR (eds): Atherosclerosis VI. Berlin, Springer-Verlag, 1983.

section **II**

section **II**

The Operations for Morbid Obesity

7

Indications for Surgery for Morbid Obesity

MERVYN DEITEL

MORBID FEATURES OF MASSIVE
    OBESITY
THE CRITERIA FOR OPERATION
    FOR MORBID OBESITY
IDEAL BODY WEIGHT
SELECTION OF PATIENTS FOR
    OBESITY SURGERY
CONCLUSION

TABLE 7.1. SEQUELAE OF MASSIVE OBESITY

Hypertension
Hyperlipidemia (usually hypertriglyceridemia)
Accelerated atherosclerosis and angina pectoris
Impaired glucose tolerance
Debilitating degenerative arthritis of weight-bearing joints and low back
Immobility
Fatigue, dyspnea, plethora, and diaphoresis
Alveolar hypoventilation and somnolence (Pickwickian syndrome)
Sleep apnea
Hepatic steatosis
Cholelithiasis
Varicose veins
Venous stasis leg ulcers
Deep vein thrombosis
Pulmonary embolism
Reflux esophagitis
Hernias
Urinary stress incontinence in women
Amenorrhea
Infertility problems (women)
Endometrial hyperplasia and carcinoma of endometrium
Carcinoma of breast
Carcinoma of prostate and colon in males
Foul intertrigos, boils and rubbing inner thighs
Accident proneness
Psychosocial and economic problems

TABLE 7.2. CRITERIA FOR OPERATION FOR MORBID OBESITY

1. Presence of serious sequelae of morbid obesity (Table 7.1).
2. > 45 kg overweight or twice ideal weight for more than 5 years.
3. Failure of sustained weight loss on exhaustive supervised dietary and conservative regimens for more than 5 years.
4. Absence of endocrine cause, e.g., subclinical hypothyroidism.
5. Will cooperate with long-term follow-up.
6. Acceptable operative risk.

The American Society for Bariatric Surgery has adopted the following guidelines.

Guidelines for Selection of Patients for Surgical Treatment of Obesity

Obesity, an increase in body weight of 20% or more above desirable weight, defined by the 1983 Metropolitan Life Insurance Company Height/Weight Tables, is an established health hazard, and weight reduction should be recommended to persons at or above this weight according to the National Institutes of Health (NIH) Consensus Development Conference of 1985[1]. Weight reduction is also highly desirable in patients with lesser degrees of overweight if they suffer from diabetes, hypertension, hyperlipidemia, coronary disease or gout. Weight reduction may be lifesaving in patients who weigh 100 lb. (45 kg.) or more over desirable weight since such patients, classified as morbidly obese, have drastically increased mortality.

Because of the documented ineffectiveness of all nonoperative methods to achieve and sustain significant weight loss for periods longer than one year in morbidly obese patients, the NIH Consensus Development Conference in 1978 affirmed the benefits of treating such patients by surgical means[2].

Based on the NIH Consensus statements of 1978 and 1985 and on guidelines recommended by the American Society for Clinical Nutrition[3], the American Society for Bariatric Surgery recognizes the following two guidelines for surgical treatment of obesity.

1. The patient should be 100 lb. (45 kg.) or more above desirable weight according to the 1983 Metropolitan Life Insurance Company Height/Weight tables (midpoint for medium frame).

2. If the patient weighs less than the amount recommended in Guideline 1, he/she should also have other serious medical obesity-related conditions known to be ameliorated by weight loss.

The American Society for Bariatric Surgery recognizes that the surgeon in charge of the individual case has the responsibility to apply the indications for operation. Pediatric patients, patients with specific endocrinological abnormalities, and patients with failure of previous operations for the treatment of obesity require special consideration.

References:
1. Annals Int Med 103:147-151, 1985.
2. Am J Clin Nutr 33 (Suppl 2):528-530, 1980, and Ann Surg 189: 455-457, 1979.
3. Am J Clin Nutr 42:904-905, 1985.

FIGURE 7.1. Guidelines for selection of patients for surgical treatment of obesity.

The operations for morbid obesity cannot guarantee that the individual patient will have successful weight loss. Furthermore, all the procedures have potential risks, both during the operation and later from postoperative sequelae. Accordingly, specific criteria must be present before the decision to operate is made.

The serious consequences of massive sustained obesity are discussed in Chapter 2. Informed consent and legal implications of the bariatric operations are presented in Chapter 27. In this chapter, we will discuss the features of morbid obesity which fulfil the criteria for selection of patients for obesity surgery.

MORBID FEATURES OF MASSIVE OBESITY

Morbid obesity is obesity which leads to significant physical disease and is disabling or life-threatening. The sequelae of massive obesity are listed in Table 7.1.[1-15] Massively obese individuals have elevated plasma low-density-lipoproteins, which transport cholesterol to tissues, and decreased plasma concentration of high-density-lipoproteins, an atherogenic combination associated with an increased incidence of ischemic heart disease.[4,16] Data confirm that morbidly obese men are prone to increased morbidity and premature death.[17] Massively obese women are also prone to considerable morbidity and mortality.[7,18] Furthermore, increased waist compared to hip circumference (i.e., excess central or upper body fat) has been found to be associated with increased hypertension and heart disease, especially in males.[4,19] Effective weight reduction can correct or markedly improve the abnormalities listed in Table 7.1. Importantly, loss of excess weight is associated with loss of increased morbidity and mortality.[1,4,15,20]

TABLE 7.3A. THE 1983 METROPOLITAN HEIGHT AND WEIGHT TABLES

Height		Weight in Pounds		
		Small Frame	Medium Frame	Large Frame
Feet	Inches	MEN		
5	2	128–134	131–141	138–150
5	3	130–136	133–143	140–153
5	4	132–138	135–145	142–156
5	5	134–140	137–148	144–160
5	6	136–142	139–151	146–164
5	7	138–145	142–154	149–168
5	8	140–148	145–157	152–172
5	9	142–151	148–160	155–176
5	10	144–154	151–163	158–180
5	11	146–157	154–166	161–184
6	0	149–160	157–170	164–188
6	1	152–164	160–174	168–192
6	2	155–168	164–178	172–197
6	3	158–172	167–182	176–202
6	4	162–176	171–187	181–207
		WOMEN		
4	10	102–111	109–121	118–131
4	11	103–113	111–123	120–134
5	0	104–115	113–126	122–137
5	1	106–118	115–129	125–140
5	2	108–121	118–132	128–143
5	3	111–124	121–135	131–147
5	4	114–127	124–138	134–151
5	5	117–130	127–141	137–155
5	6	120–133	130–144	140–159
5	7	123–136	133–147	143–163
5	8	126–139	136–150	146–167
5	9	129–142	139–153	149–170
5	10	132–145	142–156	152–173
5	11	135–148	145–159	155–176
6	0	138–151	148–162	158–179

Weights at ages 25–59 based on lowest mortality, wearing shoes with 1″ heels and indoor clothing (3 lb for women, 5 lb for men). Prepared by the Metropolitan Life Insurance Company[24] based on the 1979 Build Study.[25]

TABLE 7.3B. THE 1983 METROPOLITAN HEIGHT AND WEIGHT TABLES, CONVERTED TO METRIC SYSTEM

Height Centimeters	MEN Weight in Kilograms		
	Small Frame	Medium Frame	Large Frame
158	58.3–61.0	59.6–64.2	62.8–68.3
159	58.6–61.3	59.9–64.5	63.1–68.8
160	59.0–61.7	60.3–64.9	63.5–69.4
161	59.3–62.0	60.6–65.2	63.8–69.9
162	59.7–62.4	61.0–65.6	64.2–70.5
163	60.0–62.7	61.3–66.0	64.5–71.1
164	60.4–63.1	61.7–66.5	64.9–71.8
165	60.8–63.5	62.1–67.0	65.3–72.5
166	61.1–63.8	62.4–67.6	65.6–73.2
167	61.5–64.2	62.8–68.2	66.0–74.0
168	61.8–64.6	63.2–68.7	66.4–74.7
169	62.2–65.2	63.8–69.3	67.0–75.4
170	62.5–65.7	64.3–69.8	67.5–76.1
171	62.9–66.2	64.8–70.3	68.0–76.8
172	63.2–66.7	65.4–70.8	68.5–77.5
173	63.6–67.3	65.9–71.4	69.1–78.2
174	63.9–67.8	66.4–71.9	69.6–78.9
175	64.3–68.3	66.9–72.4	70.1–79.6
176	64.7–68.9	67.5–73.0	70.7–80.3
177	65.0–69.5	68.1–73.5	71.3–81.0
178	65.4–70.0	68.6–74.0	71.8–81.8
179	65.7–70.5	69.2–74.6	72.3–82.5
180	66.1–71.0	69.7–75.1	72.8–83.3
181	66.6–71.6	70.2–75.8	73.4–84.0
182	67.1–72.1	70.7–76.5	73.9–84.7
183	67.7–72.7	71.3–77.2	74.5–85.4
184	68.2–73.4	71.8–77.9	75.2–86.1
185	68.7–74.1	72.4–78.6	75.9–86.8
186	69.2–74.8	73.0–79.3	76.6–87.6
187	69.8–75.5	73.7–80.0	77.3–88.5
188	70.3–76.2	74.4–80.7	78.0–89.4
189	70.9–76.9	74.9–81.5	78.7–90.3
190	71.4–77.6	75.4–82.2	79.4–91.2
191	72.1–78.4	76.1–83.0	80.3–92.1
192	72.8–79.1	76.8–83.9	81.2–93.0
193	73.5–79.8	77.6–84.8	82.1–93.9

Hypoventilation results from a decreased central hypoxic and hypercapneic ventilatory drive combined with the mechanical resistance to breathing in severe obesity. Sleep in these patients may be accompanied by repeated episodes of apnea, which is defined as cessation of airflow lasting at least 10 seconds. There is a decrease in the rapid eye movement (REM) and deep sleep stages, as each apneic episode causes arousal from sleep so that deep sleep stages are hard to attain.[21,22] The sleep apnea syndrome, which occurs frequently in males, is a well-known cause of death; it is diagnosed if at least 20 apneas occur per hour of sleep. These patients have loud snoring and hypermotility during sleep, whereas during the day they have excessive sleepiness and emotional instability. With weight loss, the apneic episodes disappear, there is normalization of sleep structure, and the number of awakenings during sleep decreases.

Psychosocial problems are noted last in Table 7.1, but may be of major importance. Besides loss of self-esteem and withdrawal from society, these patients have problems with the basic activities of normal life. They cannot find clothes that fit, fit in a chair with arms (e.g. the seat on an airplane), buckle a seat-belt, get up from a lawn-chair, fit through turn-stiles, cross their legs, put on their shoes, cut their toenails, keep themselves clean, keep up with their children, engage in sexual activity, or find employment. Massive obesity can be an enormous psychological burden in the important social years of late teens and early 20's. Because of withdrawal from society, inactivity, progressive

TABLE 7.3B. THE 1983 METROPOLITAN HEIGHT AND WEIGHT TABLES, CONVERTED TO METRIC SYSTEM
Continued

Height Centimeters	WOMEN Weight in Kilograms Small Frame	Medium Frame	Large Frame
148	46.4–50.6	49.6–55.1	53.7–59.8
149	46.6–51.0	50.0–55.5	54.1–60.3
150	46.7–51.3	50.3–55.9	54.4–60.9
151	46.9–51.7	50.7–56.4	54.8–61.4
152	47.1–52.1	51.1–57.0	55.2–61.9
153	47.4–52.5	51.5–57.5	55.6–62.4
154	47.8–53.0	51.9–58.0	56.2–63.0
155	48.1–53.6	52.2–58.6	56.8–63.6
156	48.5–54.1	52.7–59.1	57.3–64.1
157	48.8–54.6	53.2–59.6	57.8–64.6
158	49.3–55.2	53.8–60.2	58.4–65.3
159	49.8–55.7	54.3–60.7	58.9–66.0
160	50.3–56.2	54.9–61.2	59.4–66.7
161	50.8–56.7	55.4–61.7	59.9–67.4
162	51.4–57.3	55.9–62.3	60.5–68.1
163	51.9–57.8	56.4–62.8	61.0–68.8
164	52.5–58.4	57.0–63.4	61.5–69.5
165	53.0–58.9	57.5–63.9	62.0–70.2
166	53.6–59.5	58.1–64.5	62.6–70.9
167	54.1–60.0	58.7–65.0	63.2–71.7
168	54.6–60.5	59.2–65.5	63.7–72.4
169	55.2–61.1	59.7–66.1	64.3–73.1
170	55.7–61.6	60.2–66.6	64.8–73.8
171	56.2–62.1	60.7–67.1	65.3–74.5
172	56.8–62.6	61.3–67.6	65.8–75.2
173	57.3–63.2	61.8–68.2	66.4–75.9
174	57.8–63.7	62.3–68.7	66.9–76.4
175	58.3–64.2	62.8–69.2	67.4–76.9
176	58.9–64.8	63.4–69.8	68.0–77.5
177	59.5–65.4	64.0–70.4	68.5–78.1
178	60.0–65.9	64.5–70.9	69.0–78.6
179	60.5–66.4	65.1–71.4	69.6–79.1
180	61.0–66.9	65.6–71.9	70.1–79.6
181	61.6–67.5	66.1–72.5	70.7–80.2
182	62.1–68.0	66.6–73.0	71.2–80.7
183	62.6–68.5	67.1–73.5	71.7–81.2

Weights at ages 25–59, wearing shoes with 2.5 cm heels and indoor clothing weighing 2.3 kg for men and 1.4 kg for women.

immobility and depression, they may turn to food, creating a vicious cycle.

THE CRITERIA FOR OPERATION FOR MORBID OBESITY

The guidelines for obesity surgery, adopted by the American Society for Bariatric Surgery October 1986, are shown in Fig 7.1. The criteria for operation are outlined in Table 7.2.[2,3,23] Patients who do not quite meet the weight criteria may still be candidates for operation under special circumstances, if medical complications are severe and progressing. Examples are debilitating degeneration of weight-bearing joints or lumbar spine with progressive immobility, diabetes, hypertension, significant reflux esophagitis, and urinary stress incontinence. Angina pectoris itself is not a contraindication to this surgery.

Bariatric surgery should generally not be performed in the young (i.e. before the epiphyses have sealed) or in the aged patient. Operative mortality increases with old age, and patients cannot attain very old age if they have had sustained true morbid obesity. The acceptable age for this surgery is 18 to 50 years, but in exceptional medical circumstances, patients outside this range may be candidates.

IDEAL BODY WEIGHT

The concept of "ideal" or "desirable" weight is derived from life insurance statistics, and is the weight for each height at which the mortality is lowest or longevity is greatest. The ideal weight is less than the average weight for a specific height in the population. The 1983 Metropolitan Height and Weight Tables are shown in Table 7.3.[24] These tables are based on the 1979 Build Study,[25] which is the result of an 18-year mortality study (1954–1972) involving 4.2 million individuals from 25 life insurance companies in U.S.A. and Canada, and is the weight associated with maximum life expectancy. These weights are given in a range for body frame (small, medium and large) which is based on elbow width (see Table 7.4).[26] The latter table was arbitrarily derived so that the 25% of the population with the smallest elbow breadth would be designated as small frame, the 25% of the population with largest elbow breadth would be designated as large frame, with the middle 50% (25th–75th percentile) of elbow breadth falling into the medium frame group. Generally, the middle point of the range of weights for medium frame is chosen as the "ideal" weight by bariatric surgeons.

There are a number of criticisms of the Metropolitan Height and Weight Tables: 1. The population consisted of a disproportionately large number of whites. 2. The weights were self-reported in 10% of the clients. 3. The insured population is a higher economic group than the general population. 4. Weights were performed wearing indoor clothing (allowing 5 lb for males and 3 lb for females) and wearing shoes with 1 inch heels for both males and females. 5. Applicants with major diseases (e.g., heart disease, cancer or diabetes) at the time of insurance policy issuance were excluded (to provide an indication of the sole effect of weight on mortality), skewing the results. 6. The individuals were from ages 25 to 59, and the weight associated with lowest mortality increased with age until the 50's.

Another criticism is that there is some evidence that obese individuals have a large body frame, as indicated by studies of metacarpal width/length. Kral and co-workers[27] found that the morbidly obese had a significantly increased bone mass, which persisted after loss of the excess weight after obesity surgery in premenopausal women.

Nonetheless, the Metropolitan Height and Weight Tables are the best estimate available of the ideal weight. Ideal weight may be calculated by a formula which gives values which correspond to the midpoint of the range for the medium frame on the 1983 Metropolitan Tables, with a margin of error of less than 1% (Fig. 7.2).[28] By using this formula, there is no need to carry around a chart.

Body mass index (BMI) is accepted as the most accurate method of comparing obesity for individuals of all heights.[29] It is calculated from the formula: W/H^2 for men and $W/H^{1.5}$ for women, where W is weight in kilograms and H is height in meters. However, the formula for women is somewhat difficult to use, and most workers use the more practical formula for men for all their patients.[4,30] A BMI of 23 indicates normal weight, ≥ 30 indicates obesity, and ≥ 47 indicates morbid obesity (Fig. 7.3). The BMI has a very high correlation with body density and skinfold thickness

TABLE 7.4. TABLE OF ELBOW BREADTH FOR MEDIUM FRAME AT VARIOUS HEIGHTS

MEN			
Height (In 1-Inch Heels)	Elbow Breadth (Inches)	Height (In 2.5-cm Heels)	Elbow Breadth (Centimeters)
5'2"–5'3"	2½"–2⅞"	158–161	6.4–7.2
5'4"–5'7"	2⅝"–2⅞"	162–171	6.7–7.4
5'8"–5'11"	2¾"–3"	172–181	6.9–7.6
6'0"–6'3"	2¾"–3⅛"	182–191	7.1–7.8
6'4"	2⅞"–3¼"	192–193	7.4–8.1

WOMEN			
Height (In 1-inch Heels)	Elbow Breadth (Inches)	Height (In 2.5-cm Heels)	Elbow Breadth (Centimeters)
4'10"–4'11"	2¼"–2½"	148–151	5.6–6.4
5'0"–5'3"	2¼"–2½"	152–161	5.8–6.5
5'4"–5'7"	2⅜"–2⅝"	162–171	5.9–6.6
5'8"–5'11"	2⅜"–2⅝"	172–181	6.1–6.8
6'0"	2½"–2¾"	182–183	6.2–6.9

Elbow breadth is an easily obtained, replicable indicator of frame size that is not affected by adiposity or age.[26] Extend arm and bend forearm upward at a 90°-angle. Keep fingers straight and turn inside of wrist toward body. Space between outer margins of the two bones at elbow (best measured with calipers) is compared to above measurements for medium frame. Measurements lower or higher indicate a small or large frame respectively.[24]

Adult female: 5 feet = 119 lb; for each additional inch,
    add 3 lb.
Adult male: 5 feet 3 inches = 135 lb; for each additional
    inch, add 3 lb.
Multiply by 2.2 to change to kg.

FIGURE 7.2. Formula for calculation of ideal weight, which corresponds to midpoint of range for medium frame of the Metropolitan Tables, with accuracy within 1%. Decreasing or increasing the result by 10% allows for small or large frame, as determined by elbow breadth (Table 7.4).

measurements, and is the best indicator of "fatness."[31]

SELECTION OF PATIENTS FOR OBESITY SURGERY

The selection process for obesity surgery consists of **four parts** (Table 7.5): 1. a **history** documenting that exhaustive conservative regimens have been tried over the years and including information from the referring doctor(s); 2. a thorough outline of the patient's **complaints** (both physical and psychological) regarding the obesity; 3. a **physical examination** verifying the degree of obesity and related physical effects, supplemented by assessment of surgical risk, indicated blood tests, pulmonary function tests and appropriate consultations, e.g., respirologist, cardiologist, endocrinologist, psychiatrist if indicated, orthopedic surgeon, gynecologist, etc. (who will also provide perioperative surveillance); and 4. an **explanation** of the operation, including hazards and sequelae, as informed consent, with the spouse and/or close relatives present.

The patient fills out a form before seeing the surgeon (Fig. 7.4 upper and lower). The form is then enlarged by discussion with the surgeon. A diagram of the operation is drawn on the back of the second page of the form while the procedure is explained to the patient.[32] The form evokes and covers intricately the criteria for operation, acts as the basis for the surgeon's consultation letter, and serves as a medicolegal document in the patient's own handwriting in the chart.

A large blood-pressure cuff is necessary, as a narrow cuff will give an erroneously elevated reading. The width of the inflatable bag should be ideally 20% greater than the diameter of the arm—usually 18–20 cm.[33,34] The inflatable bag should be long enough to encircle the arm—usually 20 cm, and should be

enclosed in a non-distensible outer cuff that measures 90 × 20 cm (36 × 8 inches).

Those who are candidates for operation have explained to them the major risks of the surgery—the potential for death, leak and reoperation, clots in legs going to lungs, pneumonia, wound infection and disruption, etc., and the sequelae, including dietary restrictions and requirements.

Further understandable literature and explanatory aids are provided to the patient. Many surgeons have developed their own printed information and booklets, and information pamphlets are available from the American Society for Bariatric Surgery, 633 Post Street, Box 639, San Francisco, California 94109. Cowan has drawn up a set of true/false questions which are filled in by the patient to determine if the patient really understands the procedure and potential sequelae (see Chapter 27).

Some super-obese patients (> 225% above ideal body weight) may have to be hospitalized for a variable period preoperatively. Adequate preoperative treatment, including supervised controlled dieting, diuretics, respiratory exercises and cleansing of intertrigos, with weight loss, may be necessary to make the operative risk acceptable. Patients suspected of having the sleep apnea syndrome should undergo preoperative sleep polysomnography to confirm the diagnosis,[21] and nocturnal nasal continuous positive airway pressure (CPAP) may be indicated.[22]

Surgery must be a well thought-out decision by the patient, and the spouse or family must be seen to be supportive. The surgeon must avoid accepting for operation the impetuous patient who has made a hasty decision on the basis of whim or who has magical expectations.

The patient must be willing to accept the risks of the operation and must agree to life-long surveillance. The follow-up recommended by the American Society for Bariatric Surgery is shown in Fig. 7.5. Alcoholics are rarely candidates because of the possible hepatic sequelae of these operations (especially the malabsorptive procedures), unless they have reformed and have acceptable liver function tests. Smokers should sincerely agree to

TABLE 7.5.   OBESITY INTERVIEW

1. *All* modalities tried.
2. Effects of the obesity.
3. Physical examination.
4. Discussion, explanation, informed consent.

NOMOGRAM FOR BODY MASS INDEX

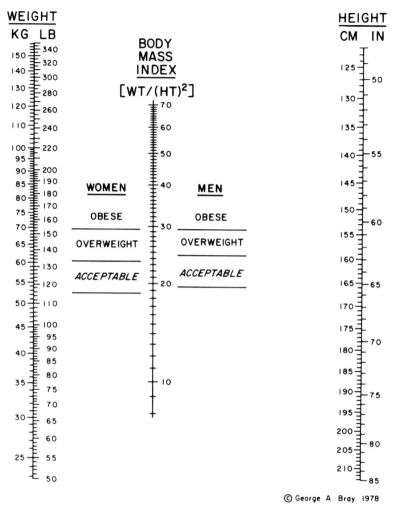

© George A Bray 1978

FIGURE 7.3. Nomogram for conversion of weight and height to BMI. To obtain BMI, draw a straight line through the appropriate points on the weight and height scales. From Bray GA (ed), Obesity in America, U.S. Department of Health, Education, and Welfare, NIH Publication No. 79–359, 1979, p 6.

quit smoking *at least* 10 days before the operation.

It has been found that psychiatric evaluation preoperatively is not necessary or helpful as a routine, but only when such evaluation and surveillance are indicated by the history. Patients who are psychiatrically unstable, totally undependable or psychotic should not be accepted for bariatric surgery. However, some of these patients who have been referred by a psychiatrist, after being under his or her care and understanding for years, are acceptable for surgery with close joint surveillance, and have benefitted markedly from the weight loss.

CONCLUSION

The conservative regimens for morbid obesity ultimately have a nearly 100% failure-rate. These include failure of diets, starvation, weight loss clinics, dieticians, exercise clinics, anorectic drugs, injections, acupuncture, hypnosis, group therapy, psychotherapy, tapes, behavior modification, teeth-wiring, etc. Surgery is indicated as a last measure. The patient must understand the risks and sequelae of the surgery, be cooperative, and agree to lifelong follow-up. It is best to decline to operate on demanding or belligerent patients.

OBESITY HISTORY   NAME:_____

(must be filled in before seeing doctor)

How long overweight? _____

All diets tried—list: _____

_____

_____

_____

_____

Weight loss clinics attended _____

Ideal weight _____

Exercise clinics attended _____

Pills tried _____

Doctors attended for weight loss _____

_____

Injections _____

Acupuncture _____

Other modalities tried, e.g. hypnosis, tapes, etc. _____

_____

_____

_____

OBESITY HISTORY—PAGE TWO

How the overweight bothers me:

Short of breath _____

Joint pains—List: _____

_____

_____

Leak of urine _____

Any blood pressure problem known _____

Other problems—diabetes, vein problems, hiatus hernia, etc. _____

_____

Social problems _____

_____

Rashes or troubles under folds; between thighs _____

Trouble fitting in chairs, finding clothes, etc. _____

Other reasons why you want weight loss surgery _____

_____

_____

Past operations & medical history _____

_____

_____

_____

FIGURE 7.4. (Upper), A form filled out by patient before entering the consulting-room, which must outline all conservative measures tried over the years. (Lower), On second page of form, the patient must describe thoroughly the effects of obesity (both physical and psychosocial). An explanatory diagram is then drawn on the back of the second page, supplemented by models and/or professional drawings.

Guidelines for Postoperative Follow-up Care

1. It is suggested that the frequency of postoperative visits should be scheduled as needed medically and at one, three, six, nine and twelve months after operation and yearly thereafter for five years, and at regular intervals thereafter for the life of the patient.

2. History:
   – interval history
   – dietary, exercise and work status
   – medications and vitamin supplements

3. Physical Exam:
   – vital signs, weight
   – supplemental exam as indicated

4. Biochemical Tests as indicated medically, and:
   – CBC, albumin (and electrolytes if vomiting)
   – B12, folate, iron and iron binding capacity in patients whose duodenum has been bypassed

FIGURE 7.5. Guidelines for postoperative follow-up care.

REFERENCES

1. Reisin E, Frohlich ED, Messerli FH, et al: Cardiovascular changes after weight reduction in obesity hypertension. Ann Intern Med 98:315–319, 1983.
2. Van Itallie, TB: Morbid obesity: a hazardous disorder that resists conservative treatment. Am J Clin Nutr 33:358–363, 1980.
3. Freeman JB, Deitel M, Anand SA, et al: Symposium: Morbid obesity. Contemp Surg 26:71–118, 1986.
4. White F, Pereira L: In search of the ideal body weight. Ann Roy Coll Phys Surg Can 20:129–132, 1987.
5. Sanderson I, Deitel M, Bojm MA: The handling of glucose and insulin response before and after weight loss with jejuno-ileal bypass. JPEN 1:274–276, 1983.
6. Adler M, Schaffner F: Fatty liver hepatitis and cirrhosis in obese patients. Am J Med 67:811–816, 1979.
7. Deitel M, Bojm MA, Atin MD, et al: Intestinal bypass and gastric partitioning for morbid obesity: a comparison. Can J Surg 25:283–289, 1982.
8. Maybee TM, Myer P, DenBesten L, et al: The mechanism of increased gallstone formation in obese human subjects. Surgery 79:460–468, 1976.
9. Deitel M, Petrov I: Incidence of symptomatic gallstones after bariatric operations. Surg Gynecol Obstet 164:549–552, 1987.
10. Hagen J, Deitel M, Khanna RK, et al: Gastroesophageal reflux in the massively obese. Int Surg 72:1–3, 1987.
11. Deitel M, Stone E, Kassam HA, et al: Gynecologic-obstetric changes after loss of massive excess weight. J Am Coll Nutr 7:147–153, 1988.
12. To TB, Deitel M, Stone E, et al: Sex hormonal changes after loss of massive excess weight. Surg Forum 38:465–467, 1987.
13. Donegan WL, Wharton JT: Carcinoma of the endometrium: a survey of practice. ACS Bulletin 69:5–7, 1984.
14. Burton BT, Foster WR, Hirsch J, et al: Health and implications of obesity: an NIH consensus development conference. Int J Obes 9:155–169, 1985.
15. Cowan GSM Jr, Murray G, Golden E, et al: Exercise induced wall motion abnormalities and resting left ventricular dysfunction in the morbidly obese as assessed by first pass radionuclide ventriculography (RNV). Int J Obes 11:214, 1987 (abstract).
16. Kesaniemi YA, Grundy SM: Overproduction of low density lipoproteins associated with coronary heart disease. Arteriosclerosis 3:40–46, 1983.
17. Drenick EJ, Bale GS, Selzer F, et al: Excessive mortality and causes of death in morbidly obese men. JAMA 243:443–445, 1980.
18. Noppa H, Bengtsson C, Wedel H, et al: Obesity in relation to morbidity and mortality from cardiovascular disease. Am J Epidemiol 111:682–692, 1980.
19. Hartz AJ, Rupley DC, Rimm AA: The association of girth measurements with disease in 32,856 women. Am J Epidemiol 119:71–80, 1984.
20. Alpert MA, Terry BE, Kelly DL: Effect of weight loss on cardiac chamber size, wall thickness and left ventricular function in morbid obesity. Am J Cardiol 55:783–786, 1985.
21. Charuzi I, Ovnat A, Reiser J, et al: The effect of surgical weight reduction on sleep quality in obesity-related sleep apnea syndrome. Surgery 97:535–538, 1985.
22. Sugerman HJ, Fairman RP, Baron PL, et al: Gastric surgery for respiratory insufficiency of obesity. Chest 90:81–86, 1986.
23. Rabinovitz D: Some endocrine and metabolic aspects of obesity. Ann Rev Med 21:241–258, 1970.
24. 1983 Metropolitan Height and Weight Tables. Metropolitan Life Foundation, Statistical Bulletin 64(1):2–9, 1983.
25. Build Study, 1979. Society of Actuaries and Association of Life Insurance Medical Directors of America. Philadelphia, Recording and Statistical Corporation, 1980.
26. Frisancho AR, Flegel PN: Elbow breadth as a measure of frame size for US males and females. Am J Clin Nutr 37:311–314, 1983.
27. Kral JG, Wang J, McKeon E, et al: Large frame in morbid obesity: bone mass maintained after weight loss. Int J Obes 11:204, 1987.
28. Miller MA: A calculated method for determination of ideal body weight. Nutritional Support Services 5(3):31–33, 1985.
29. Keys A, Fidanza F, Karvonen MJ, et al: Indices of relative weight and obesity. J Chron Dis 25:329–342, 1972.
30. Abraham S, Johnson CL: Prevalence of severe obesity

in adults in the United States. Am J Clin Nutr 33:364–369, 1980.

31. Womersley J, Durnin JVGA: A comparison of skinfold method with extent of "overweight" and various weight-height relationships in the assessment of obesity. Br J Nutr 38:271–284, 1977.

32. Deitel M: 26. Selection of patients for gastric partitioning. Can J Surg 27:237, 1984.

33. Kirkendall WM, Burton AC, Epstein FH, et al: Recommendations for human blood pressure determinations by sphygmomanometers. Circulation 36:980–983, 1967.

34. King GE: Taking the blood pressure. JAMA 209:1902–1904, 1969.

8

Jejunocolic and Jejunoileal Bypass: An Historical Perspective

MERVYN DEITEL

The earliest operations for massive intractable obesity were based on malabsorption techniques. Intestinal bypasses had their beginnings in the 1950's, and developed through the 1960's. They produced significant sustained weight loss in a high percentage of patients. Approximately 100,000 jejunoileal bypasses were performed in the U.S.A.,[1] and the majority of these patients reached their weight loss goals. However, serious sequelae were a potential, and the mandatory close surveillance and need for availability were a full-time responsibility for the bariatric surgeon. It is our contention that if the gastric restrictive operations had not developed, we would still be performing the jejunoileal bypass today.

JEJUNOCOLIC BYPASS

Jejunocolic bypass (Fig. 8.1) was reported by Payne, Lewis, Shibata and colleagues.[2-4] All patients showed dramatic weight losses. The procedure was abandoned because of uncontrollable diarrhea, severe fluid and electrolyte disturbances and hepatic failure, which required reversal of the bypass. When intestinal continuity was restored, these patients regained all the previously lost weight.[2]

JEJUNOILEAL BYPASS

Jejunoileal (JI) bypass was reported by Payne and DeWind[5] and was widely adopted. Payne reduced his original end-to-side 15″ to 5″ (37.5 cm to 12 cm) anastomosis to 14″ to 4″ (35 cm to 10 cm), in order to prevent weight gain after the adaptations had occurred in the in-continuity bowel (Fig. 8.2). However, almost 10% of patients did not have significant weight loss due to variable degrees of reflux

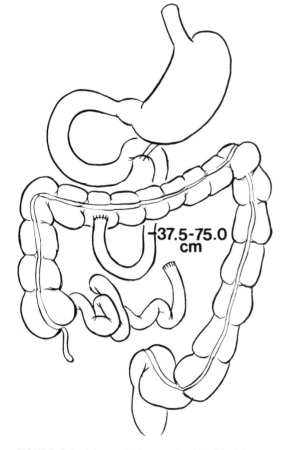

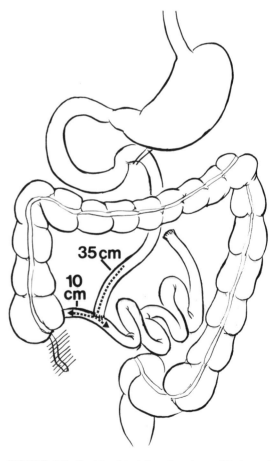

FIGURE 8.1. Jejunocolic bypass (end-to-side jejunocolostomy); Payne and colleagues[2] anastomosed the proximal 15″ (37.5 cm) and Lewis and colleagues[3] anastomosed the proximal 30″ (75 cm) of jejunum to transverse colon.

FIGURE 8.2. End-to-side jejunoileostomy (T-shaped anastomosis), popularized by Payne.[5]

of nutrients into the bypassed ileum where they were absorbed. Thus, Scott and associates,[6] Salmon[7] and Buchwald and associates[8] used an end-to-end JI bypass, and drained the bypassed small bowel into the transverse colon, sigmoid or cecum (Fig. 8.3).

The jejunal stump was tacked to the root of the transverse mesocolon to prevent intussusception, and the appendix was removed in all JI bypasses. Palmer and Marliss[10] modified the Payne T-shaped end-to-side anastomosis to a Y-shaped anastomosis, which directed food to the cecum without reflux; furthermore, they simply tacked the jejunal stump to the adjacent ileum (Figs. 8.4-A to D). After mobilization of the cecum, the jejunoileal anastomosis could be performed readily at the level of the anterior abdominal wall.

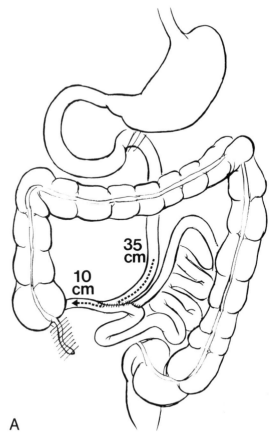

A

FIGURE 8.4. *A,* Modification of the simpler Payne JI bypass by Palmer.[10]

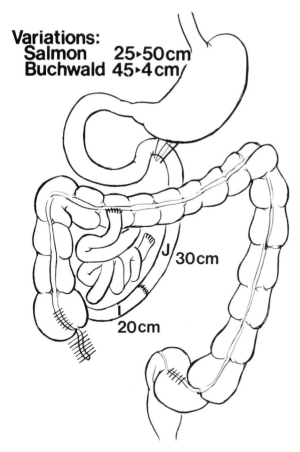

FIGURE 8.3. Scott end-to-end JI bypass (30 cm to 20 cm); Scott and associates[6] and Salmon[7] drained the bypassed bowel into transverse or sigmoid colon; Buchwald and colleagues[8] chose cecum. Subsequently, Salmon altered his lengths to 25 to 37.5 cm and Buchwald to 40 to 4 cm. Reproduced with permission from Can J Surg 25:283–289, 1982.[9]

All the derived lengths for the JI bypasses were measured (using a pre-cut umbilical tape) on the stretched *mesenteric border* precisely, as there are one million absorptive villi per square inch of small bowel. If these measurements were taken accurately, weight loss (after the compensatory bowel adaptations to the short-bowel syndrome) remained in the long-term at about 80% of excess body weight.[5,6,9,11–15] Most of the weight loss occurred in the first year following the JI bypass, and weight usually stabilized at 18 months postoperatively. The JI bypass had a less than 1% operative mortality.

Weight loss resulted not only from malabsorption due to the decreased absorptive surface of the small intestine, but also from a decrease in food intake.[16,17] The adaptations in the in-continuity bowel consisted of dilatation, elongation, prominence of the intestinal folds, and elongation of the villi due to hyperplasia of mucosal cells (Fig. 8.5). The

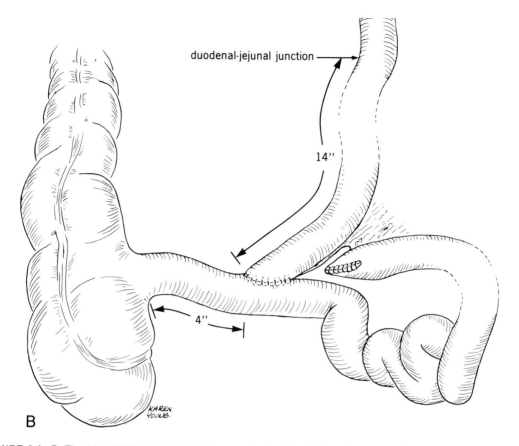

FIGURE 8.4. *B,* The 14 to 4″ (35 to 10 cm) JI bypass, showing the Y-shaped anastomosis and the blind end of the bypassed loop. At the site of jejunal division, a small wedge of jejunum (with its apex on the mesenteric side) is resected between bowel clamps. The jejunum is turned at the anastomosis so that its *mesenteric border is on the patient's right,* and a Y-shaped anastomosis is achieved.

mucosa in the bypassed bowel became atrophic.[9]

The end-to-side JI bypass gave equal weight loss to the end-to-end bypass,[9,18,19] with one instead of two anastomoses, and avoided fecal backwash from the colon into the excluded small bowel. This anastomosis could easily be shifted more distally or proximally if revision was necessary for inadequate or excessive weight loss or electrolyte abnormality.

REVERSAL

Reversal of the Payne JI bypass is generally a simple procedure. Bowel prep including oral antibiotics is instituted. The JI bypass is first dismantled, using the TA (or RL or PI) or GIA (or PLC or ILA) stapler to close the side of the ileum. The antimesenteric borders of the proximal and distal limbs of jejunum are then approximated with stay sutures. The forks of the GIA stapler are inserted into the excised antimesenteric corner of each limb,

closed, and fired to create a functional end-to-end anastomosis. The common opening is closed with a TA stapler, with care that the anterior and posterior GIA staple-lines are not in apposition.[20] Optionally, increased safety may be achieved by inverting the staple-lines with interrupted seromuscular silk sutures.

Reversal of the bypass is generally followed by inexorable rapid regain of weight, despite attempts at dietary control. To maintain the weight loss achieved by the JI bypass, take-down requires a concomitant gastric restrictive operation if the patient is in satisfactory condition or a later bariatric operation if the patient is severely malnourished, electrolyte-depleted, or cirrhotic.

MANAGEMENT OF THE COMPLICATIONS OF THE JI BYPASS

The adverse long-term sequelae of JI bypass are listed in Table 8.1. In 60% of patients,

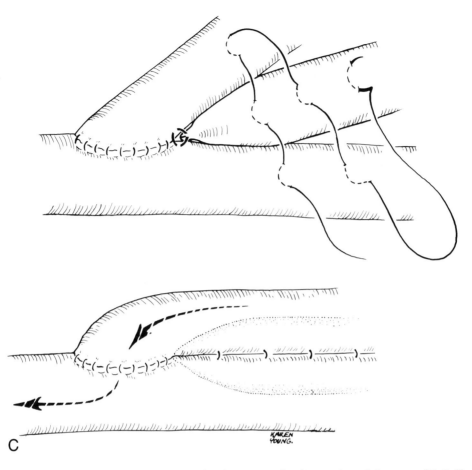

FIGURE 8.4. *C,* The blind end of the bypassed loop has been sutured to the anastomosis by a row of 3–0 silk sutures. Interrupted silk sutures are then placed to approximate the jejunum, the proximal end of the bypassed loop and the ileum. Reproduced with permission from Nutrition in Clinical Surgery, Baltimore, Williams & Wilkins, 1980, Chapter 29.[10]

there have been few if any undesirable sequelae. Problems in most of the remaining patients can be effectively treated.[9,13]

ELECTROLYTE ABNORMALITIES

Hypokalemia is treated by liquid potassium (Kaon Elixir®). Enteric-coated potassium pills were often not absorbed.[21] **Hypomagnesemia**[22] was treated by oral magnesium glucoheptonate (Magnesium Rougier®). **Hypocalcemia** was treated by Calcium Sandoz® and vitamin D.[8] A chronic **metabolic acidosis** with **elevated serum chloride** (hyperchloremic acidosis) persists in most patients due to excessive alkaline stools, and generally is of no consequence.

MIGRATORY ARTHRALGIAS

Transient or recurrent joint pains, usually of fingers, wrists, knees, ankles, feet, shoulders and neck, appear to be a hypersensitivity reaction to systemically absorbed antigenic products of anaerobic bacterial growth in the bypassed bowel. They resolve with metronidazole or broad-spectrum antibiotics (e.g. deoxycycline—Vibramycin®, a long-acting tetracycline).[23] However, prolonged very high doses of metronidazole can cause a peripheral neuropathy, which is generally reversible.[24] Cutaneous lesions ranging from urticaria to pustular necrosis have occurred rarely,[25] and immune deposits have been found in the skin lesions.[26]

BYPASS ENTERITIS

Bypass enteritis manifests as abdominal bloating and malodorous flatus. This condition is due to fecal backwash into the bypassed intestine with stasis and bacterial colonization.[27] Bypass enteritis was more

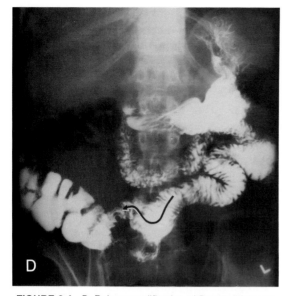

FIGURE 8.4. *D*, Palmer modification of Payne JI bypass. Barium meal 2 years postoperatively shows rapid transit to cecum. Reflux into bypassed ileum is negligable.

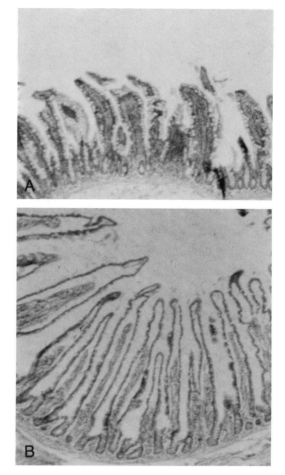

FIGURE 8.5. *A*, Normal jejunum 30 cm distal to ligament of Treitz at the time of a Scott JI bypass (30 cm of proximal jejunum anastomosed end-to-end to 20 cm of distal ileum) (× 25). *B*, Jejunum 30 cm distal to ligament of Treitz in same patient 5 years later, after adaptations which were able to maintain ideal weight. Note the elongated villi, due to hyperplasia (not hypertrophy) of mucosal cells (× 25).

common when the bypassed bowel was anastomosed to the colon, especially the sigmoid, rather than to the distal ileum, due to the higher pressure in the colon.[28] The contents of the blind loop, consisting of bacterial overgrowth with a large population of anaerobes, drain into the colon and produce colonic dilatation. This is relieved quickly by metronidazole or doxycycline or related broad-spectrum antibiotics. Many of these patients have been maintained beneficially on one doxycycline capsule (100 mg) daily.

Various attempts were made to construct a one-way valve near the distal end of the bypassed bowel to prevent reflux,[29–32] but these procedures were problematic. Gourlay's modification, draining the bypassed bowel into the low pressure upper stomach, is presented in Chapter 9; his method removed the blind-loop syndrome and these sequelae.

DIARRHEA

Anal irritation occurred due the effect of unabsorbed digestive enzymes on perianal skin, and was a problem in the early months postoperatively. The initial diarrhea of eight to 15 liquid stools per day decreased, so that by the end of the first year, patients usually had two to five soft, formed stools per day. However, dietary indiscretion, particularly greasy and oily foods, still resulted in steatorrhea. The diarrhea was controlled with di-

phenoxylate HCl (Lomotil®) or loperamide (Imodium®). However, if the intestinal transit-time was slowed, the weight loss was decreased.

Diarrhea was due to the short bowel, steatorrhea, mucosal irritation by unabsorbed bile salts in the colon (where bacteria deconjugated the bile acids), bypass enteritis from bacterial overgrowth and inflammation in the bypassed bowel, and/or intake of milk with inadequate lactase enzyme at the brush border in the remaining short bowel, permitting bacterial fermentation of lactose in the colon. Activated charcoal (Charcocaps®, 260 mg/capsule, Requa Manufacturing Inc., Greenwich, CT) 30 minutes before meals which is devoid of side-effects,[33] bismuth subgallate (Pepto

TABLE 8.1.   LONG-TERM COMPLICATIONS OF JEJUNOILEAL BYPASS[9,14,15]*

		Percent of Patients
Persisting electrolyte abnormality requiring replacement		20
Hypokalemia	15	
Hypomagnesemia	6	
Hypocalcemia	5	
Symptomatic calcium oxalate nephropathy		10†
Migratory polyarthralgia		9
Excess flatus, bloating and cramps or bypass enteritis		17
Incisional hernia		8
Intussusception of jejunal stump		1
Mechanical obstruction of bypassed ileum		1

*Hepatic failure, diarrhea and proctitis are generally not long-term sequelae, and have varied in series with patient selection (no alcoholics) and dietary indiscretion.
†Major reason for reversal.

Bismol™), and low lactose in the diet reduced gas in the lower intestinal tract, foul flatus, and abdominal bloating.

RENAL STONES

All patients show oxalate crystals on urinalysis postoperatively. Recurring calcium oxalate kidney stones are a long-term problem, occurring in 10% of patients, with the potential for diffuse interstitial oxalate nephropathy.[9,11,34–36] In the normal person, calcium and oxalate in the diet combine in the gut to form insoluble nonabsorbable calcium oxalate, which is excreted in the stool. After JI bypass, however, calcium combines with the unabsorbed fatty acids to form insoluble soaps; thus dietary oxalate is left free and is absorbed by simple passive diffusion in the right colon. Oxalemia and hyperoxaluria result. Diarrhea with resulting dehydration contributes.

Treatment consists of a low oxalate diet (avoiding cocoa, beets, carrots, celery, spinach, gelatin, nuts, plums and strawberries) and large amounts of oral calcium carbonate (as powder or tablets, e.g. Titralac™), which binds with oxalate before it can be absorbed. Oxalate nephropathy has been the major long-term complication which required takedown of the JI bypass in some series.[9]

HEPATIC DISEASE

At the time of the JI bypass operation, liver biopsies have shown hepatic steatosis in 90% of morbidly obese patients (Fig. 8.6).[8,9,37,38] The fatty changes were usually centrilobular, centrilobular-midzonal or diffuse. The 10% with normal livers tended to be the younger patients.

After JI bypass, percutaneous needle liver biopsies were performed for supervision.[39]

These appeared worse at 12 months, but generally were improved by 30 months over the biopsy taken at the time of operation.[9,38,40] The fatty metamorphosis of the liver decreased toward normal as protein absorption improved while the bowel adapted to the bypass. There were transient elevations of SGOT and alkaline phosphatase, which generally returned to normal after 24 months. Hepatic cirrhotic changes developed if there was deficient protein intake,[37,40] and were reversed by intravenous infusion of amino acids or by exteriorization of the jejunal stump with infusion of amino acids down the bypassed bowel.[8,41–43] However, hepatic deterioration was prevented by predigested collagen capsules (three capsules three times daily, containing lipotropic factor L-methionine 3.9 mg/capsule), with larger doses taken when the results of liver function tests or needle liver biopsy were abnormal.[9] Methionine permits the body to synthesize choline, a lipotropic factor needed to prevent the development of fatty liver.[44]

In selection of patients for JI bypass, no chronic alcoholics were accepted because of potential ongoing hepatic damage. Late deaths have occurred due to progressive liver damage,[15,43] again indicating obligatory follow-up for properly-timed takedown.

DECREASED BONE DENSITY

Bone demineralization has been noted, associated with low levels of 25-hydroxyvitamin D after JI bypass. This is the result of malabsorption of fat-soluble vitamin D[13] and loss of sterols secreted in the bile which normally re-enter the enterohepatic circulation. The multiple vitamin preparation given to all patients must include a vitamin D supplement.

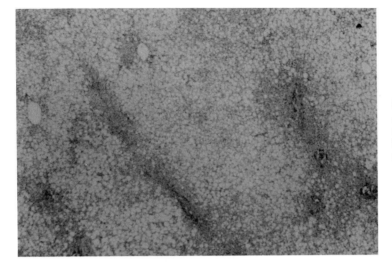

FIGURE 8.6. Liver biopsy at time of JI bypass shows severe diffuse fatty metamorphosis (>75% of liver infiltrated). Some portal areas are spared (× 25).

MECHANICAL PROBLEMS

Twists, adhesions or internal hernias involving the bypassed bowel were possible, with resulting mechanical obstruction. Intussusception of the jejunal stump was a possibility, if the stump was not suitably anchored. These mechanical complications were rare.

POSTOPERATIVE FOLLOW-UP

Multiple vitamin (both water-soluble and fat-soluble vitamins, especially A and D) and mineral supplementation was important, with the awareness that only a variable portion of ingested medications was absorbed due to the rapid transit.[21,45] A diet high in protein and low in fat was strongly recommended. In a minority of patients, serum levels of vitamin B_{12}, depending on the length of distal ileum left in continuity, were low, and parenteral vitamin B_{12} is occasionally indicated. Infrequently, serum levels of folate were slightly diminished.[11] Pregnancies were hopefully delayed until 18 months after JI bypass because of the "starvation" period. Newborn infants weighed slightly less (0.5 kg) than their pre-bypass siblings.[46,47] Gastric hypersecretion was not a feature after JI bypass, although it is known to occur for a period following massive *resection* of small bowel.[48]

The diseases associated with the morbid obesity (e.g., hypertension, pulmonary insufficiency, debilitating osteoarthritis of weight-bearing joints) resolved or improved with the weight loss.[9,12] Diabetes was cured immediately by the malabsorption of glucose, with a fairly flat glucose tolerance curve.[49] Serum cholesterol fell significantly, due to loss of bile salts. Normally, circulating cholesterol enters the liver where it is degraded to bile salts and secreted in the bile; when bile salts reach the distal ileum, almost all are reabsorbed and returned to the liver, where they exert a negative feedback on the rate of degradation of cholesterol. Serum triglycerides also fell to low levels as weight was lost.[9,15] Serum carotene remained low as a lasting indicator of impaired intestinal fat absorpton. Permanent follow-up, with surveillance of serum electrolytes (especially potassium, calcium and magnesium), SGOT, alkaline phosphatase, hemoglobin and urinalysis is mandatory.

BILIO-INTESTINAL BYPASS

A modification of the end-to-side JI bypass involves anastomosis of the fundus of the gallbladder to the proximal end of the bypassed jejunum. Stasis with bacterial overgrowth in the excluded bowel is reduced, eliminating the blind loop syndrome. Furthermore, bile salt reabsorption is increased, maintaining the enterohepatic circulation of bile. Bile loss is 50% of that with the standard JI bypass, diminishing the bile-acid-provoked watery diarrhea. The operation also avoids intussusception of the blind jejunal stump.

Both Eriksson and Hallberg have combined a Payne end-to-side JI bypass with a cholecystojejunostomy in patients who still have gallbladders.[51-52] Eriksson performs a 30-cm jejunum to 12.5-cm ileum end-to-side JI bypass,[53] and for the cholecystojejunal anastomosis, he uses the end or, in extremely obese patients, the side of the jejunal loop.[50] The anastomosis is large (2 cm wide), enclosed with two rows of polyglycolic acid sutures. Although 50% of the enterohepatic circulation of bile and cholesterol is maintained, serum cholesterol is decreased postoperatively.

Eriksson reports a series of 167 patients over an 11-year period, with 55 patients now followed more than 4 years, with no mortality.[53] Maximum weight reduction occurred within the first 2 years and then leveled, with loss at 4 years being 84% of excess weight. Gallstones were present and extracted before the cholecystojejunal anastomosis was performed in four patients, and no new gallstones have formed thus far. No gallstones, cholangitis or bacterial growth in the gallbladder have resulted. Vitamin B_{12} absorption is usually reduced but still in the normal range, while serum folate shows no significant changes over 10 years. No liver insufficiency has occurred. Serum potassium and magnesium may require replacement in the first year, but are normal by 4 years.

Eriksson also uses cholecystojejunostomy as a secondary procedure in patients who have side-effects from a previous Payne JI bypass, with marked stool frequency. The procedure results in two to eight loose stools at 6 months, which decreases to one to five soft stools per day at 1 year. One-third of patients have had occasional abdominal distention, foul-smelling stools and excess flatulence in the first year, mostly after large fatty meals. Renal oxalate stones occurred in seven patients, all within the first year only, during the catabolic phase of rapid weight loss. There have been four reversals.

CONCLUSION

The JI bypass has largely been superseded by other bariatric operations. The procedure generally gave good weight loss when performed by skilled hands. There were potential serious side-effects, which could be kept to a minimum or treated, if patient cooperation and close follow-up were maintained. Careful and assiduous supervision and follow-up management remain essential, so that complications many years after the JI bypass can be reduced. A commitment of time by a physician or group knowledgeable in JI bypass and the short-gut syndrome is mandatory. An active support group is a major advantage after this operation. Takedown is necessary for intractable diarrhea, malnutrition unresponsive to conservative measures, advancing cirrhosis and renal disease. JI bypass may still be indicated in highly selected patients on fully informed decision who claim that under no circumstances could they accept the dietary restrictions of a gastric restrictive procedure. Modifications of the original JI bypasses may help to prevent the untoward sequelae.

REFERENCES

1. Mason EE: Development of gastric bypass and gastroplasty. In: Surgical Management of Obesity. New York, Academic Press, 1980, p 29.
2. Payne JH, DeWind LT, Commons RR: Metabolic observations in patients with jejunocolic shunts. Am J Surg 106:273–289, 1963.
3. Lewis LA, Turnbull RB Jr, Page IH: Effects of jejunocolic shunt on obesity, serum lipoproteins, lipids and electrolytes. Arch Intern Med 117:4–16, 1966.
4. Shibata HR, MacKenzie JR, Long RC: Metabolic effects of controlled jejunocolic bypass. Arch Surg 95:413–428, 1967.
5. DeWind LT, Payne JH: Intestinal bypass surgery for morbid obesity: long term results. JAMA 236:2298–2301, 1976.
6. Scott HW Jr, Dean RH, Shull HJ, et al: Results of jejunoileal bypass in two hundred patients with morbid obesity. Surg Gynecol Obstet 145:661–673, 1977.
7. Salmon PA: The results of small intestinal bypass operations for the treatment of obesity. Surg Gynecol Obstet 132:965–979, 1971.
8. Buchwald H, Schwartz MZ, Varco RL: Surgical treatment of obesity. Adv Surg 7:235–255, 1973.
9. Deitel M, Bojm MA, Atin MD, et al: Intestinal bypass and gastric partitioning for morbid obesity: a comparison. Can J Surg 25:283–289, 1982.
10. Palmer JA, Marliss EB: The present status of surgical procedures for obesity. In Deitel M (ed): Nutrition in Clinical Surgery, Baltimore, Williams & Wilkins, 1980, pp 281–292.
11. Hocking MP, Duerson MC, O'Leary JP, et al: Jejunoileal bypass for morbid obesity. Late follow-up in 100 cases. New Engl J Med 308:995–999, 1983.
12. Montorsi W, Doldi SB, Klinger R, et al: Surgical therapy for morbid obesity. Int Surg 71:84–86, 1986.
13. Thorlakson TK: Overview of jejunoileal bypass. Can J Surg 27:127–128, 1984.
14. Zollinger RW, Coccia MR, Zollinger RW 2nd: Critical analysis of jejunoileal bypass. Am J Surg 146:626–630, 1983.
15. Rucker RD Jr, Chan EK, Horstmann J, et al: Searching for the best weight reduction operation. Surgery 96:624–631, 1984.
16. Bray GA, Barry RE, Benfield JR, et al: Intestinal bypass surgery for obesity decreases food intake and taste preferences. Am J Clin Nutr 29:779–783, 1976.
17. Condon SC, Janes NJ, Wise L, et al: Role of caloric intake in the weight loss after jejunoileal bypass for obesity. Gastroenterology 74:34–37, 1978.
18. Gaspar MR, Movius HJ, Rosenthal JJ, et al: Comparison of Payne and Scott operations for morbid obesity. Ann Surg 184:507–515, 1976.

19. Baddeley RM: The management of gross refractory obesity by jejuno-ileal bypass. Br J Surg 66:525–532, 1979.

20. Chassin JL, Rifkind KM, Turner JW: Errors and pitfalls in stapling gastrointestinal tract anastomosis. Surg Clin North Am 64:441–459, 1984.

21. Bojm MA, Deitel M: Malabsorption of medications after bypass surgery (correspondence). Can Med Assoc J 124:681–684, 1981.

22. Lipner A: Symptomatic magnesium deficiency after small-intestinal bypass for obesity. Br Med J 1:148, 1977.

23. Wands JR, La Mont JT, Mann E, et al: Arthritis associated with intestinal bypass procedure for morbid obesity. N Engl J Med 294:121–124, 1976.

24. Karlsson IJ, Hamlyn AN: Metronidazole neuropathy (correspondence). Br Med J 2:832, 1977.

25. Stein HB, Schlappner OL, Boyko W, et al: The intestinal bypass: arthritis-dermatitis syndrome. Arthritis Rheum 24:684–690, 1981.

26. Halverson JD, Teitelbaum SL, Haddad JG, et al: Skeletal abnormalities after jejunoileal bypass. Ann Surg 189:785–790, 1979.

27. Drenick EJ, Ament ME, Finegold SM, et al: Bypass enteropathy: an inflammatory process in the excluded segment with systemic complications. Am J Clin Nutr 30:76–89, 1977.

28. Martyak SN, Curtis LE: Pneumatosis intestinalis. A complication of jejunoileal bypass. JAMA 235:1038–1039, 1976.

29. Starkloff GB, Stothert JC, Sundaram M: Intestinal bypass: a modification. Ann Surg 188:697–700, 1978.

30. Hubbard TB Jr: The prevention of bypass enteritis after jejunoileal bypass for morbid obesity. Ann Surg 187:502–509, 1978.

31. Wiklund B, Hallberg D: Experiences with antireflux valves in jejunoileal bypass surgery. Acta Chir Scand 151:159–162, 1985.

32. Forestieri P, De Luca L, Mosella G, et al: An antireflux system in end-to-side jejunoileal bypass for high degree obesity. Int Surg 65:119–121, 1980.

33. Jain NK, Patel VP, Pitchumoni CS: Efficacy of activated charcoal in reducing intestinal gas: a double-blind clinical trial. Am J Gastroenterol 81:532–535, 1986.

34. Gregory JG, Starkloff EB, Miyai K, et al: Urologic complications of ileal bypass operation for morbid obesity. J Urol 113:521–524, 1975.

35. Stauffer JQ: Hyperoxaluria and calcium oxalate nephrolithiasis after jejunoileal bypass. Am J Clin Nutr 30:64–71, 1977.

36. Clayman RV, Williams RD: Oxalate urolithiasis following jejunoileal bypass. Surg Clin North Am 59:1071–1077, 1979.

37. Adler M, Schaffner F: Fatty liver hepatitis and cirrhosis in obese patients. Am J Med 67:811–816, 1979.

38. Juhl E, Christoffersen P, Baden H, et al: Liver morphology and biochemistry in eight obese patients treated with jejunoileal anastomosis. N Engl J Med 285:543–547, 1971.

39. Kondi ES, Gallitano AL: The anterior approach to percutaneous liver biopsy. Surg Gynecol Obstet 140:422–424, 1975.

40. Moxley RT 3rd, Pozefsky T, Lockwood DH: Protein nutrition and liver disease after jejunoileal bypass for morbid obesity. N Engl J Med 290:921–926, 1974.

41. Heimburger SL, Steiger E, Lo Gerfo P, et al: Reversal of severe fatty hepatic infiltration after intestinal bypass for morbid obesity by calorie-free amino acid infusion. Am J Surg: 129:229–235, 1975.

42. McClelland RN, De Shazo CV, Heimback DM, et al: Prevention of hepatic injury after jejunoileal bypass by supplemental jejunostomy feedings. Surg Forum 21:368–370, 1971.

43. Brown RG, O'Leary JP, Woodward ER: Hepatic effects of jejunoileal bypass for morbid obesity. Am J Surg 127:53–58, 1974.

44. Best CH, Hartroft WS, Lucas CC, et al: Effects of dietary protein, lipotropic factors and re-alimentation on total hepatic lipids and their distribution. Br Med J 1:1439–1444, 1955.

45. Alexander MA, Deitel M: Complication of jejunoileal shunt (correspondence). Can Med Assoc J 117:129, 1977.

46. Hey H, Niebuhr-Jorgensen U: Jejunoileal bypass surgery in obesity. Gynecological and obstetrical aspects. Acta Obstet Gynecol Scand 60:135–140, 1981.

47. Wong KH, Leader A, Deitel M: Maternal nutrition in pregnancy. Part II: The implications of previous gastrointestinal operations and bowel disorders. Can Med Assoc J 125:1328–1334, 1981.

48. Deitel M, Wong KH: Short bowel syndrome. In Deitel M (ed): Nutrition in Clinical Surgery, 2nd Edition, Baltimore, Williams & Wilkins, 1985, pp 255–275.

49. Sanderson I, Deitel M, Bojm MA: The handling of glucose and insulin response before and after weight loss with jejuno-ileal bypass: a preliminary report. JPEN 7:274–276, 1983.

50. Eriksson F: Biliointestinal bypass. Int J Obes 5:437–447, 1981.

51. Hallberg D: A survey of surgical techniques for treatment of obesity and a remark on the bilio-intestinal bypass method. Am J Clin Nutr (Suppl) 33:499–501, 1980.

52. Hallberg D, Holmgren U: Bilio-intestinal shunt. A method and a pilot study for treatment of obesity. Acta Chir Scand 145:405–408, 1979.

53. Eriksson F: Bilio-intestinal bypass—long term follow-up. Fifth Annual Symposium, Surgical Treatment of Obesity, Universal City, CA, Feb. 11–14, 1987.

9

Jejunoileal Bypass with Drainage of the Bypassed Small Bowel into Stomach (Ileogastrostomy)

ROBERT H. GOURLAY
IAIN G.M. CLEATOR

In 1971 Salmon's jejunoileal (JI) bypass[1] for the treatment of morbid obesity was selected for a study, because it provided more ileum than either the Payne[2] or Scott[3] bypasses, in order to avoid B_{12} deficiency and reduce bile salt loss into the colon with associated problems.[4] Subsequent review revealed an effective weight loss,[5] similar to that of Salmon's. In 1978 our group found the arthralgia and dermatitis to be due to bacterial overgrowth in the defunctioned ileum[6]—a blind loop syndrome[7,8] accompanied by malodorous flatus, bloating and foul stools. A "bypass enteritis" with mucosal erosions and chronic inflammation accompanied massive overgrowth of bacteria in the stagnant bypassed bowel with toxic breakdown products.[9,10] The blind loop syndrome could also contribute to more serious renal[11] and hepatic complications.[4,12,13] Barium swallows with 24-hr follow-up films demonstrated reflux of colonic contents and retention in the defunctioned ileum. Metronidazole or tetracycline resulted in a significant improvement in the symptoms, but usually transient.

We performed 874 of the Salmon JI bypasses with good weight loss (Fig. 9.1), but various modifications in the ileocolostomy were ineffective in preventing a significant incidence of blind loop syndrome.[9] The basic problem was high pressure in the colon (100 cm of water)[14] and low pressure in the ileum (5–25 cm of water), as recorded in several defunctioned ileostomies. Ileostomy of the defunctioned ileum was effective in treating or preventing blind loop syndrome,[15] but was

not acceptable to patients. Construction of an ileal valve near the distal end of the bypassed intestine could prevent reflux and bypass enteritis, but was a problematic procedure.[16]

In September 1982 a decision was made, on the suggestion of I.G.M. Cleator, to drain the bypassed bowel into the stomach where the pressure is low and the contents of stomach are essentially sterile. Ulcers rarely, if ever, develop in the afferent loop of a gastroenterostomy. Therefore, with compensatory hypertrophy of the functioning bowel and elimination of the blind loop syndrome, the JI bypass would be an effective, safe operation for treatment of morbid obesity. To June 1, 1986, 213 such primary operations have been performed, and the first 51 patients followed for >1 year have been reviewed.

Our selection of patients follows the criteria of Payne, Scott and others. However, we increasingly strive to treat only those patients who have "earned the operation": i.e., they have seriously dieted, are intelligent, and are prepared to commit themselves to our instructions and protocol for the basic 2-yr period. Patients must avoid alcohol for 2 yr and thereafter consume it only in sensible moderation. We will not operate upon those who practice gluttony. We demand that we direct their care for 2 years and continue to see them intermittently thereafter, particularly if they have any problem. As a result, since 1982 we have had a 100% 2-yr follow-up of those living in British Columbia.

OPERATIVE PROCEDURE

No bowel preparation is used. One hour pre-operatively, 2,500 units of heparin are administered subcutaneously. Metronidazole and an aminoglycoside are given intravenously. Polyglycolic acid sutures 2-0 or 3-0 are used throughout the intra-abdominal procedure. No. 2 polyglycolic acid sutures are used for the incisional closure.

A supraumbilical midline incision is made and the abdomen is explored (Fig. 9.2). The ileocecal area is examined, and if the ileum cannot be readily measured it is mobilized to facilitate later measurement. The small bowel is delivered. From the duodenojejunal junction, using a milliner's tape and Babcock forceps, stretching the antimesenteric border in stages, 10 inches (25 cm) of jejunum is measured. Between Glassman clamps the jejunum is divided between vessels and to avoid bleeding if possible, only a few millimeters into the

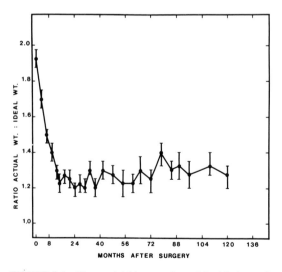

FIGURE 9.1. 10-yr weight loss on the original Salmon JI bypass.

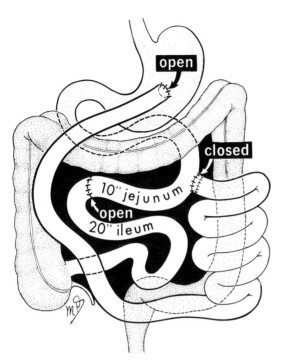

FIGURE 9.2. JI bypass (Salmon-type), with drainage of the bypassed small bowel into upper stomach.

mesentery. The proximal end of the distal jejunum is closed by running locking suture, forceps being applied to the end of the suture for easy delivery later. The ileum is then delivered, and in a similar manner with milliner's tape and Babcock forceps, 20 inches (50 cm) of ileum is measured from the ileocecal valve. The ileum is divided between Glassman clamps. The peritoneum is divided in front and behind as far down as possible, following which the mesentery is divided between forceps and the bleeders ligated. All the vessels are usually within 3 inches of the bowel. With blunt dissection, the remaining mesentery can be divided to mobilize the ileum adequately for the anastomoses. The distal ileum is trimmed and then anastomosed end-to-end with a single layer of interrupted sutures to the proximal jejunum. The proximal end of the defunctioned bowel (which has already been closed) is then anchored to the inferior surface of the proximal functioning jejunum with 3 or 4 interrupted sutures about 2 inches above the anastomosis.

The distal end of the bypassed bowel is then brought up anterior to the functioning jejunum and ileum in an antecolic manner, if necessary through an opening in an avascular area in the greater omentum. The stomach is delivered and, as high up as is conveniently

possible in the parietal cell area, a wedge of muscle and mucosa is excised between Babcock forceps, from the anterior wall of the stomach. The distal end of the defunctioned bowel is anastomosed to the stomach with a single layer of interrupted sutures.

If there is cholelithiasis, cholecystectomy is next performed. A liver biopsy is routinely taken. The peritoneal cavity is washed out with saline, and the incision is closed with figure-of-8 No. 2 sutures in the rectus sheath.

POSTOPERATIVE CARE

EARLY

The patients are fully heparinized 6 hours postoperatively, unless there has been excessive bleeding during the operation or a cholecystectomy, in which case full heparinization is postponed for 24 hr. Full heparinization is maintained until the day before discharge—usually the 7th to 10th postoperative day. Care has to be taken with follow-up for possible bleeding and any bleeding controlled by stopping heparin and other measures. Once controlled, heparinization is resumed.

A nasogastric tube is rarely required at operation but if used is removed the following day. On the third postoperative day oral fluids are started, and before discharge the dietitian instructs the patient, who has received a booklet of instructions and advice. The booklet contains a list of oxalate-rich foods to be avoided for 18 months and a list of potassium-rich foods to be included with diet.

If there is nausea, it is helped by metaclopromide or sucralfate and reassurance, or occasionally mild sedation is required. The patients are discharged on a high protein, very low fat diet, to be followed according to verbal and written instructions. They are warned that fluid intake must be restricted to 2 to 3 ounces every half hour to prevent severe diarrhea with dehydration. They are put on multiple vitamins and discharged on diphenoxylate or loperamide or codeine to assist in the control of diarrhea.

LATE POSTOPERATIVE

There is a 2-yr follow-up, which is directed by the surgeon with complete cooperation by the patient. The referring doctor receives the protocol plus a standard letter of instructions, and is advised to phone if any problems arise and to forward the laboratory tests to the surgeon (RHG). These patients should be seen at 3-month intervals by the surgeon. Those within the geographical area of the surgeon are followed by him.

The protocol requires monthly visits to the family doctor or surgeon, with appropriate laboratory tests, until diarrhea is controlled without drugs, when visits can be reduced to 6 weeks and then 8 weeks. This goes on for the full 2 yr. During the first 12 to 14 months any deficiencies encountered in the laboratory tests are corrected by appropriate measures.

The 2-yr protocol is necessary for the following reasons:

1. Compensatory hypertrophy of the functioning jejunum and ileum takes between 12 and 18 months, and there is a period when bile salt loss into the colon can create such complications as electrolyte and calcium loss and oxaluria with renal calculi. Bile salts in the colon cause increased permeability of the colonic mucosa to oxalate.

2. Weight loss continues for 18 to 24 months, and it is during this long period that the liver is under stress as shown by liver function tests and biopsy. This is dealt with by increasing protein intake and rarely, if necessary, by intravenous amino acids.[17] Needless to say, there must be no hepatotoxic agents, particularly alcohol, consumed during this period, and patients are warned that afterwards alcohol should be consumed in sensible moderation.

3. Patients' dietary habits are directed to assist them to reach a normal intake of 2,000–3,000 kcal/d according to requirements.

At the end of 2 years with stability of the bowel and the liver, the patient should be able to lead a normal, healthier life, maintaining the lost weight on a normal diet. However, as this depends on bowel compensatory hypertrophy and liver function, should there be evidence after 12–18 months that there is insufficient functioning jejunum as indicated usually by the laboratory tests, then this can be readily corrected by adding a further 12–18 inches of jejunum without regaining all the lost weight (which almost inevitably occurs if there is complete restoration of bowel continuity).

RESULTS AND DISCUSSION

The first 51 patients with ileogastrostomy were studied. There were no deaths. One pa-

tient, a native Indian, vomited repeatedly when she returned home and was not eating. This did not occur while she was in Vancouver. Because of the problem of long-range management of this lady, bowel continuity was restored. The other 50 patients are now discussed.[18,19]

WEIGHT LOSS

This was very satisfactory (Fig. 9.3). At 24 months the patients were 125% of ideal weight—reduced from 213% pre-operatively. Of the total weight loss, 45% occurred in the first 3 months. The cause of this massive weight loss is not clear, and cannot be accounted for by the conventional suggestion of malabsorption, since such a weight loss does not appear to occur even in fasting. The intriguing features are that the patients are eating a normal diet (2,000–3,000 kcal) while losing this weight and have a healthy color and feel well. We are currently looking into the metabolic changes that occur at this time.

PATIENT SATISFACTION

On a scale of 1 (bad) to 10 (excellent), the mean satisfaction of the patients with the operation was 9.9 (range 7–10). Of the patients, 96.8% had higher self-esteem following the operation, with 82.6% working and 97.7% significantly more active than before. It is difficult to overestimate the effect of improvement in body image. Before the operation, many were reluctant or unable to work or even go outside their homes.

A sequela was that 28.1% had gas problems regularly and 59.4% occasionally, with only 12.5% having no such problems. The characteristic complaint was of passage of exceptionally foul flatus. We have since discovered that a lactose-restricted diet may relieve this problem considerably.

EARLY COMPLICATIONS

The complications that occurred within 3 months were: 6.6% had wound infections; 2.2% had respiratory complications due to an atelectasis which responded to physiotherapy; 6.8% developed electrolyte disturbances which required correction. Nausea was present much of the time in 11.1%, with 4.5% occasionally nauseated. This was probably due to the outpouring of succus entericus from the defunctioned loop into the stomach

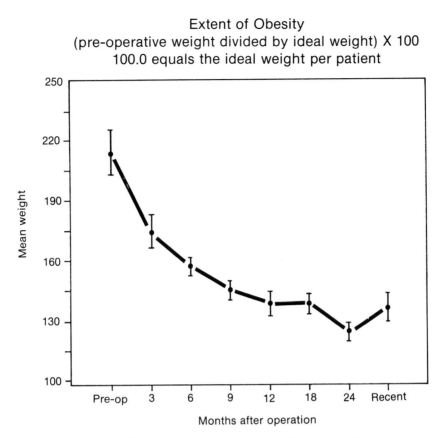

FIGURE 9.3. Weight loss curve after JI bypass with ileogastrostomy. The Y-axis shows the mean percent of ideal body weight.

during the early weeks and may contribute to reduced appetite and, in a few patients, electrolyte disturbances due to decreased fluid intake.

LATE COMPLICATIONS

Electrolyte disturbances were present in 15.9% at 3 months, due presumably to the same cause as early electrolyte disturbance. Sometimes this required only dietary advice, but on other occasions admission to hospital for 2–3 days and intravenous fluids were required. By 12 months only 9% had electrolyte disturbances, and by 18 and 24 months there were no electrolyte disturbances. We explain the resolution of the electrolyte disturbances by the reduction in flow of succus entericus to the stomach from the bypassed bowel, with resumption of more normal intake of fluid and food.

Bowel Movements

At 3 months, 69.7% of patients had loose bowel movements, with increased frequency in most patients (mean of 7 per day with a range of 3–20). Antidiarrheal medication was required regularly in 40%, with 27% requiring the medications occasionally.

After the 3-month period, the loose frequent stools rapidly settled. At 24 months, 10% had loose movements regularly and 30% occasionally. There was a mean of 2.9 movements per day (range 0.5–9) at 24 months, with 3% taking antidiarrheal medication regularly and 10% taking the medication occasionally.

The cause of the loose frequent bowel movements could be reduced absorption of bile salts, which improves with time. The severity and frequency of the loose bowel movements were not sufficient to upset this group of patients. We have since discovered that improvement can be achieved by a lactose-restricted diet.

At 3 months, foul stools occurred in 7.3% regularly and 24% occasionally. This did not alter substantially over the 24-month period.

Bloating

Bloating occurred in 10% at 6 months, with 35% having occasional bloating. These figures stayed the same in the one- to two-year periods. Dietary indiscretion may cause this problem. Again, a lactose-restricted diet often improves this situation.

Liver Function

Liver function tests were monitored carefully. Severe abnormalities (jaundice, liver failure) did not occur. At 3 months, moderate abnormalities (enzymes >10% above upper limit of normal) occurred in 12.8%, with 37% having mild disturbances (<10% increase in liver enzymes). At 12 months, none had severe or moderate liver function disturbance, but 20.5% had mild disturbance. By 18 months, mild disturbance had fallen to 13.6%, with 86.3% having normal liver function. The disturbance could be related to the effect of massive weight loss on a liver which is generally fatty to begin with.

Stomal Ulcer

Patients were endoscoped at 3, 6, 12 and 24 months. Stomal ulcer occurred in 6.2% at 3 months, falling to zero at 6, 12 and 24 months. The ulcer was always small (<3 mm) and always at the anastomotic line of ileum and stomach. Dyspepsia always occurred and the ulcer was sometimes associated with use of anti-arthritic drugs. A drop in hemoglobin occurred on one occasion. No transfusion of blood was required. One patient had a pre-existing unsuspected ulcer in the second part of duodenum, which was recognized by review of pre-operative films after the ulcer was seen on routine endoscopy; she did not develop a stomal ulcer. All ulcers resolved within 4 weeks on H2-blockers. This is a specific complication of the operation and must be looked for.

We have earlier demonstrated no change in fasting serum gastrin in 50 bypassed patients with the Salmon operation. However, in this operation (ileogastrostomy), there is a large outpouring of alkaline succus entericus in the first days and weeks of the postoperative period. This could result in alkalinization of the antrum with increased gastrin secretion and consequent increase in acid secretion. Additionally, the suture-line would be more vulnerable in the early days to such an increased acid and pepsin. This would account for the development of ulcer in 3 patients at the 3-month time interval. As the volume of succus entericus declines to an insignificant amount, the fasting gastrin would be expected to fall to normal (as in the earlier Salmon bypass)

and that would explain the absence of ulcer at 6, 12 and 24 months. On this hypothesis, we would not expect ulcer to occur in subsequent years.

Nausea

Severe nausea was present in 11.1% at 3 months, with 4.5% having mild nausea. The incidence rapidly decreased over the first year, and at 18 and 24 months 100% of patients had no nausea. We ascribe this to the large amount of succus entericus entering the stomach in the early months and then declining. Encouragement of regular fluid and food intake is essential.

Serum Protein and Albumin

Serum proteins were lower than normal in 21% at 3 months, with 7.9% having a low albumin. This gradually improved, with only 4.3% having decreased serum proteins at 18 months and none having a low albumin. We ascribe these changes to increased fatty change in the liver during the early months, with some impairment of function in some patients.

Renal Function

Renal function tests were abnormal in 2.2% pre-operatively, 2.8% at 3 months, 8.1% at 6 months, 0% at 12 months and 2.0% at 18 months. The patient at 18 months developed the nephrotic syndrome following a long period of travel. This resolved spontaneously and renal function was maintained. No patients developed calculi, but a history consistent with passage of gravel occurred in a few patients. Further studies on this important aspect are in progress.

Iron and Folate Deficiency

At 3 months 6.7% had iron deficiency and 8.7% had folate deficiency. Iron deficiency increased to 22.7% at 18 months, but folate deficiency decreased to 5.3%. Supplemental iron and folate are required in this group of patients.

Skin Lesions

Skin lesions were present in 2% of patients pre-operatively and 4% postoperatively and did not change thereafter. The complaints were of dry skin, and no erythema nodosum or other severe skin problems of the type seen in the blind loop syndrome[6] occurred.

Joint Pains

These were present in 8.7% pre-operatively and fell to 2.4% at 6 and 12 months, rising slightly to 6.9% at 18 months. Occasional joint pains occurred in 4.4% pre-operatively, rising at 12 months to 9.5% and at 18 months to 13.8%. None of these were the arthralgias associated with the blind loop syndrome. Rather, they were osteoarthritic symptoms related to the stresses from high pre-operative weight.

ASSESSMENT OF THE OPERATION

This operation has progressed from an experimental to developmental phase. Further elucidation of the mechanisms of weight loss and monitoring of the liver and renal function are essential. The complications which occurred in the prior JI bypass operations were serious (see Chapter 8), and would spell the failure of our operation if they were found. To date these have not occurred, but long-term studies including liver biopsy are in progress.

The nausea, bloating and electrolyte disturbances are of a different order to those in the earlier JI bypasses. A critical index is the number of patients' telephone calls with problems, which is at an all-time low.

The decrease in electrolyte disturbances from those in the earlier JI bypass operations is probably due to the succus entericus going into the stomach rather than the colon. The use of antidiarrheal medication falls off dramatically at 3 months, when there is less stool frequency than in the earlier operations. The improvement may be related to 1) avoidance of bacterial overgrowth and 2) succus entericus of the defunctioned loop entering stomach and not colon. The arthralgia and skin lesions associated with earlier operations did not occur, likely due to the avoidance of bacterial overgrowth in the blind loop.

IMPROVEMENTS

Encouragement of fluid and protein intake during the early months is essential, and should lower nausea, bloating and electrolyte disturbances. Monitoring of iron and folate levels suggests supplements of these are required in some patients.

POSSIBLE FURTHER APPLICATIONS

Patients with a previous problematic result from a JI bypass may benefit from **conversion to ileogastrostomy.** Many such patients have considerable morbidity from bacterial overgrowth in the blind loop, but are resolved not to have reconnection of the bowel because of the inevitable recurrence of their morbid obesity. In addition to the primary operations reported herein, in October 1982 we began revisions to an ileogastrostomy on patients with the blind loop syndrome, and 265 such revisions have been performed, with resulting decrease in stool frequency and features of the blind loop syndrome. Metronidazole or a broad-spectrum antibiotic is given for the first week postoperatively to eliminate the remaining bacteria in the bypassed bowel. Revision to an ileogastrostomy must in our view include an ileal segment of 20 inches (50 cm) in the functioning bowel. In such revision operations, we have found the recovery is slow but steady over the first year.

CONCLUSION

With 20 inches (50 cm) of functioning ileum in continuity and the elimination of the blind loop syndrome, the intestinal bypass operation has been a safe, effective treatment for morbid obesity in selected patients. Arthralgias, dermatitis and other side-effects of the blind loop syndrome have not occurred to date. We now have produced an effective weight-loss operation in which the small bowel makes an adequate compensatory recovery over 1½ years. Deficiency to compensate can be corrected by adding to the functioning bowel an appropriate length (several more inches of jejunum) without re-establishment of total bowel continuity and the inevitable regain of all the lost weight.

The blind loop syndrome is the cause of many of the serious sequelae of JI bypass. Defunctioning the bypassed bowel into the upper stomach avoids these complications and may make this procedure an operation of choice for morbid obesity.

REFERENCES

1. Salmon PA: The results of small intestine bypass operations for the treatment of obesity. Surg Gynecol Obstet 132:965–979, 1971.
2. Payne JH, DeWind L, Schwab CE, et al: Surgical treatment of morbid obesity: sixteen years of experience. Arch Surg 105:432–437, 1973.
3. Scott HW, Law DH, Sandstead HH, et al: Jejunoileal shunt in surgical treatment of morbid obesity. Ann Surg 171:770–782, 1970.
4. Mason EE: Surgical Treatment of Obesity: Major

Problems in Clinical Surgery, vol 26. Philadelphia, WB Saunders, 1981, pp 78–136.

5. Gourlay RH, Reynolds C: Complications of surgery for morbid obesity. Am J Surg 136:54–60, 1978.

6. Stein HB, Schlappner OL, Boyko W, et al: The intestinal bypass: Arthritis-dermatitis syndrome. Arthritis Rheum 24:684–690, 1981.

7. King CE, Toskes PP: Bacterial overgrowth syndromes. In Berk JE (ed): Bockus Gastroenterology, 4th ed. Philadelphia, WB Saunders, 1985, pp 1781–1802.

8. Faloon WW: Surgical treatment of morbid obesity. In Berk JE (ed): Bockus Gastroenterology, 4th ed. Philadelphia, WB Saunders, 1985, pp 4390–4399.

9. Gourlay RH, Evans KG: Jejunoileal bypass and the defunctioned bowel syndrome. Surg Gynecol Obstet 148:844–846, 1979.

10. Drenick EJ, Ament ME, Finegold SM, et al: Bypass enteropathy: an inflammatory process in the excluded segment with systemic complications. Am J Clin Nutr 30:76–89, 1977.

11. Drenick EJ, Stanley JM, Wills CM: Renal damage after intestinal bypass. Internat J Obes 5:501–508, 1981.

12. O'Leary JP: Liver failure after jejunoileal bypass: an appraisal. Internat J Obes 5:531–535, 1981.

13. Christophi C, Hughes ER: Hepatobiliary disorders in inflammatory bowel disease. Surg Gynecol Obstet 160:187–193, 1985.

14. Code CJ (ed): Handbook of Physiology, vol IV. Washington, DC, American Physiological Society, 1968, pp 2075–2091.

15. Preston FW, Svoboda AJ Jr, Horvath SM: Ileostomy of the distal end of the bypassed intestine in a patient with jejunoileal bypass for obesity. Am J Surg 135:710–713, 1978.

16. Hubbard TB Jr: The prevention of bypass enteritis after jejunoileal bypass for morbid obesity. Ann Surg 187:502–509, 1978.

17. Heimburger SL, Steiger E, LoGerfo P, et al: Reversal of severe fatty hepatic infiltration after intestinal bypass for morbid obesity. Am J Surg 29:229–237, 1975.

18. Cleator IGM, Gourlay RH: Ileogastrostomy for morbid obesity. Can J Surg 31:114–116, 1988.

19. MacFarlane JK: Important modification of the jejunoileal bypass procedure for morbid obesity. Can J Surg 31:75, 1988.

10

Duodenoileal Bypass

JOHN G. KRAL

Surgical methods to treat obesity rely on two basic principles: gastric restriction or malabsorption, although some procedures employ both. Since the etiology of the eating disorder in obesity is not known, treatment is essentially symptomatic. Successful long-term maintenance of significant weight reduction should ideally incorporate principles that reinforce a reduction in food intake. Such regulatory effects can be achieved by surgically induced aversiveness (negative reinforcement or conditioning) or preferably by reducing "hunger" or the drive to eat.

Restrictive procedures rely on the ability of the operation to limit energy intake and withstand abusive eating behavior or on the ability of the patient to follow a diet and modify eating behavior. Malabsorptive procedures rely on dissipation of calories, although reduced food intake also contributes to the weight loss.[1] It is unclear whether this is achieved by reducing "hunger" or by causing aversion.

Failure of gastric restriction is being reported increasingly and significant numbers of patients spontaneously elect not to have such procedures or are turned down for gastric procedures (50% of potential candidates according to estimates by several active surgeons). It is possible that gastric restriction as a principle has strong conceptual limitations, since it essentially represents "just another diet" for the majority of patients, once the initial aversive effects have worn off.

Since the abandonment of the traditional Payne and Salmon/Scott jejunoileal bypass operations, several malabsorptive alternatives have been developed. Biliointestinal bypass[2] uses an anastomosis of the blind loop of jejunum to the gallbladder in an attempt to prevent blind loop overgrowth and toxicity. End-to-end jejunoileostomy with ileogastrostomy[3] reduces blind loop overgrowth, by anastomosing the bypassed bowel antiperistaltically into the relatively less colonized stomach. Biliopancreatic bypass[4] creates a long Roux-Y limb with intact biliary and pancreatic secretions, while the alimentary limb is deprived of acid.

Several attempts have been made to improve the classical jejunoileal bypass, e.g. by creating antireflux valves in the bypassed segment[5] or by lengthening the ileal segment[6] to reduce the risk for bacterial overgrowth closer to the ileocecal valve. New knowledge concerning the management of patients with jejunoileal bypass, recognition of side-effects, the importance of liver biopsies, and specific methods for treating and preventing kidney stones, liver failure and arthritis might "legitimize" a renewed interest in malabsorptive procedures.[7]

The findings of significant reduction in food intake in rats with ileal interposition into the proximal jejunum[8] suggested the existence of "satiety" signals elicited from the terminal ileum when it is stimulated by food. This concept prompted H.E. Dorton in Lexington, Kentucky, to perform a modification of jejunoileal bypass in 1981. It was called "duodenoileal bypass" (DIB) to indicate the exclusion of virtually all jejunum, to distinguish it from the classical jejunoileal bypass.

PROCEDURES

The abdomen is entered through a transverse or midline incision. Needle or knife biopsy of the liver is performed after routine exploration of the abdomen. Taking great care to identify the ileocecal junction and Treves' fold, 50 cm of terminal ileum is measured with cotton tape four times along the mesenteric border, choosing the spot for construction of the antireflux nipple valve just proximal to the 50 cm point (Fig. 10.1).

After clearing a 5-cm isosceles wedge of mesenteric fat on both sides of the mesentery as required to facilitate invagination, 3 cm of proximal ileum is invaginated into the distal portion. The ensuing "lip" is stapled axially with three applications of Premium TA-30 4.8-mm AutoSuture® staplers with the pin removed to avoid piercing the intestinal wall. Four interrupted 3-0 silk sutures are sewn circumferentially to tack down the lip and to secure the invagination. Patency of antegrade flow and resistance to retrograde flow are tested by milking intestinal contents and gas towards the nipple valve from both directions.

The ligament of Treitz is identified and, if necessary, mobilization of the duodenojejunal junction is performed to allow alignment of the ileal segment to facilitate stapling the anastomosis. Two interrupted 3-0 silk sutures are placed 5–7 cm apart for approximation of the two limbs of intestine, prior to stapling with a GIA cutting stapler (AutoSuture®). After closure of the combined stabwound through which the jaws of the GIA stapler had been introduced, a new GIA cutting stapler is used to transect the jejunum just distal to the anastomosis. The stumps are oversewn for hemostasis and to bury stapled

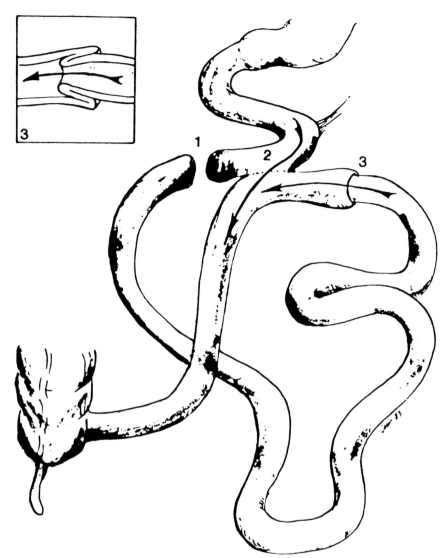

FIGURE 10.1. Duodenoileal bypass. Side-to-side anastomosis (2) of terminal ileum to jejunum at the ligament of Treitz. Transection of jejunum (1). Antireflux intussusception valve in terminal ileum (3), detailed in insert. (From Kral JG: Obesity surgery: state of the art. In Hirsch J, Van Itallie TB (eds): Recent Advances in Surgical Research IV. London, John Libbey, 1985, p 241.)

mucosa, and are then tacked to each other to prevent intussusception and facilitate possible future localization. After irrigation with antibiotic solution, the abdomen is closed with running #2 Dexon® in the linea alba.

The nasogastric tube can be removed after 1–2 days. The patient is started on a regular diet minus liquids upon resumption of bowel function, maintaining intravenous fluids depending on stool output. Most patients are discharged passing 3–5 liquid stools/day. Every patient is prescribed 1.5 g of calcium and a therapeutic dose of multivitamins daily, upon leaving the hospital on the sixth post-

operative day on an average. The patient is also furnished with a prescription for diphenoxylate and potassium in the event of increased stool frequency.

RESULTS

Primary duodenoileal bypass as described above has been performed in 64 patients (58 women) in Lexington, Kentucky and 44 (32 women) in New York as of December 1, 1986. An additional 26 operations each have been performed in Lexington and New York, bringing the total experience to 160 operations, including cases with prior and concomitant gastric procedures and with modifications such as varying lengths of intestinal segments and methods of valve construction.

This text will summarize the results in the 44 patients in New York who had primary duodenoileal bypass. Two patients have died. A 42-year-old hypertensive woman, weighing 106.9 kg (235.1 lbs) at 161 cm (5'3½"), who smoked but had no cardiac history and normal EKG died within 14 hours of the operation. She had ≈ 90% occlusion of the left main coronary artery with no other findings on postmortem examination. The other patient was 43 years old and weighed 193 kg (424.7 lbs) at 168.9 cm (5'6½"). She had cholecystectomy, panniculectomy and duodenoileal bypass. She was readmitted to the hospital with overwhelming sepsis from wound infection one month postoperatively, dying after one month in the intensive care unit. Two patients are lost to follow-up and an additional three have been observed less than 6 months. Table 10.1 summarizes the results of the 26 women and 11 men available for follow-up for 6–36 months (mean: 16 ± 2.2 s.e.m.).

The women lost less weight than the men in both absolute (32.9 vs 59.4 kg) and relative (26 vs 35% of initial weight) terms, as is usually the case in obesity surgery. However, the observation period was shorter for women and their initial relative weight was lower (BMI = 46.6 vs 51.2 in men). Ten of the women and four of the men lost weight prior to surgery, with mean losses of 12 and 50 kg respectively. Six of the women gained a mean of 6.4 kg preoperatively, while none of the men gained. Weight loss from the time of operation until follow-up was greater in patients who had lost preoperatively. Seven of 10 patients observed for more than 2 years have had slight increases in weight after reaching a nadir between 15–18 months postoperatively.

COMPLICATIONS AND SIDE-EFFECTS

These are presented in Table 10.2. The two deaths have been described earlier in this chapter. It is noteworthy that only 4 patients have a stool frequency of >3/day requiring diphenoxylate or loperamide after the first 3 months. Quantitatively the dominating side-effect is flatulence, which in the majority of cases is dietarily induced. The significant carbohydrate malabsorption presents large amounts of carbohydrate to the colonic flora, which causes fermentation and flatulence. A five-day treatment with 0.5 g metronidazole three times daily is effective in all cases and must occasionally be repeated at varying intervals.

The most troublesome effect of the operation is the occurrence of liver pathology disclosed by routine biopsy (Table 10.3). One patient with cirrhosis did not have baseline biopsy but admitted to regular moderate consumption of wine, in spite of being advised of the importance of abstinence. The other patient is a non-alcoholic 42-yr-old man who had lost 140 kg by preoperative dieting, having had a maximum weight of 374 kg. It is difficult to assess the combined impact of massive weight loss, cardiac cirrhosis and the effect of the operation causing cirrhosis in this patient. The third patient with cirrhosis is a non-alcoholic 45-yr-old woman with a strong family history of cirrhosis. Serial biopsies during 2 years' observation have revealed essentially unchanged histopathology with a decrease in fatty infiltration.

COMMENT

This relatively small series with short follow-up does not permit conclusions about the ultimate efficacy or safety of duodenoileal bypass. Most of the women in the series have not reached their nadir weight and the length of observation for all patients is too short to predict possible regain of weight with this operation. The observation of regain in 7 of the patients is troublesome in this respect.

In comparing with conventional jejunoileal bypass, it is obvious that several of the complications and side-effects are similar, e.g. hypokalemia, hypocalcemia, flatulence and di-

TABLE 10.1. WEIGHT LOSS IN PATIENTS AVAILABLE FOR FOLLOW-UP MORE THAN 6 MONTHS AFTER DUODENOILEAL BYPASS (MEANS ± S.E.M.)

Sex	Race W/B	Age	Height (cm)	Weight (kg)	BMI[1] (kg/m²)	IBW[2] (%)	Follow-up (mos)	Wt Loss (kg)	Loss of Excess Wt (%)
F	15/11	35.3±2.1	163.1±1.3	125.5±3.6	46.6±1.1	205±5	14.2±1.2	32.9±2.2	52±3
M	11/0	36.0±2.3	180.3±2.4	167.5±14.1	51.2±3.9	227±17	21.8±2.6	59.4±3.9	66±6

[1]Body mass index
[2]Ideal body weight—1983 Metropolitan Life tables[9]

TABLE 10.2. COMPLICATIONS AND SIDE-EFFECTS IN 44 PATIENTS WITH PRIMARY DUODENOILEAL BYPASS

Surgical complications (11/44)		Systemic complications (12/44)	
Postop. obstruction (non-op)	3	Hypokalemia (hospitalized)	7
		Hypocalcemia	2
Wound complications	8	Cholangitis	2
		Hypoalbuminemia	1
Infection	2		
Seroma	2	Side-effects (23/44)	
Incisional hernia	2	Flatulence	18
Dehiscence/hernia	1	Diarrhea >3/day	4
Seroma/hernia	1	Hemorrhoid flare-up	1

TABLE 10.3. HISTOPATHOLOGY OF LIVER BIOPSIES IN 24 PATIENTS MORE THAN 1 YEAR AFTER PRIMARY DUODENOILEAL BYPASS

	Increase	Unchanged	Decrease
Steatosis	5	12	7
Fibrosis	3	1	
Cirrhosis	3		
Regeneration	2		

arrhea. Furthermore, the appearance of liver abnormalities is a potentially serious side-effect which certainly limits the applicability of the operation to only the most well motivated of the patients. However, in comparing with jejunoileal bypass, it is noteworthy that the complications are fewer and less severe. Urolithiasis, cholelithiasis, arthritis and enteritis have not been seen as yet, as they had been after similar lengths of observation in series of jejunoileal bypass patients in this author's experience and in other published series. The longer segment of terminal ileum (50 vs 12.5 cm) and the construction of an antireflux valve probably make duodenoileal bypass a safer operation.

The preliminary experience with duodenoileal bypass in 16 patients (12 females) who had had failure of prior gastric restriction (vertical banded gastroplasty) observed for 12–30 months after duodenoileal bypass, has revealed a lower incidence of complications and side-effects than in the patients who underwent primary duodenoileal bypass. Longer follow-up in a greater number of patients is required to verify these preliminary findings.

CONCLUSION

Duodenoileal bypass is a variant of jejunoileal bypass which is prone to similar side-effects and complications, albeit fewer and less severe. The operation should only be performed if strict surveillance can be guaranteed, including periodic liver biopsies and continuous supplementation of multivitamins and minerals. The ultimate role of this operation as a primary procedure or in cases with failure of gastric restriction is as yet not defined.

REFERENCES

1. Pilkington TR, Gazet JC, Ang L, et al: Explanations for weight loss after ileojejunal bypass in gross obesity. Br Med J 1:1504–1505, 1976.
2. Eriksson F: Biliointestinal bypass. Int J Obes 5:437–447, 1981.
3. Gourlay RH: Jejunoileal bypass with ileogastrostomy: an operation free of the complications associated with intestinal bypass. Proceedings of the American College of Surgeons Postgraduate Course 2: Problems in Obesity Surgery. Vancouver, April 1986, pp 35–37.
4. Scopinaro N, Gianetta E, Civalleri D, et al: Partial and total bilio-pancreatic bypass in the surgical treatment of obesity. Int J Obes 5:421–429, 1981.
5. Wiklund B, Hallberg D: Experience with antireflux valves in jejunoileal bypass surgery. Acta Chir Scand 151:159–162, 1985.
6. Dano P, Christiansen C: Calcium absorption and bone mineral contents following intestinal shunt operation in obesity. Scand J Gastroenterol 9:775–779, 1974.
7. Zollinger RW, Coccia MR, Zollinger 2d RW: Critical analysis of jejunoileal bypass. Am J Surg 146:626–630, 1983.
8. Koopmans HS, Sclafani A, Fichtner C, et al: The effects of ileal transposition on food intake and body weight loss in VMH-obese rats. Am J Clin Nutr 35:284–293, 1982.
9. Metropolitan Life Foundation. Height and weight tables. Metropolitan Life Insurance Co., New York, Statistical Bulletin 64:2–9, 1983.

11

Biliopancreatic Bypass

DARWIN K. HOLIAN

Developing a malabsorption syndrome that would correct morbid obesity without creating the innumerable undesirable side-effects of the jejunoileal (JI) bypass has been the goal of many surgeons. While pursuing that goal Scopinaro of Italy confirmed other studies which showed that the absorption of toxins from bacterial overgrowth in the unused, excluded bowel was the cause of most of the JI bypass' undesirable side-effects. He was one of the first to show that if the entire intestine in a bypass procedure could be utilized, with no portion set aside as a "blind loop", major complications could be avoided. The operation that now bears his name is unique in that it accomplishes this end.

Initially working in his laboratory at the University of Genoa using dog models, and later transferring this knowledge to patients at his hospital, Scopinaro eventually published his first 4-year study on both dogs and humans in the same journal in 1979.[1,2] In describing his numerous trials using varying bowel-lengths for different functions, he showed how he eventually arrived at the most acceptable procedure for the vast majority of obese patients. Since that time only minor variations of the initially described procedure have been recommended.[3]

The operation is based on the physiological fact that, if one cannot digest the food that one consumes, the intestine will not be able to absorb it. This is accomplished by diverting bile and pancreatic juice away from the food that is ingested. The majority of carbohydrates, fat and protein consumed is passed through the bowel in an unchanged state. Two years postoperatively following compensatory bowel hypertrophy, as little as 30% of food becomes digested.

PREOPERATIVE MANAGEMENT

Selecting patients for surgery follows telephone qualification and extensive consultations. The same criteria for selection as required by other bariatric surgeons are utilized. Medical evaluation by an internist is requested when deemed necessary. After insurance coverage has been verified so that patients are not required to make large hospital deposits, they are admitted to the hospital the day before scheduled surgery. Cholecystograms are not done, as the gallbladder is removed in all patients because 80% of patients would develop cholesterol stones following the procedure. This appears to be due to gallbladder bile stasis from lack of cholecystokinin stimulation in the biliopancreatic tract and due to increased hepatic cholesterol excretion in the bile accompanying mobilization of fat stores with weight loss. Upper G.I. series is not routinely obtained.

After blood has been drawn for chemistries which include lipid profiles, and chest x-rays and electrocardiograms have been obtained, bowel lavage with Ringer's solution is begun through a small nasogastric tube. Bowel sterilization follows, utilizing a combination of neomycin and erythromycin base. Spirometry lessons are given and postoperative walks planned. A shower using chlorhexidine is taken the morning of surgery.

Patients are placed in a comfortable, minimally flexed position on the operating-table with knees slightly bent and lower legs elevated. At no time during the operation is the patient placed in an upright position. No anticoagulants are used, as no thromboses or pulmonary emboli have been observed. Subclavian infusion catheters are inserted in all patients, with position of the catheter confirmed by x-ray. Only in unusual circumstances do we employ arterial lines.

PROCEDURE AND TECHNIQUE

As proposed by Scopinaro and as utilized by the majority of proponents of the operation today, the procedure closely resembles a Billroth II gastrectomy with a long Roux-en-Y loop (Fig. 11.1). Cholecystectomy is routinely performed before any bowel lumen is exposed. The size of the gastric remnant varies somewhat from surgeon to surgeon, but most believe that a gastric pouch of 150–200 mL is essential in order to allow adequate food intake. This pouch size results when the greater curvature length is made 15 cm long and the lesser curvature is cut 2–3 cm below the gastroesophageal junction. Creating this size pouch produces a parietal cell mass sufficiently small to reduce hydrochloric acid secretion to a minimum. The short gastric arteries are divided, so that the remaining gastric pouch can be brought sufficiently caudad to meet the ileum which will be placed retrocolic. A good-sized branch of the left gastric artery is preserved. A 75% distal gastric resection is performed, using the TA90, reinforced with running 2–0 Dexon, leaving the approximately 150 mL pouch. Duodenum is closed with the TA55 stapler.

Initially, in 1979 bowel length for the new

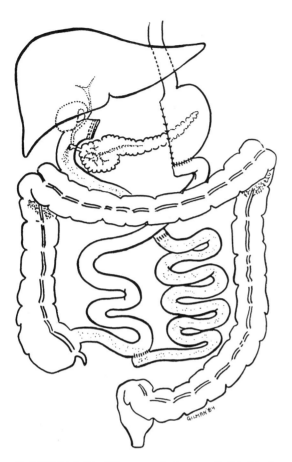

FIGURE 11.1 The biliopancreatic bypass. Gallbladder is removed. A 75% gastrectomy (approximately 150 mL pouch) is done, with stapled closure of the duodenal stump. Ileum is divided 250 cm proximal to the ileocecal valve. The proximal segment is placed on the left side and the distal segment on the right side of the peritoneal cavity. The distal 250 cm of ileum (**alimentary limb**) is brought retrocolic and anastomosed to the remaining stomach, and the transverse mesocolon tacked to stomach. The jejuno-proximal ileal segment (**biliopancreatic conduit**) is anastomosed to the side of the terminal ileum 50 cm from the ileocecal value (**common ileal segment** for digestion and absorption of food), and the mesenteric defect is closed. The new alimentary tract is about one-half the length of the biliopancreatic conduit.

alimentary tract was recommended to be half of the total length of the bowel. Approximately a year later, in order to improve weight loss Scopinaro recommended that the tract length be reduced to 250 cm. In our experience this shortening resulted in an overall improvement in excess weight loss of only 3%. The most critical measurement, however, is the distance one allows from the ileocecal valve to the place where the intestine containing bile and pancreatic digestive juice is anastomosed to the new alimentary or food tract. That length, where bile and pancreative juice mix with food, was originally established at 50 cm and remains as such today. Shorter distances have been found to cause increased stool frequency, reduce protein digestion and also result in too much weight loss. A longer distance can produce inadequate weight loss, as it allows too much food digestion to take place.

Ileocecal bowel is mobilized initially, and ileum is marked with a silk suture 50 cm and 250 cm proximal to the ileocecal valve, measuring along the anti-mesenteric border of the ileum. The mesentry is divided without dividing a major mesenteric artery at the point 250 cm proximal to ileocecal valve, and the ileum is divided with a GIA apparatus, placing the jejunum and proximal ileum (bile and pancreatic juice conduit) on the left side of the abdominal cavity and the distal ileum (new alimentary tract) on the right side.

The distal enteroenterostomy is made relatively small, as only bile and pancreatic juice need flow through it. The side-to-side anastomosis of the distal end of the proximal bowel is made to the previously marked 50-cm site on the terminal ileum. The mesenteric defect or hernia between the two limbs of bowel is appropriately and carefully closed.

A defect is created in the transverse mesocolon to the left of the middle colic vessels and posteriorly so that Petersen's hernia will be able to be closed with ease, and the ileum is brought up retrocolic. The retrocolic side-to-side gastroileostomy is constructed by hand or with the GIA apparatus, between the antimesenteric side of the ileum and the greater curvature side of the stomach. A stoma at least 4 cm in diameter is made, to prevent retention of gastric acid secretions and to permit an unobstructed path to propel food into the bowel. The nasogastric tube is brought down to the anastomosis. The hole left by the GIA is closed with running 3–0 Dexon reinforced with interrupted 3–0 silk. The anastomosis is then tacked below the colon mesentery, by suturing the edge of the mesenteric rent to the serosal surface of the stomach just cephalad to the anastomosis. Petersen's hernia is carefully closed by approximating the cut edge of the small bowel mesentry to the posterior abdominal peritoneum with interrupted sutures, so as to prevent volvulus formation.

A right upper quadrant suction catheter drain is brought out from Morison's pouch, draining the gallbladder bed, duodenal stump and gastric edge. The wound fascia is closed with widely placed interrupted sutures of No. 2 polyglycolic acid. Despite this careful closure our incidence of postoperative hernia is 14%. When repaired later we always employ an onlay covering of Marlex mesh.

Use of a third generation cephalosporin effective against anaerobes is begun in the operating-room and is continued for 48 hours. Gastric suction is removed in 48 hours and oral liquids permitted on the third postoperative day. By the fifth day soft foods are started, with most patients leaving the hospital on the sixth postoperative day.

MORBIDITY AND MORTALITY

To date we have operated upon more than 400 patients. Morbidity includes two duodenal stump leaks, three cases of iatrogenic splenectomy, five subphrenic abscesses (all after revision operations), one postoperative peritonitis from an enteroenterostomy leak and one wound infection. Operative mortality in our hands is 0.5%. Both of the postoperative deaths were patients who were in their late fifties and had complicating problems of diabetes and advanced arteriosclerosis. Despite the length of operative time and number of anastomoses, these complications are no greater than those reported following lesser operations.

WEIGHT LOSS

The prime purpose of any obesity operation is to achieve a weight loss significant enough and permanent enough to render a patient no longer in jeopardy from his or her obesity. Most gastric restrictive procedures done today can achieve a 60% excess weight loss, but few make this loss permanent. The biliopancreatic bypass like the JI bypass causes a loss of almost 80% of excess weight with permanence of that loss extending at least 10 years. Our studies which now extend beyond 7 years show a 53% excess weight loss in 6 months. This loss increases to 69% at one year and 79% at two years. Our 98% follow-up substantiates the claim that there is little tendency to regain weight after this procedure.

HYPERACIDITY

When the Scopinaro procedure was initially described, it was apparent that the operation resembled the Mann-Williamson experimental dog model designed at the Mayo Clinic in 1923, which produced peptic ulcers in almost 100% of dogs.[4] In 1950 Dragstedt's group[5] had protected this model from ulcers either by doing a subtotal gastrectomy or by performing a truncal vagotomy. Appreciating this fact Scopinaro's first procedures utilized a partial gastrectomy. An incidence of symptomatic hyperacidity of 7% has, however, been observed and an incidence of ulcers of 2% has been confirmed. Creation of a 4-cm-diameter large gastroileostomy (as opposed to the stoma initially described by this author using a 25-mm EEA stapler[6]) has decreased hyperacidity symptoms dramatically. Hydrogen ion blocking agents are required by a small percentage of patients, but none has ever required reversal of the operation for this reason alone.

At present, there are two series being done in which the stomach is left in place and not resected.[7,8] Wittig, in his last 150 biliopancreatic bypass operations, has stapled across the proximal stomach, similar to the technique commonly used in the gastric bypass operation, with the gastroileostomy in the upper segment.[7] Wittig tacks the distal stomach to anterior abdominal wall, using a radiopaque silastic ring to enable later identification if necessary, e.g. to percutaneously insert a needle, guidewire, dilator and gastrostomy tube or take a gastric biopsy. No significant increase in ulcer problems has been noted. Biron and co-workers[8] reported a small series of biliopancreatic bypasses combining highly selective vagotomy with stapled closure of the first part of duodenum, but with no gastric resection or segmentation.

If long-term studies verify that the stomach may be simply stapled with the TA90B without distal resection with no increase in ulcer problems, it will make the biliopancreatic bypass operation less in magnitude and probably result in its greater acceptance. However, Flickinger and associates,[9] using retrograde duodenogastrostomy after the Roux-en-Y gastric bypass found unexplained bile reflux, atrophic gastritis and intestinal metaplasia in the distal gastric segment. The possibility of these gastric mucosal changes and their long-term significance in the bypassed stomach will then have to be pondered.[10]

FLUID AND ELECTROLYTE IMBALANCE

Because there is no comparable diarrhea associated with this procedure as with the JI bypass, fluid and electrolyte abnormalities are rarely seen. Only when a patient neglects treating an intestinal flu have we observed imbalance. Our patients are strongly encouraged to keep antidiarrheal medications on hand at all times in order to stem this problem before it becomes serious.

HEPATIC ABNORMALITIES

With no "blind loop" to permit overgrowth of bacteria, toxic deterioration of the liver has never been observed. During the first 6 months after surgery because of the severe deprivation of nutrition, elevation of liver enzymes is commonly seen. These enzymes then return to normal except in 10% of patients who continue an elevation of their alkaline phosphatase. When fractionated, this enzyme has been found to be primarily from bone and not of liver origin. Scopinaro's group has done over 400 liver biopsies, almost all of which showed improvement or stability of liver architecture when compared with preoperative studies.[11] Our smaller experience agrees with this finding.

LIPID STUDIES

Enterohepatic and extrahepatic lipid absorption is markedly reduced by this operation, with the result that both cholesterol and triglyceride values are significantly decreased. Our ongoing studies show that total cholesterol values are reduced an average of 37%. Measurements of desirable HDL increase 8%; LDL values decrease 48%. Triglycerides lower by over 300%. Although extensive angiographic studies have not been done, based on the fact that only 7% of patients continue cholesterol values >170 mg/dl (>4.3 mmol/L), and relying on DePalma's studies,[12] it is safe to assume that reduction of cholesterol deposits in their vessels is occurring.

KIDNEY STONES

Determination of oxalate levels in the urine reveals values 2 to 3 times normal. This is similar to that seen in JI bypass patients. Unabsorbed fatty acids in the colon compete with oxalate for calcium. This leaves free oxalate which is absorbed by the colon, resulting in high urinary output of the substance. Without diarrhea to cause dehydration, patients with biliopancreatic bypass have little trouble handling this oxalate. Only those patients who have had gastroenteritis leading to dehydration have ended up with stones. To date this is a total of 9 patients or an incidence of 3%.

HYPOPROTEINEMIA

With any malabsorption procedure there is always the risk of nutritional abnormalities. Reduced protein digestion and absorption have been seen both early and late following the biliopancreatic diversion. Since enlarging the gastroileostomy to facilitate better early intake of food, we have seen very few early protein problems.[13] When detected during the first 6 months, hypoproteinemia usually responds to amino acid supplements and pancreatic enzymes. The late type seen 2–3 years after surgery is much more difficult to correct. At that time it is seen only in patients who for many and various reasons are not eating properly nor enough. This circumstance has been the main reason for reversals. We believe that a bulimia or anorexia nervosa type of personality is usually involved.

CALCIUM

Much criticism of the biliopancreatic bypass centers about the fact that many patients demonstrate reduced serum calcium. Compston's report on a group of Scopinaro's patients pointed out that metabolic bone disease is common after the operation.[14] Responding to this report at a recent obesity symposium, Scopinaro stated that the disease process, whatever its cause, disappears after 4 years.

There appear to be two causes for the reduced serum calcium. First, the majority of lactase enzyme which is necessary for milk digestion is present on the surface of the proximal jejunum. Because this portion of the bowel is not in contact with food following the biliopancreatic diversion, little lactase is available. Most patients, therefore, have a significant milk intolerance, i.e. milk lactose reaches the colon where fermentation produces excess hydrogen (H_2) with intestinal discomfort. Lactaid milk or milk digestants can be prescribed, e.g. Lactaid®* tablets (beta-galactosidase lactase enzyme which hydrolyses lactose to glucose and galactose).[15] However, most patients avoid milk. As a result, calcium intake is often insufficient. Second,

*Lactaid Inc., Pleasantville, NJ 08232, U.S.A.

most calcium is absorbed in the bypassed duodenum and proximal jejunum. Thus, calcium depletions can occur. Calcium supplements in the form of calcium salts (carbonate, citrate) are prescribed for everyone, e.g. calcium carbonate antacid tablets (Tums®) eight per day. We insist that our patients consume at least 1500 mg of elemental calcium daily, and taking calcium in the evening assures better absorption. Increase in calcium levels and reduction in alkaline phosphatase (bone fraction) have been observed with this regimen. Vitamins must include D.

ANEMIAS

An 8% incidence of anemia has been observed both in males and females. For this reason a well absorbed iron product consisting of ferrous fumarate with vitamin C is recommended for all patients. Menstruating females especially require iron supplements on a regular basis, as iron, like calcium, is normally absorbed primarily in the bypassed gut. Only three cases of vitamin B_{12} deficiency have been observed by us to date, and we continue to search for it. In treating iron deficiencies in biliopancreatic bypass patients, one must be aware that most available iron compounds are enteric-coated and pass directly through the patient's gut without even the coating being dissolved.

PREGNANCY

Return to normal menstrual cycles is common several months after surgery. Fortunately, only two patients have found that they were surprised by pregnancy within 6 months after their initial surgery. Both required insertion of central venous catheters and "home hyperalimentation" during the last 3 months of gestation. Significant reduction in the albumin fraction of their proteins as well as reduction of iron stores were the primary reasons for implementing this therapy. We warn our patients of the difficulty of early pregnancy. Except for anemia, later pregnancies have been without nutritional problems, and all our ten babies have been healthy although small.

BOWEL ACTIVITY

Most patients have two to three, soft, mushy, very foul-smelling stools per day. Liquid or diarrhea stools are seen only with infectious enteritis, excess milk and milk product intake, and unusual intake of fats. We have been impressed with the effectiveness of two 50 mg zinc tablets per day to reduce the foul odor of the stools.

SUPPLEMENTS

We have determined based on full chemistry panels done every 6 months as well as clinical evaluations at this same interval, that all patients need certain basic vitamin and mineral supplements. We prescribe two multivitamins per day and have still seen occasional vitamin A, D and K deficiencies. New, water-soluble A, D and K vitamin preparations are available and are very effective in preventing and correcting deficiencies. Vitamin B_6 is recommended as it is essential for protein synthesis by the liver. As mentioned above, calcium supplements in good amounts are critical for maintaining good bone structure. Iron tablets to prevent anemias are given early postoperatively. This number of pills is usually less than most patients were taking before their surgery.

REVISIONS AND REVERSALS

During the past 7 years only 12 patients have required reversal of their diversion because of intolerance to the procedure. This represents an incidence of 3%, which is far below the nearly 50% reversal-rate following the JI bypass.[16] All patients who were reversed had become malnourished from a combination of factors including hyperacidity with stenosis of the gastroenterostomy, persistent nausea or anorexia, intolerance of stool consistency and odor, and psychological problems. There are two ways to effect reversal. Complete restoration of the alimentary tract requires reanastomosis of the stomach to the duodenum and an end-to-end enteroenterostomy. It is always possible and has been done several times. An easier procedure and the one recommended for the ill and malnourished patient is a high enteroenterostomy. Physiologically this maneuver returns digestion to an almost normal state. Whether the reversal was accomplished by the first or second method, all reversed patients are regaining their original obesity.

Revisions of gastroenterostomy stenoses which followed use of the 25-mm EEA apparatus used to be fairly common. Since enlarging the gastroileostomy, such revisions have no longer been necessary.

Revision of bowel length to either improve digestion or reduce digestion has been done on only a few patients. In our experience, shortening of the bowel in association with reduction in the size of the stomach has not improved weight loss. Likewise, lengthening the bowel to improve nutrition has met with mixed results.

ASSESSMENT OF THE OPERATION

The magnitude of this very effective procedure has no doubt been a stumbling block to its greater acceptance. Although in our hands the mortality rate is low and the morbidity less than that reported by many gastric bypass proponents, there is great objection to the operative time of 3 to 4 hours and the removal of three-fourths of the stomach. The original division of the intestine at the halfway mark made creation of the gastroenterostomy simple, since mesenteric length increases the farther up the bowel one goes. With an increase in weight loss of only 3%, it would seem that the return to the original length of the alimentary limb might be appropriate. The longer alimentary tract could well improve calcium absorption as well as decrease stool activity. In addition, if studies confirm that the stomach can be left in with no increase in the incidence of ulcer problems, many objections to the procedure will be circumvented.

This operation because of its malabsorption component has continued successful after 10 years of observation. All proposed gastric restrictive procedures introduced during this same era have ultimately failed and have required some form of modification.[17] The Roux-en-Y gastric bypass, because of its element of malabsorption, alone remains popular as a long-term procedure.[18]

For those who wish to convert a failed gastric restrictive procedure to a biliopancreatic-diversion type diversion it must be remembered that a good sized gastric pouch must be created so as to allow adequate food intake. The Scopinaro procedure is very effective, but if made too severe will result in patients with significant malnutrition.[19]

REFERENCES

1. Scopinaro N, Gianetta E, Civalleri D, et al: Biliopancreatic bypass for obesity: I. An experimental study in dogs. Br J Surg 66:613–617, 1979.
2. Scopinaro N, Gianetta E, Civalleri D, et al: Biliopancreatic bypass for obesity: II. Initial experience in man. Br J Surg 66:618–620, 1979.
3. Scopinaro N, Gianetta E, Civalleri D, et al: Two years of clinical experience with biliopancreatic bypass for obesity. Am J Clin Nutr 33:506–514, 1980.
4. Mann FC, Williamson CS: Experimental production of peptic ulcer. Ann Surg 77:409–422, 1923.
5. Storer EH, Woodward ER, Dragstedt LR: The effect of vagotomy and antrum: resection of the Mann-Williamson ulcer. Surgery 27:526–530, 1950.
6. Holian DK: Biliopancreatic bypass for morbid obesity. Contemp Surg 21:55–65, 1982.
7. Wittig JH, Clinical Assistant Professor of Surgery, UCLA Medical Center, 18370 Burbank Blvd., Tarzana, California: personal communication.
8. Biron S, Plamondon H, Bourque, R-A, et al: Clinical experience with biliopancreatic bypass and gastrectomy or selective vagotomy for morbid obesity. Can J Surg 29:408–410, 1986.
9. Flickinger EG, Sinar DR, Pories WJ: The bypassed stomach. Am J Surg 149:151–156, 1985.
10. Orlando R III, Welsh JR: Carcinoma of the stomach after gastric operation. Am J Surg 141:487–491, 1981.
11. Gianetta E, Vitali A, Civalleri D, et al: Liver morphology and function after biliopancreatic bypass. Clin Nutr 5:207–214, 1986.
12. DePalma RG: Control and regression of atherosclerotic plaques: A commentary. In Dale, WA (ed): Management of Arterial Occlusive Disease. Chicago, Yearbook Medical Publishers, 1971, pp 64–64.
13. Holian DK, Clare MW: Biliopancreatic Bypass for morbid obesity: Late results and complications. Clin Nutr 5:133–136, 1986.
14. Compston JE, Vedi S, Gianetta E, et al: Bone histomorphology and vitamin D status after biliopancreatic bypass for obesity. Gastroenterology 87:350–356, 1984.
15. Solomons NW, Guerro A-M, Torun B: Effective in vivo hydrolysis of milk lactose by beta-galactosidases in the presence of solid foods. Am J Clin Nutr 41:222–227, 1985.
16. Halverson JD, Scheff RJ, Gentry K, et al: Jejunoileal bypass: late metabolic sequelae and weight gain. Am J Surg 140:347–350, 1980.
17. Knol JA, Strodel WE, Eckhauser FE: Critical appraisal of horizontal gastroplasty. Am J Surg 153:256–261, 1987.
18. Rucker RD, Chan EK, Chute EP, et al: The use of jejunoileal bypass, loop gastric bypass and Roux-en-Y gastric bypass to achieve similar weight reduction in morbidly obese individuals. Clin Nutr 5:101–105, 1986.
19. Scopinaro N, Gianetta E, Friedman D, et al: Evolution of biliopancreatic bypass. Clin Nutr 5:137–146, 1986 (Supplement).

12

Gastric Bypass Procedures

DAVID K. MILLER
GERALD N. GOODMAN

HISTORY AND DEVELOPMENT

With few successful medical cures, surgeons began performing surgical procedures for the treatment of morbid obesity—Bariatric Surgery. Surgeons initially performed malabsorption-type operations classified as jejunoileal (JI) bypass. However, many patients had significant side-effects such as hepatic failure, renal stones, electrolyte imbalance, arthritis, bloating, uncontrolled diarrhea, flatulence and malnutrition. Because of the long-term sequelae, many patients required reversal of the JI bypass. Thus, the public, medical community and medical insurance companies had an unenthusiastic attitude towards bariatric surgery.

In the 1940's and 1950's, the standard operation for complicated peptic ulcer was subtotal gastrectomy with Billroth II anastomosis. In 1966, Mason began restrictive gastric surgery for morbid obesity with the gastric bypass, using a loop gastrojejunostomy[1,2] (Fig. 12.1-A). Initially, Mason divided the proximal 10% of stomach producing a 100–150 ml pouch and performed a Billroth II-type retrocolic, short-afferent-loop, end-to-side gastrojejunostomy with a stoma 12-mm in diameter. The limited storage capacity of the proximal gastric segment and the narrow outlet produced early satiety. Overdistension caused distress and vomiting, promoting a change in eating behavior. Subsequently, the size of the pouch was reduced (Fig. 12.1-B), still preserving blood supply high on the lesser curvature.[3]

Mason's operation was not readily accepted by surgeons because of skepticism caused by the prior JI bypasses. However, Mason persisted with research studies and showed the effectiveness and safety of the loop gastric bypass, including the following: (a) ideal pouch size 50 ml or less, in order to assist weight loss and include acid-secreting mucosa in the distal segment to avoid marginal or duodenal ulcer;[3–5] (b) low serum gastrin levels despite residual distal stomach;[3,6] (c) optimal diameter of the gastrojejunostomy anastomosis 12 mm;[3] (d) midline epigastric incisions through the linea alba.[3]

Mason subsequently shifted to other gastric restrictive operations such as gastroplasties and gastric partitionings, in the quest for an operation that would allow effective weight loss with less complications than the loop gastric bypass. In the late 1970's, because of their effectiveness and safety, gastric restrictive operations became the operations of choice of most bariatric surgeons.

In 1977, John Alden introduced the use of one application of a 90-mm automatic stapling device to cross-staple the stomach in continuity without transection.[7] Alden also simplified the loop gastric bypass by performing

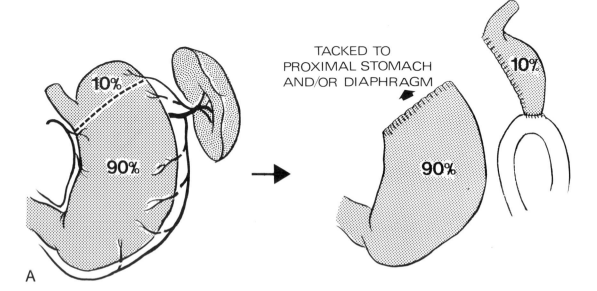

A

FIGURE 12.1-A. Original loop gastric bypass of Mason, 1966. Several 2–0 silk sutures were taken between the two gastric segments at the lesser and greater curvature, to prevent torsion or intussusception of the distal stomach.

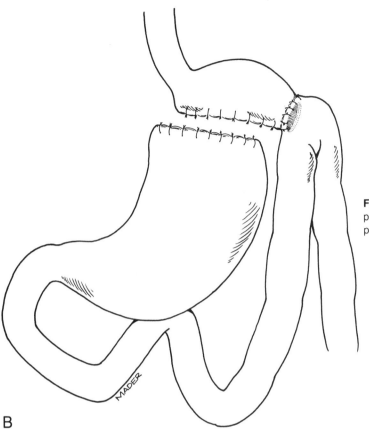

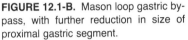

FIGURE 12.1-B. Mason loop gastric bypass, with further reduction in size of proximal gastric segment.

an antecolic gastrojejunostomy to the small proximal segment.

Anastomotic leakage was a dreaded complication, manifested by tachycardia, tachypnea, high white count, oliguria, left upper quadrant pain and left shoulder pain. Prompt re-operation and drainage were mandatory. Ward Griffen modified Mason's divided-stomach loop gastric bypass by performing a retrocolic Roux-en-Y gastrojejunostomy[8] (Fig. 12.2). This diverted bile and pancreatic juice from the gastrojejunostomy, so that if a leak occurred, there was only some saliva present. Furthermore, the Roux-loop facilitated technically the movement of the jejunum in a retrocolic fashion to a high position.

In the 1970's, a common general surgical operation was the conversion of the Billroth II gastrectomy into a Roux-en-Y anastomosis, in order to cure bile reflux esophagitis and gastritis. Cimetidine became available at that time and peptic ulcer surgery was becoming less frequent. In 1978, the most common gastric operation in our hospital became this conversion operation. Griffen and Alden modified their techniques and recommended an undivided gastric bypass with Roux-en-Y gastrojejunostomy (Fig. 12.3),[9] as this decreased contamination, facilitated bringing up the jejunum, decreased threatening leaks and avoided bile reflux and bilious vomiting. For security of the in-continuity partition, Griffen later used two applications of the TA-90 mm stapler. Stapling techniques were then variously applied to the performance of the Roux-en-Y gastric bypass (Fig. 12.4).[10]

In order to prevent staple-line breakdown, in addition to two applications of the TA-90 (U.S. Surgical) or PI-90 (3 M) stapler with 4.8-mm staples, some surgeons inserted non-absorbable sutures around the staple-lines. A proximal 50 ml pouch was constructed.[9,11–13] Halverson noted that weight loss was inversely related to pouch size.[14] In an attempt to prevent expansion of the stoma, many surgeons used a continuous 3–0 polypropylene suture circumferentially,[11,15] often between the rows of inner catgut and outer silk.[9] Reported operative mortality was <1% and morbidity 4%,[9,13] and more than 90% of patients had lost more than 50% of excess weight at 3 years.[9,13–17]

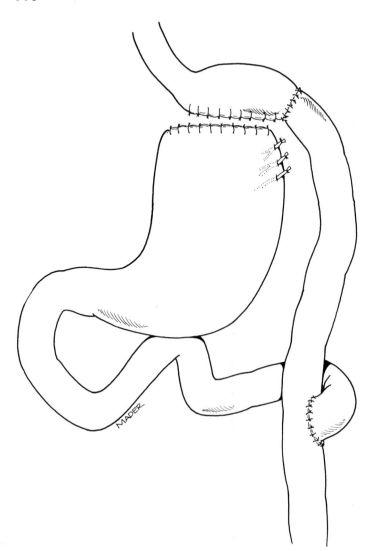

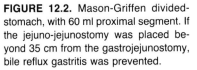

FIGURE 12.2. Mason-Griffen divided-stomach, with 60 ml proximal segment. If the jejuno-jejunostomy was placed beyond 35 cm from the gastrojejunostomy, bile reflux gastritis was prevented.

CURRENT PROCEDURES

THE AUTHORS' METHOD

In 1979, we began performing the divided gastric bypass with Roux-en-Y gastrojejunostomy-jejunojejunostomy (Fig. 12.5). Two 90-mm staplers are placed parallel from the lesser curvature, preserving the ascending branch of the left gastric artery and the nerve of Latarjet, to the greater curvature, proximal to the short gastric vessels. The staples are then fired and the stomach is divided. This technique preserves blood supply to the proximal and distal stomach pouches and does not require the ligation of any of the greater curvature vessels. In undivided gastric bypasses, the short gastric vessels need to be ligated, possibly compromising the blood supply to the stomach.

The proximal gastric pouch is approximately 50 ml. Because the gastric pouch tissue thickness and distensibility are so varied in patients, we do not believe that it is essential or necessary to have pressure measurements of the gastric pouch in a gastric bypass.* The subsequent size of the proximal pouch varies in long-term follow-up, depending on type and quantity of intake and tissue distensibility. The estimated visual measurement of the proximal pouch in patients is extremely effective. In some patients, the proximal pouch size may be reduced to as little as 30 ml. An example is in conversions of previous gastroplasties where the remaining size of the proximal stomach can only be 30 ml. The variation

---

*For pressure measurement after the stapler has been closed but prior to firing,[3,18] see Chapter 16.

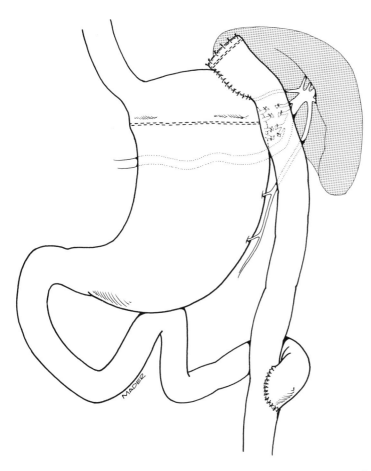

FIGURE 12.3. Subsequent Roux-en-Y stapled undivided gastric bypass. Many surgeons used 2 applications of the linear stapler (4 rows) and some workers over-sewed the staple-line with non-absorbable suture material. Most surgeons changed from a 35 to a 60 cm Roux-en-Y limb to ensure that there was no reflux.

of pouch size from 50 ml to 30 ml does not seem to significantly affect food quantity or ability of patients to eat after gastric by-pass. The actual pouch size is probably most significant during the early post-operative period when the patient is forced to change eating habits and ingest only small amounts of food. A significant benefit of the divided proximal gastric pouch is the prolonged feeling of satiety that the patients experience. Upper gastrointestinal barium studies in later years have continued to demonstrate a small proximal gastric pouch. However, all of these studies are performed on patients in a fasting state with a contracted stomach. To our knowledge, pressure studies of the proximal gastric pouch in years following surgery have not been reported.

The most important measurement at surgery is the size of the gastrojejunal anastomosis. To ensure the size of the gastrojejunostomy, a 12-mm diameter bougie (36 F) is placed through the anastomosis by the anesthesiologist after an inner 3–0 Vicryl row is completed. Two outer rows of interrupted,

mattressed, 3–0 silk sutures are then placed tightly against the bougie. These three rows create significant tensile strength and thickness of the anastomosis, preventing dilatation and resulting in good long-term weight loss. Excessive scarring or stricturing is rare. The diameters of stapled gastrojejunal anastomoses are often inaccurate and inconsistent, and usually result in incomplete staple-rings requiring suture closure and reinforcement. Studies have shown that stapled anastomoses have less edema and scarring than sutured anastomoses,[19] which may allow the anastomosis to dilate more readily. Some scarring of the anastomosis is necessary for long-term effectiveness in preventing stomal dilatation.

The proximal divided gastric pouch is free of splenic attachments, allowing the greater curvature to move caudally and anteriorly. The tip of the jejunal limb is attached with 3–0 silk fixation sutures to the stapled edge of the proximal pouch for 2 cm on the medial side of the gastrojejunostomy. The greater curvature side of the proximal gastric staple-line is excised and anastomosed to the side

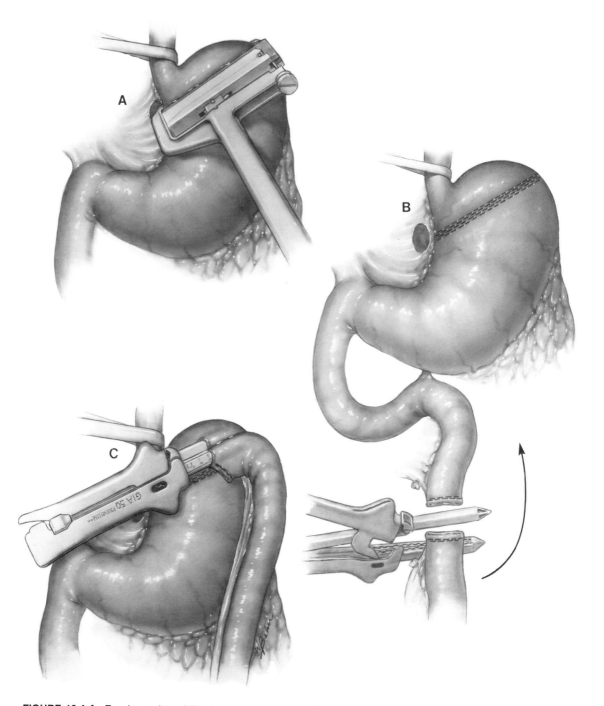

FIGURE 12.4-A. Esophagus is mobilized on a Penrose drain. Opening is made in lesser omentum, and linear stapler (here TA-90B) is applied from lesser greater curvature and closed. Pouch volume is measured. Instrument is fired and removed. **B.** GIA distal to ligament of Treitz is fired, transecting the jejunum between two double staggered staple-lines. **C.** Antimesenteric border of jejunum is approximated to fundus of stomach with stay sutures 2.5 cm from gastric staple-lines and 2.5 cm from greater curvature, to ensure adequate gastric vascularity. Stab-wound is made into lumen of stomach and antimesenteric corner of jejunum is excised. GIA instrument is inserted and fired.

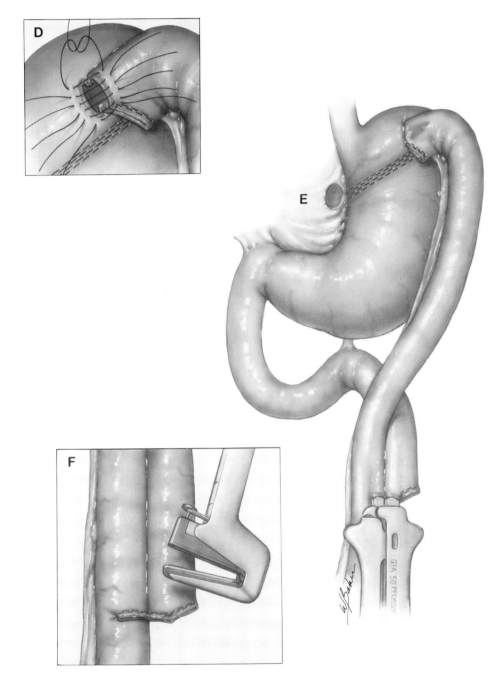

FIGURE 12.4-D. Inner surface of anastomosis is inspected for hemostasis, and common stab-wound closed manually. **E.** Antimesenteric corner of proximal jejunal segment is excised and stab-wound is made into antimesenteric border of apposed jejunal segment. GIA is inserted and fired. **F.** Inner surface of anastomotic staple-lines are inspected for hemostasis. GIA introduction site is closed transversely with TA-55. (Figs. 12.4A–F: Copyright United States Surgical Corporation, 1986. Used by permission.)

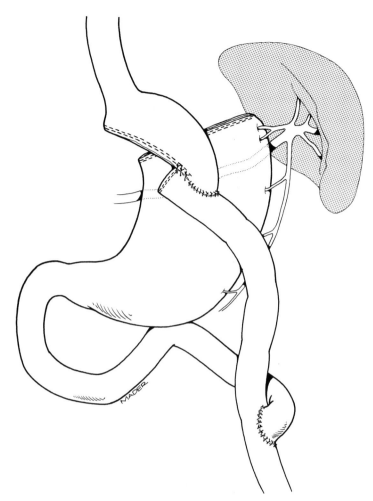

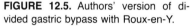

FIGURE 12.5. Authors' version of divided gastric bypass with Roux-en-Y.

of the jejunal limb with a 12-mm anastomosis. The tapering into the gastrojejunostomy allows the funneling of gastric contents into the dependent anastomosis. This permits better emptying and prevents pooling of gastric contents that could otherwise obstruct or distort the outlet. The jejunal limb places anterior and caudal traction on the proximal gastric pouch. The combination of the small proximal stomach, the funneling, and the traction completely eliminates most symptoms of reflux esophagitis and hiatus hernia, which are common problems in the morbidly obese. Other gastric restrictive procedures have frequently aggravated reflux esophagitis. The Roux-en-Y divided gastric bypass should be the procedure of choice for reflux esophagitis and hiatus hernia in the morbidly obese patient.

The divided proximal pouch is mobile and moves anteriorly to allow the gastrojejunal suturing to be completed closer to the wound surface. With no ligated vessels, less manipulations, and better visualization and expo-

sure, the divided gastric bypass surgery is safer, technically easier, and has less complications than the stapled stomach that has not been divided. Alden and Griffen stopped dividing the stomach because of potential leaks and infection. However, for the past 2 years our average subdiaphragmatic abscess incidence is 0.8%, and only three patients have demonstrated a leak. The divided stomach avoids late staple-line disruption, which may occur in all the undivided gastric restrictive operations. Staple-line disruption has had variable rates of occurrence in the other operations, but the highest was in the horizontal partitioning gastroplasty. Carey and Martin have revised many of their failed horizontal partitioning gastroplasty patients with divided gastric bypasses and Roux-en-Y anastomoses similar to our procedure.[20]

Distal pouch disruption in the post-operative period has been reported by some surgeons, deterring them from dividing the stomach.[14] To prevent early post-operative distention with potential perforation of the distal gastric pouch, some surgeons decompress the distal pouch with a tube gastrostomy, which is removed before discharge from hospital.[13] Some surgeons only use a distal Stamm gastrostomy when there were distal adhesions, increased chance of ileus or in revision operations.[3,21]

The Roux-en-Y limb of our patients is made by dividing the jejunum 20 cm from the ligament of Treitz with a GIA stapler. Then, a 60-cm limb of jejunum is measured and a side-to-side jejunojejunostomy is performed. The side-to-side anastomosis is accomplished with a GIA stapler, followed by a TA-55 stapled closure of the enterotomy. The mesenteric inside GIA staple-line (i.e. inner aspect of the staple-line anastomosis) is often reinforced with a running 3–0 Vicryl suture to avoid post-operative excessive bleeding from the stapled anastomosis. Large amounts of blood in the jejunum from the jejunojejunostomy may obstruct the outflow of fluids from the duodenum and the distal gastric pouch, leading to acute distal pouch distention. Since we began over-sewing the mesenteric inside GIA staple-line and prevented excessive bleeding at the jejunojejunostomy, distal pouch distention is rarely seen. Thus, the distal tube gastrostomy is not used in our divided gastric bypasses. The mesenteric window is closed with running 3–0 Vicryl suture.

We originally brought the Roux-en-Y limb over the transverse colon in an antecolic position. We chose to perform an antecolic gastrojejunostomy until five of our first 3000 patients developed internal herniae through the opening where the jejunal limb crossed anterior to the transverse colon. Three of these patients required small-bowel resection because of infarction. The other two patients required only reduction of the small-bowel obstruction and closure of the hernial window. These same complicating internal hernias have occurred in patients treated with gastric resections with Billroth II loop gastrojejunostomy or Roux-en-Y antecolic anastomoses. Because of the possibilities of internal hernias, we now tunnel the jejunal limb through the omentum and over the colon (Fig. 12.6), or preferably retrocolic through the transverse mesocolon and anterior to the distal stomach if the transverse mesocolon is very long (Fig. 12.6—inset). These are short routes creating no tension on the gastrojejunostomy, even in heavy men with a short mesentery. We have seen no ileus or obstruc-

tion in any patients since using these tunneling techniques. These tunnelings adhere the jejunal limb to the transverse colon area in such a way that hernial complications have not occurred. This fixation is one all surgeons should consider in other gastric operations where gastrointestinal anastomoses are performed. On the other hand, the retrocolic retrogastric tunnel brings the jejunal limb through the root of the transverse mesocolon behind the distal pouch and requires the gastrojejunostomy to be accomplished deep in the wound, cephalad to the distal gastric pouch. This method was difficult and is rarely performed by us.

After the gastrojejunal anastomosis has been completed, the bougie is removed and a nasogastric tube is then passed by the anesthesiologist through the gastrojejunostomy for approximately 5 cm into the jejunal limb. This tube is left in for approximately 24 hours on suction.

Other surgical procedures performed in association with the gastric bypass have not demonstrated significant increased morbidity or mortality. Pelvic operations, such as tubal ligation, ovarian cystectomy, cyst drainage and oophorectomy have been combined occasionally. Ventral and umbilical hernias are frequently repaired. Cholecystectomies have been performed either before the gastric bypass or simultaneously in at least 50% of our patients. For over 5 years, we have advocated the removal of questionably diseased gallbladders and especially gallbladders showing cholesterolosis (Table 12.1). We have improved in our gross acuity and accuracy in identifying cholesterolosis on the mucosa of the gallbladder without opening it. Willbanks and others have advocated routine removal of all gallbladders of morbidly obese patients.[22,23] Subsequent cholecystectomies in our series of at-risk patients has dropped to as low as 0.8%; therefore, we have been more selective and do not remove normal appearing gallbladders.

Five percent of our gastric bypass operations are performed for revision of other failed surgical obesity procedures. Most frequently, the failed operation has been some type of gastroplasty. The divided gastric bypass with Roux-en-Y is the operation of choice of some surgeons for revising failed obesity operations.[24] Complication rates for revisions into gastric bypasses are slightly higher than those for primary gastric bypasses.

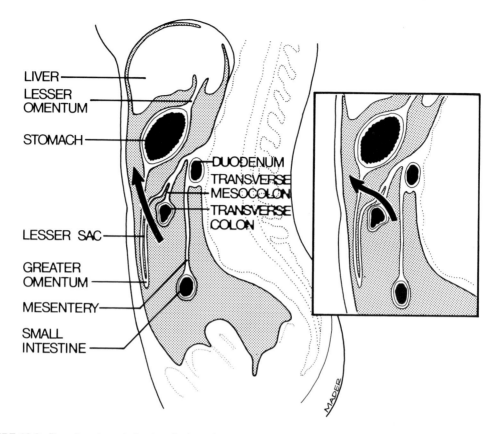

FIGURE 12.6. Roux-loop tunneled antecolic through greater omentum. Inset: Roux-loop tunneled retrogastric and antecolic.

ANTERIOR POUCH WITH FASCIAL BANDING OF OUTLET (LINNER)

Linner and Drew make a measured anterior pouch of volume 10–15 ml, by using Babcock clamps to bring a 2 × 5-cm segment of anterior wall of the stomach (containing a 30F Pingree-Jack tube) through the jaws of a PI-55 stapler (Fig. 12.7). This method requires no division of vasa brevia. In their earlier patients they cross-stapled the stomach wihout division.[18,21] However, because of staple-line disruptions, they now transect the stomach between two 55-mm linear staplers, and oversew the pouch staple-line with interrupted 3–0 silk sutures and the distal stomach

TABLE 12.1.   GALLBLADDER SURGERY (GB) WITH GASTRIC BYPASS (GBP)*

	1882 Primary Patients									
	Jan 1979 to Sept 1982		Oct 1982 to Sept 1983		Oct 1983 to Sept 1984		Oct 1984 to Sept 1985		Oct 1985 to Sept 1986	
Previous GB	96	12%	42	14%	21	8%	47	17%	24	10%
Surgery GB	126	16%	79	26%	101	38%	102	38%	87	37%
Later GB	79	14%	17	9%	3	2%	5	4%	1	0.8%
	Re-do Partitioning 62 Patients				JI Bypass to GBP 15 Patients					
Previous GB	14	22%			5	33%				
Surgery GB	10	16%			1	7%				
Later GB	0				0					

*Patients of Dr. D.K. Miller.

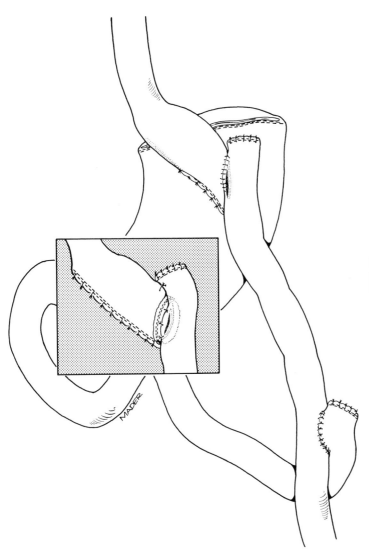

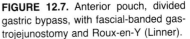

FIGURE 12.7. Anterior pouch, divided gastric bypass, with fascial-banded gastrojejunostomy and Roux-en-Y (Linner).

with running 2–0 Vicryl for reinforcement and hemostasis.[25,26] The level of transection on the lesser curvature is 3–4 cm below the esophagogastric junction to ensure adequate vascularity of the pouch. At least one of the superior branches of the left gastric artery to the upper pouch is left intact. The jejunum is brought up retrocolic and antegastric, and the defect in the mesentery is closed around the jejunum with interrupted fine silk. The anterior pouch facilitates the gastrojejunostomy. Through gastric and jejunal adjacent stab incisions, the PLC or ILA is inserted to the 1.8-cm mark, and a side-to-side gastrojejunostomy is performed. Hemostatic sutures are placed through the inner posterior wall of the gastrojejunostomy, before the anterior wall is sutured. The anastomosis is completed with

interrupted Lembert 3–0 silk sutures. Using the PLC and PI-55, a side-to-side jejunojejunostomy is made 60 cm from the gastrojejunostomy.

To prevent late dilatation of the gastrojejunal stoma and weight gain, Linner and Drew formerly used a circumferential continuous no. 1 polypropylene pursestring and later a radioopaque 12F Silastic band containing a polypropylene suture. Both eroded into the lumen in a high percentage of patients.[21,25,26] They now use a 9 × 1-cm strip of midline abdominal wall (linea alba) fascia, marked longitudinally by PI-90 4.8-mm staples for yearly radiographic identification on flatfilm. The fascial strip is sutured to itself, but not tightly, over a 1-cm diameter Pingree-Jack tube with 3–0 silk, overlapping 1.5–2.0

cm. This produces an 11-mm diameter outlet. A few silk sutures are passed through the fascial band to the jejunal side of the anastomosis to prevent slippage. A tube gastrostomy is routine and usually removed on the day of discharge.

LESSER CURVATURE GASTROJEJUNAL ANASTOMOSIS (TORRES AND OCA)

Many surgeons who perform gastric bypass operations continue to report gastrojejunal stapled anastomoses.[27] Jose Torres and Clemente Oca[16] make an opening in the lesser curvature 4 cm from the cardioesophageal junction, which preserves the upper branch of the left gastric artery to the upper pouch (Fig. 12.8). They apply the TA-55 or RLG-60 stapler from the lesser curvature to the angle of His, almost vertically. The pouch is more muscular in this location. They make two applications of the stapler as close to each other

as possible, and reinforce the staple-line with interrupted non-absorbable sutures of 4–0 Surgilon. The stomach is not transected. The greater curvature is not mobilized and there is no division of blood vessels on the greater curvature. Their pouch has a volume of about 35 ml. If an hiatal hernia is present, they approximate the crura to avoid reflux in this procedure which does not have a fundal reservoir.

They divide the jejunum 18″ (45 cm) from the ligament of Treitz. The distal segment of the divided jejunum is brought up retrocolic and antegastric to the lesser curvature of the upper pouch. The ILS or EEA-21 (i.e. the outside diameter of the staple cartridge is 21 mm) is inserted though a transverse jejunotomy on the Roux-en-Y gastric limb and through a gastrotomy within a carefully placed pursestring suture in the anterior wall of the upper gastric pouch. The gastrojejunostomy is imbricated to an internal diameter of 10–12 mm over a 28F catheter at the anastomosis by figure-of-

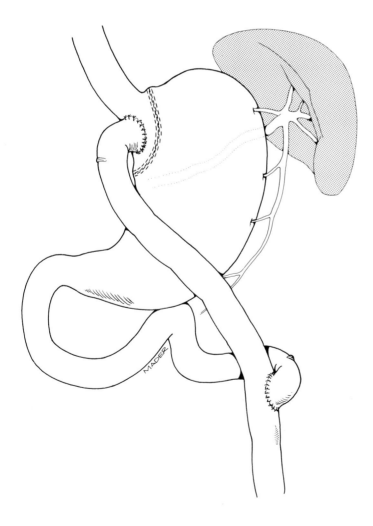

FIGURE 12.8. Torres and Oca make a lesser curvature pouch and perform a lesser curvature gastrojejunal anastomosis, using a circular stapler with a 21-mm cartridge, which is passed through a jejunal enterotomy. The jejunal enterotomy is closed transversely with a TA-30 stapler.

eight non-absorbable 4–0 sutures. The naso-gastric tube is positioned above the stoma for 6–8 hours postoperatively.

The jejunojejunostomy of the Roux-en-Y is done end-to-side 36–40″ (90 cm) from the stoma through a transverse jejunotomy using an ILS or EEA-25 stapler. The jejunal enterotomies are closed with the TA-30 stapler. Reinforcement with fine nonabsorbable sutures is done in all anastomoses and enterotomies.

DISTAL ROUX-EN-Y MODIFICATION (TORRES AND OCA)

Torres and Oca found that some of their patients regained significant weight 4 to 5 years after gastric bypass. Reoperation with suture reinforcement of the outlet was not found to produce uniformly successful weight loss. For failed gastric bypasses, they developed a modification of the JI or bilio-pancreatic bypass to their lesser curvature gastric bypass (gastric bypass, lesser curvature, gastroileostomy, Roux-en-Y) (Fig. 12.9). They also advocate their procedure as the primary operation in selected patients.[28] The small bowel is measured with a calibrated umbilical tape. From the gastroenterostomy to the ileocecal valve, a total of 8 feet (3 and 5 feet) is used for sweet snackers and 10 feet (4 and 6 feet) is used for big eaters.

The jejunum or ileum is divided 8–10 feet from the ileocecal valve. The distal end of the bowel is brought up retrocolic, antegastric and anastomosed to the upper pouch using ILS 21-mm stapler. The gastroenterostomy anastomosis is reinforced and imbricated with fine interrupted sutures to about 12–15 mm in diameter, using a 28F catheter as a stent. The Roux-en-Y is constructed with the liga-

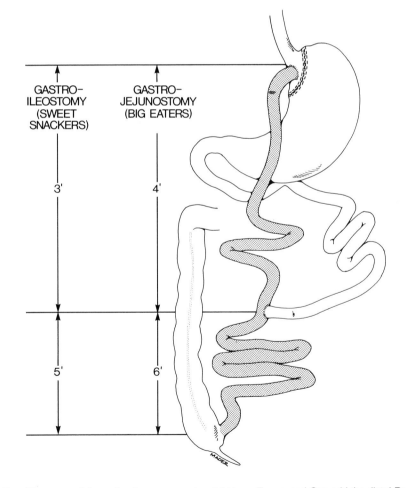

FIGURE 12.9. To add some malabsorption for permanent weight loss, Torres and Oca add the distal Roux-en-Y to their lesser curvature gastric bypass. The alimentary limb from gastroenterostomy to ileocecal valve is measured at 8′ for sweets nibblers and 10′ for gorgers.

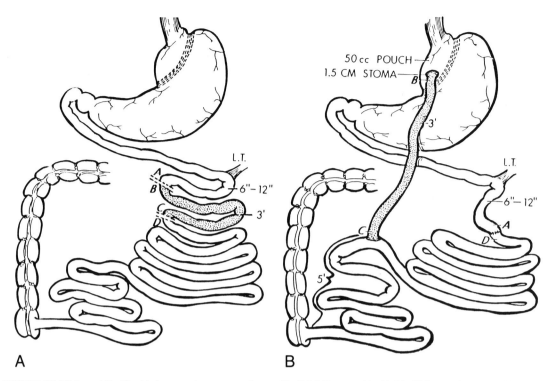

FIGURE 12.10-A and B. Gastric bypass, lesser curvature, with distal Roux-en-Y with 3′ of jejunum interposed between the stomach and the ileum 5–6′ from the ileocecal valve.

ment of Treitz bowel limb and anastomosed end-to-side 3–4 feet from the stoma, using the ILS-21 or 25-mm stapler.

At the point of anastomosis, pancreatic juice and bile for the first time come in contact with the partially digested food, and the 5–6 foot common channel prevents malnutrition. The patient has three to five soft stools per day, occasional lactose intolerance, and must take multivitamins, iron and injections of B_{12}. Because of the increased risk of stomal ulcer following this procedure, Torres and Oca performed truncal vagotomies at the same time.

DISTAL ROUX-EN-Y WITH JEJUNAL INTERPOSITION (TORRES AND OCA)

In patients with the distal Roux-en-Y with gastroileostomy, there was a 4% incidence of marginal ulcer. Thus, bilateral truncal vagotomy was added, but subsequently 7.5% of these patients developed dumping syndrome. Due to the side-effect of dumping syndrome, Torres and Oca have designed a new procedure of gastric bypass, distal Roux-en-Y with 3 feet of jejunal interposition without the vagotomy (Fig. 12.10-A).

A 50-cc pouch is constructed at the lesser curvature and anterior wall of the stomach using a double application of the RLG-60-mm staple cartridge. The 3 feet of jejunum shown with dark shadow is divided between A and B (6–12″ from the ligament of Treitz) and C and D; this segment is used for the interposition (Fig. 12.10-B). The proximal jejunum A is anastomosed to the distal jejunum D end-to-end to maintain continuity and drainage of the gastro-biliopancreatic system, using the ILS-21-mm or 25-mm depending on the size of the jejunum.

The Roux-en-Y is constructed with the 3 feet of B to C jejunal interposition; the proximal jejunum B is anastomosed to the upper pouch end-to-side with the ILS-21. The stoma is imbricated to about 1.5 cm in diameter with fine interrupted figure-of-eight and simple sutures. The distal jejunum C is anastomosed to the common channel of ileum 5–6 feet from the ileocecal valve end-to-side using the ILS-21 stapler.

With this procedure, weight loss is comparable or better than the distal Roux-en-Y with gastroileostomy and the early and late complications have been reduced. This procedure has been used in 57 patients, with average weight loss at 9 months 62 kg, representing a loss of 83% of excess weight.

PATIENT SELECTION

The primary criterion for gastric bypass is morbid obesity, which is 100 lb (45 kg) above ideal weight by the Metropolitan Life Insurance Tables[29] (Table 12.2). Recently, with such minimal surgical risks, good long-term weight loss and improved health, many centers have changed their criteria to 80 lb of excess weight. Exceptions to the weight criteria include patients with sequelae of JI bypasses and serious obesity-associated diseases requiring special consideration.[30] JI bypass reversal operations need to be combined with gastric restrictive operations or else the patients will regain weight.

Most studies show a ratio of 7–10 women for each man operated on for obesity. Our studies have found no significant difference in the amount of weight lost or regained in long-term follow-up between men and women. Men seem to lose weight more rapidly at first than women, but tend to stabilize sooner.

Pulmonary restrictive diseases (asthma, sleep apnea, Pickwickian syndrome), diabetes, hypertension, gouty arthritis and hyperlipidemias have been cured by the weight loss after gastric bypass. Several patients with previous coronary artery bypasses have had excellent results from gastric bypass. The complication rate has become so low that very few medical diseases contraindicate gastric bypass. Contraindications include drug dependency, alcoholic cirrhosis and psychoses.

The outcome of psychiatric problems is unpredictable. We have found that routine psychiatric evaluations prior to surgery are rarely helpful. However, seriously mentally impaired or disturbed patients require psychiatric evaluations before gastric bypass. Patients with poor self-image and mental inadequacies usually develop marked improvement in their mental health after the weight loss.

Patents with severe arthritic or low-back pain are improved. However, post-operative antiarthritic medication or aspirin should preferably not be administered. The small proximal pouch develops ulcers readily with ingestion of ulcerogenic medications. Of our combined 3000 gastric bypass patients, six developed intractable ulcer disease which required revision of the gastrojejunal anastomosis, usually precipitated by excess ingestion of antiarthritic medication.

PRE- AND POST-OPERATIVE CARE

Our standard pre-operative work-up consists of patient interviews with discussions of indications for surgery, operations and techniques, alternative procedures, possible risks, complications, and finances. An administrative assistant also interviews and educates the patient in the areas of work-up, insurance and scheduling, and is available to respond to general questions and concerns.

Before surgery, the patient has in-hospital teaching involving educational videos and question-answer sessions with nurses experienced in surgical treatment of morbid obesity. Additionally, an internist with special training in obesity management performs a complete medical evaluation including: chest X-ray, upper GI and gallbladder studies, EKG, urinalysis, SMAC, CBC, T3, T4, and any other indicated evaluations to ensure quality care. If medical problems are encountered, they are treated, resolved or controlled before surgery.

An infectious disease study conducted at our hospital revealed that the least wound infections occurred when patients came to the operating-room with the least number of bacteria on the skin. Patients receive Hibiclens showers the night before and the morning of surgery.

Prophylactic cephalosporins are given 1 hour before surgery and continued for 30 hours post-operatively.[31] In complicated cases, such as revisions of other gastric restrictive procedures to gastric bypass, we utilize gentamycin and clindamycin if additional antibiotic support is deemed necessary. This additional antibiotic support is continued until 48 hours of an afebrile state. Heparin 4000 units is given subcutaneously 1 hour before surgery and continued every 8 hours for 4 days. Heparin therapy is occasionally discontinued in patients who bleed excessively during surgery, usually because of pre-operative use of aspirin or aspirin-like drugs. We rarely need to transfuse patients. Only two out of 3000 patients have developed pulmonary emboli, and both patients developed the pul-

TABLE 12.2. PATIENT CHARACTERISTICS*

	1979–1983	*1984*	*1985*	*1986*
No. of Patients	1130	276	288	237
Average age	36 yr	36 yr	36 yr	35 yr
Average height	5'4"	5'4"	5'4"	5'4"
Average weight	266 lb	252 lb	245 lb	253 lb
F:M ratio	9:1	14:1	8:1	8:1

*Patients of Dr. D.K. Miller.

monary emboli after heparin had been discontinued for other reasons. When we first began performing gastric bypass surgery, we used 5000 units of heparin subcutaneously every 12 hours. However, we have determined that 4000 units every 8 hours results in fewer complications and has been equally effective in the prevention of deep vein thrombosis or pulmonary emboli.

Post-operatively, patients are treated with oxygen by nasal prongs for 48 hours or longer if clinically indicated. This is supported by studies performed by Taylor.[32] Incentive spirometry instructions and care are given before and continued after surgery. Pre-operative screening spirometry is not indicated routinely in morbidly obese patients.[33] We vigorously use bronchodilators or extensive respiratory therapy in patients with asthma, atelectasis, pneumonia or other pulmonary diseases when indicated. Patients rarely need to be in an intensive care unit.

The nasogastric tube placed during surgery through the gastrojejunostomy is usually removed within 24 hours, unless there is excessive drainage.

Post-operative pain control is usually accomplished using patient controlled analgesia (PCA) pumps with morphine sulfate or Demerol. Within 3 days, patients are usually converted to an oral pain medication that is free of aspirin and not ulcerogenic.

On the third post-operative day, clear liquids are started orally at the rate of 2 ounces per hour. Advancement to full liquids begins on the fourth day. Patients at discharge, usually on the fifth day, are placed on a soft bland gastric bypass diet. After one month, diet restrictions are removed and patients are encouraged to eat a balanced diet of proteins, dairy products, grains, fruits and vegetables. Multivitamins, especially containing B_1 (thiamine), calcium and iron supplements are prescribed as appropriate. Patients are also advised initially not to drink liquids 30 minutes before meals, during meals or for 30 minutes after meals. Should the patients consume sugars, sweets or high-caloric liquids, they may experience dumping syndrome. Dumping symptoms are usually mild and can be alleviated by restricting sugars, sweets and high caloric liquids, although mild dumping symptoms are beneficial in patients' long-term weight control and behavior modification. Dumping is rarely severe enough to necessitate any treatment changes or revisions of the gastric bypass, as also noted by Linner.[18] Patients are encouraged to permanently avoid high caloric liquids and carbonated beverages for more effective and long-term weight loss.

Patients are strongly advised to begin a gradual and regular life-time exercise program following recovery. The program should begin with walking and/or swimming and then may be increased to more vigorous activities. The physical activity should be scheduled and followed faithfully.

Patient follow-up is mandatory. One week after discharge, the patient returns for suture

TABLE 12.3. COMPLICATIONS*

	Before Sept 1983		Oct 1983 to Sept 1984		Oct 1984 to Mar 1985		Apr 1985 to Dec 1985		Dec 1985 to Oct 1986
No. of patients	1130		276		154		200		237
Leak with abscess (1 thoracotomy)	18	1.5%	3 (1 thoracotomy)	1.1%	2	1.3%	1	0.5%	
Other abscesses (only 1 abscess drained surgically in 6 years)	10	0.8%	1	0.4%	2	1.3%			
Wound infections	3	0.2%	3	1.1%					
Splenectomy (10 in first 363 patients)	11	0.9%							
Arterial line thrombosis	3	0.2%							
Pleural effusion	3	0.2%							
Ileus	3	0.2%							
Miscellaneous	3 (pancreatitis, colitis, colon infarct)	0.2%	2 (pancreatitis, GI bleed)	0.8%					
Distal pouch distention (drained)									1 0.5%
Total	4.2%		3.4%		2.6%		0.5%		0.5%

*Patients of Dr. D.K. Miller.

removal. One month after operation, the patient visits the surgeon for further general and diet instructions. Patients are followed-up with monthly office visits for the first 6 months, bimonthly visits for the next 6 months, and semiannual visits are recommended thereafter. A yearly follow-up questionnaire is mailed to all post-gastric bypass patients. Follow-up may be accomplished through either patient office visits or by telephone. We have maintained a 90% long-term follow-up in spite of half of our patients not being within travel convenience to our office.

COMPLICATIONS

The significant early post-operative complication incidence is 0.5% now (Table 12.3), and the death-rate is 0.4% overall (Table 12.4). There have been less complications and deaths since we no longer participate in a resident-teaching service. Later deaths and their causes are shown in Table 12.5.

The 0.5% early post-operative complication incidence does not include the occasional early atelectasis, insignificant fevers, tape blisters, seromas, IV infiltrations, etc. Diabetics, asthmatics, patients on corticosteroids and older patients are at greater risk for complications than the average morbidly obese patient.

The most common serious complication is subdiaphragmatic abscess. Early recognition and treatment of subdiaphragmatic abscesses usually only require a few days of extra hospitalization. Early signs of subdiaphragmatic abscess are tachycardia, fever and elevated white cell count. Hypoxemia, dyspnea and left pleural effusion may occur as sepsis progresses. Late signs are decreased urine output, hypotension, extreme hypoxemia and severe tachycardia. CT scan allows early and accurate diagnosis. If an abscess or leak is suspected, we do not delay the CT scan with a Gastrografin study first, but proceed directly with a CT scan. CT drainage of the abscess with continuous saline irrigation and more vigorous antibiotic coverage have nearly eliminated the need for surgical exploration and drainage. Competent and experienced radiologists may provide CT-guided percutaneous abscess drainage. We believe that complications of abscess, leak and infection treated with CT drainage and irrigation have much less morbidity and mortality than with re-exploration and drainage.

The re-operation rate due to late complications, such as narrowing of the gastrojejunostomy, bowel obstructions, marginal ulcers or other reasons has been 0.7% (Table 12.6). It has been found by others that stomal and duodenal ulcers do not occur after gastric bypass if the proximal gastric segment is ≤50 ml,[3,4,12,34] and those that occurred previously responded to medical therapy, e.g. ranitidine. A late post-operative complication is slight narrowing or stricturing of the gastrojejunostomy.[35] Endoscopy with balloon dilatation is needed in approximately 0.8% of patients and is usually performed in the office 6 to 8 weeks post-operatively, and resolves the outlet narrowing.

Small-bowel obstructions from adhesions or internal hernias have been extremely rare. As discussed previously, we recommend fixation of the jejunal limb where it crosses the transverse colon. Associated with many of the other restrictive operations is a high rate of re-operation. Some series of the horizontal partitioning gastroplasty have had over 50% re-operations. The gastric bypass operation rarely fails enough to require re-operations. Panniculectomies and body contouring procedures are the most common operations performed after gastric bypass.

TABLE 12.4. DEATHS*

Jan 1979 to Sept 1983	Oct 1983 to Sept 1984	Oct 1984 to Mar 1985	Apr 1985 to Dec 1985	Dec 1985 to Dec 1986
1 Infection—became well, then died of pulmonary embolism	1 peritonitis	1 sepsis	1 arrhythmia	0
3 Infections and complications				
1 Pancreatitis				
2 Cardiac arrhythmias				
7 0.6%	1 0.4%	1 0.6%	1 0.5%	0

*Patients of Dr. D.K. Miller.

TABLE 12.5.   LATER DEATHS*

3 Suicides (2 yr, 3 yr, 4 yr)
1 Accident (2 yr)
3 Cancer (2 yr, 2 yr, 1 yr)
2 Heart attack (1 yr, 4 yr)
1 Chronic nephritis (1 yr)
1 Toxic shock syndrome (2 yr)
1 Embolism (5 yr)
1 Unknown (lost)

*Patients of Dr. D.K. Miller.

RESULTS

Table 12.7 illustrates the short and long-term weight losses, percent of weight lost and percent of excess weight lost. Results in different series vary in the last two columns, depending on levels used for ideal weights. Approximately 95% of our patients experience permanent significant weight loss and improvement in overall health.

Early in the series frequent laboratory studies were performed and nearly all results were within good health parameters. Serum calcium levels were within normal range, whether or not calcium or multivitamins were supplemented. Of significance was a routine drop in uric acid, cholesterol and triglyceride levels often to subnormal.[36] Adult onset diabetes, which has a high incidence in the morbidly obese, was nearly 100% cured by the successful weight loss and restricted sugar intake following gastric bypass.

The need for routine follow-up by x-ray has been so unproductive that only those studies indicated are performed on a timely basis.

Our studies indicated that female patients who have successful weight loss following gastric bypass tend to be healthier during pregnancy and bear healthier infants with fewer complications than morbidly obese patients.[37]

Most women who have had a hysterectomy will have mild elevation of their hematocrit from the low forties to the mid-forties after gastric bypass. Premenopausal women will occasionally become anemic but this is usually corrected with iron and vitamin B_{12} therapy, although hysterectomy may be necessary with menorrhagia. Because the duodenum is bypassed, there is an incidence of iron deficiency anemia, which can be prevented by oral iron supplementation.[9] In particular, following gastric bypass, pregnant women should take an oral iron supplement. Subnormal serum B_{12} concentration may occur due to deficiency of intrinsic factor, gastric acid and pepsin, and dietary animal protein.[38] Some series have found significant numbers of patients with anemia correctable with oral iron and parenteral B_{12} therapy.[9,14] We have found oral combined iron-B_{12} supplements effective. The metabolic complications of gastric bypass are discussed in Chapter 28.

Pre- and post-operative support groups are organized and managed by post-gastric bypass patients. We encourage the patients' participation and support these groups in any way possible.

Flickinger used the 140-cm pediatric colonoscope for retrograde duodenogastroscopy with biopsies. He observed superficial gastritis in 87% of patients, which was found histologically in 42%. Intestinal metaplasia was present in 10% of biopsies.[39] The mucosa of the proximal pouch was normal. Although gastric bypass procedures have been done on a large scale for more than 15 years, there have been no reports of carcinoma. Linner and Drew developed a method of visualizing the distal stomach by the percutaneous instillation of contrast medium into the excluded stomach that has been deliberately distended by the insufflation of air into the

TABLE 12.6.   LATER SURGERIES RELATED TO THE GASTRIC BYPASS*

	Jan 1979 to Sept 1983	Oct 1983 to Sept 1984	Oct 1984 to Sept 1985	Oct 1985 to Sept 1986
No. of patients	1130	276	288	237
Bowel obstructions	5			2
Outlet obstructions (re-do)	2			
Marginal ulcers with revision (learning curve)	3			
Later splenectomy	1			
Colectomy	1			
Thoracotomy	1	1		
Gastric bypass revision	1	1 (re-do)	2	
Total	14 2%	2 0.7%	2 0.7%	2 0.7%

*Patients of Dr. D.K. Miller.

TABLE 12.7. PRIMARY GASTRIC BYPASS WITH ROUX-EN-Y*

Mean age 37
Mean Ht 5'4"
Mean Wt 258 lb

Follow-up	No. of Patients Recorded	Mean Wt Loss (lb)	Mean % of Wt Lost	Mean % of Excess Wt Lost
8 yr	1	92	35%	69%
7 yr	35	94	36%	70%
6 yr	183	82	31%	61%
5 yr	452	84	32%	63%
4 yr	461	91	35%	68%
3 yr	955	93	36%	69%
2 yr	1150	100	38%	75%
1 yr	1148	99	38%	74%
6 mo	1386	74	28%	55%
3 mo	1555	50	19%	37%

*Patients of Dr. D.K. Miller.

Previous Stapling
Mean age 38
Mean Ht 5'4"
Mean Wt 257 lb

Follow-up	No. of Patients Recorded	Mean Wt Loss (lb)	Mean % of Wt Lost	Mean % of Excess Wt Lost
5 yr	4	89	34%	67%
4 yr	14	81	31%	61%
3 yr	15	89	34%	67%
2 yr	34	82	31%	62%
1 yr	48	88	34%	66%
6 mo	52	65	25%	49%
3 mo	50	46	17%	34%

JI Bypass to Gastric Bypass
Mean age 42
Mean Ht 5'4"
Mean Wt 257 lb

Follow-up	No. of Patients Recorded	Mean Wt Loss (lb)	Mean % of Wt Lost	Mean % of Excess Wt Lost
5 yr	5	73	28%	55%
4 yr	7	75	29%	56%
3 yr	7	60	23%	45%
2 yr	11	78	30%	59%
1 yr	13	73	28%	55%
6 mo	9	60	23%	45%
3 mo	12	38	14%	28%

afferent jejunum following a routine gastroendoscopy, and then obtaining an excellent contrast gastroradiograph.[26]

CONCLUSION

Until medicine can find safe, effective, noninvasive control of massive obesity, divided gastric bypass with Roux-en-Y anastomosis is our operation of choice. The divided stomach procedure provides better exposure, less manipulation and less interference with blood supply. With such a high success rate of curing obesity and many of its associated diseases with minimal morbidity and mortality, it would appear that gastric bypass should be more widely applied. Etched in the progress of medicine are some milestones that have drastically aided quality health and life, such as polio vaccine, antibiotics, cyclosporins, sterilization, safe surgical techniques, lithotripter, and other surgical operations. Unless some way is found to alter genes to prevent obesity or a safe medical cure is found for obesity, we believe that gastric bypass may someday take its place with the milestones. Very few other medical treatments improve the present and future health of patients so drastically. Physicians, insurance companies, quality assurance boards and the public should be made aware of the safety and effectiveness of gastric bypass for obesity. We believe that the rules limiting application of the surgery should be less restrictive, with younger and lighter patients as acceptable candidates. Dietz and Gortmaker have shown a rapid increase in obesity in the younger generations;[40] this suggests a greater need in the future for an effective, safe and persistent surgical cure for obesity.

Patient satisfaction and cure of the medical complications of obesity are so gratifying that we continue to do bariatric surgery despite the skepticism and prejudice of an uninformed portion of the medical community and the insurance companies. Happy patients have been the major referral basis for future patients.

ACKNOWLEDGEMENT

The authors are grateful to Drs. Mervyn Deitel, John H. Linner, Jose C. Torres and Clemente F. Oca for their input.

REFERENCES

1. Mason EE, Ito C: Gastric bypass in obesity. Surg Clin N Am 47:1345–1352, 1967.
2. Mason EE, Ito C: Gastric Bypass. Ann Surg 170:329–339, 1969.
3. Mason EE, Printen KJ, Hartford CE, et al: Optimizing results of gastric bypass. Ann Surg 182:405–413, 1975.
4. Mason EE, Ito C: Graded gastric bypass. World J Surg 2:341–349, 1978.
5. Mason EE, Printen KJ, Blommers TJ, et al: Gastric bypass and morbid obesity. Am J Clin Nutr (Suppl) 33:395–405, 1980.
6. Mason EE, Munns JR, Kealey GP, et al: Effect of gastric bypass on gastric secretion. Am J Surg 131:162–168, 1976.
7. Alden JF: Gastric and jejuno-ileal bypass: a comparison in the treatment of morbid obesity. Arch Surg 112:799–806, 1977.
8. Griffen WO, Jr, Young VL, Stevenson CC: A prospective comparison of gastric and jejunoileal bypass procedures for morbid obesity. Ann Surg 186:500–509, 1977.
9. Griffen WO, Jr, Bivins BA, Bell RM, et al: Gastric bypass for morbid obesity. World J Surg 5:817–822, 1981.
10. Surgical Stapling Techniques with Auto Suture® Instruments: Bariatric Surgery. US Surgical Corp, Norwalk, CT 06856, 1986, pp 10–13.
11. Pories WJ, Flickinger EF, Meelheim D, et al: The effectiveness of gastric bypass over gastric partition in morbid obesity: consequence of distal, gastric and duodenal exclusion. Ann Surg 196:389–399, 1982.
12. Knecht BH: Mason gastric bypass. Am J Surg 145:604–608, 1983.
13. Anand SV, William CN: 16. Gastric bypass in Nova Scotia: an analysis of 100 patients. Can J Surg 27:228–229, 1984.
14. Halverson JD, Zuckerman GR, Koehler RE, et al: Gastric bypass for morbid obesity: a medical-surgical assessment. Ann Surg 194:152–160, 1981.
15. Linner JH: Comparative effectiveness of gastric bypass and gastroplasty: a clinical study. Arch Surg 117:695–700, 1982.
16. Torres JC, Oca CF, Garrison RN: Gastric bypass: Roux-en-Y gastrojejunostomy from the lesser curvature. South Med J 76:1217–1221, 1983.
17. Sugarman HJ, Wolper JL: Failed gastroplasty for morbid obesity: revised gastroplasty versus Roux-en-Y gastric bypass. Am J Surg 148:331–339, 1984.
18. Linner JH: Surgery for Morbid Obesity. New York, Springer-Verlag, 1984, pp 65–80.
19. Stapling Techniques: General Surgery. 2nd Edition U.S. Surgical Corporation, 1980, p 81.
20. Mojzisik C: Gastric partitioning. Presentation at the Fourth Annual Symposium on Surgical Treatment of Obesity, Anaheim, CA, March 6th, 1986.
21. Linner JH, Drew RL: Technique of anterior wall Roux-en-Y gastric bypass for the treatment of morbid obesity. Contemp Surg 26:46–59, 1985.
22. Calhoun R, Willbanks O: Coexistence of gallbladder disease and morbid obesity. Am J Surg 154:655–658, 1987.
23. Amaral JF, Thompson WR: Gallbladder disease in the morbidly obese. Am J Surg 148:550–558, 1985.
24. Panel Discussion: State of the Art—Surgical Treatment of Obesity. Fifth Annual Symposium on Surgical Treatment of Obesity, Universal City, CA, Feb 11–14, 1987.
25. Linner JR, Drew RL: New modification of Roux-en-Y gastric bypass procedure. Clin Nutr 5:33–34, 1986.
26. Linner JH, Drew RL: Roux-Y gastric bypass for morbid obesity. Scientific Exhibit, American College of Surgeons 73rd Clinical Congress, San Francisco, October 11–16, 1987.
27. Brolin RE: Calibrated gastrojejunostomy for gastric bypass using the EEA stapler. Contemp Surg 26:40–44, 1985.
28. Torres J, Oca C: Gastric bypass lesser curvature with distal Roux-en-Y. Bariatric Surgery 5:10–15, 1987.
29. Height and Weight Tables, Metropolitan Life Foundation, Statistical Bulletin 64(1):2–9, 1983.
30. Guidelines for selection of patients for surgical treatment of obesity. American Society for Bariatric Surgery, October 1986.
31. Pories WJ, van Rij AM, Burlingham BT, et al: Prophylactic cefazolin in gastric bypass surgery. Surgery 90:426–432, 1981.
32. Taylor RR, Kelly TM, Elliott CG, et al: Hypoxemia after gastric bypass surgery for morbid obesity. Arch Surg 120:1298–1302, 1985.
33. Crapo RO, Kelly TM, Elliott CG et al: Spirometry as a preoperative screening test in morbidly obese patients. Surgery 99:763–768, 1986.

34. Shamos RF, Menguy RB: Effect of gastric bypass on serum gastrin. Surg Forum 30:350–351, 1979.

35. Kretzschmar CS, Hamilton JW, Wissler DW, et al: Balloon dilation for the treatment of stomal stenosis complicating gastric surgery for morbid obesity. Surgery 102:443–446, 1987.

36. Kelly T, Jones S: Changes in serum lipids after gastric bypass surgery. Int J Obese 10:443–452, 1986.

37. Richards KR, Miller DK, Goodman GN: Pregnancy after gastric bypass for morbid obesity. J Reproductive Med 32:172–176, 1987.

38. Crowley LV, James S, Mullin G: Late effects of gastric bypass for obesity. Am J Gastroenterol 79:850–860, 1984.

39. Flickinger EG, Sinar DR, Pories WS, et al: The bypassed stomach. Am J Surg 149:151–157, 1985.

40. Dietz WH, Gortmaker SL: Increasing pediatric obesity in the United States. Am J Children 141:535–540, 1987.

13

Horizontal Gastric Partitionings: An Historical Review

MERVYN DEITEL
SUNDARAM V. ANAND

Horizontal gastric partitioning theoretically was an excellent concept which unfortunately had a high failure rate. The intent was to make a small fundal pouch with a tiny outlet in order to produce satiety and delayed emptying, by a relatively simple operation. However, the enlargement of the thin-walled fundal pouch, the dilatation of the outlet and the disruption of the staple-lines led to further searches for gastric restrictive techniques. The experience showed that results must not be given significance early but must be evaluated instead in the long-term.

HORIZONTAL GASTRIC STAPLING WITH CENTRAL OUTLET

Pace and colleagues[1] described the simple technique of gastric partitioning, removing three central staples (two from the upper row and one from the lower row) before a single application of the TA-90 stapler across the proximal stomach, producing a $\leq$50-ml pouch (Fig.13.1). This left a 9-mm central opening. Cohn and associates,[2] using this method, had a mean loss of only 20% of initial body weight at 16 months. There was a high incidence of disruption of the singly-applied staggered staple-line, and a failure-rate in 71% of patients was reported.[3–5]

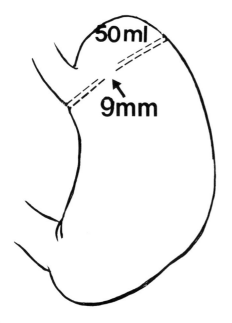

FIGURE 13.1. Gastric partitioning by a single application of the TA-90 (with cartridge containing 4.8-mm staples), after 3 central staples had been removed.[1] A nasogastric tube was threaded through the opening in the staple-line and left in place for 4 days postoperatively.

Carey's group[6,7] and others[5] modified the operation by applying the stapling instrument twice, with the two openings aligned. They permitted only a liquid diet for the first 8 weeks postoperatively, so that the staple-lines would not disrupt. Following this, a dietician-coordinated small-feeding diet containing minced solids was instituted. Using this method, a mean of 28% of body weight was lost at 1 year, but following this, weight gain occurred almost uniformly. The use of reinforcing sutures[6] or a Teflon pledget[5] on each side of the channel did not prevent failure.

ANTERIOR GASTROGASTROSTOMY

LaFave and Alden,[8] Pories and associates,[9] Smith[4] and Buckwalter and Herbst[10,11] performed a 1.2 cm-diameter anterior gastrogastrostomy after two applications of the TA-90 stapler across the proximal stomach, leaving a tiny pouch (Fig. 13.2). This operation was followed not infrequently by initial obstruction and, after 3–6 months, enlargement of the channel. The latter occurred despite continuous nonabsorbable suture anteriorly.[4,8,9] Pories' group[9] found in a group of 45 gastrogastrostomy patients at 18 months that there were 28 failures (62%) (i.e. loss <25% of initial body weight), whereas the Roux-en-Y gastric bypass group had no failures. After finding that 77% of patients failed following gastrogastrostomy,[4,12] other workers reinforced the channel, both anteriorly and posteriorly, by a pledget of Teflon felt, and experimented with the anterior gastrogastrostomy closer to the greater curvature.[4,5]

The gastrogastrostomy was followed occasionally by bezoar formation in the upper pouch, due to failure to chew well, eating quickly, and stasis. The bezoar usually responded to enzymatic disintegration with meat-tenderizer, papain or cellulase. Buckwalter reported that one-half teaspoon of meat-tenderizer (containing proteolytic enzyme papain) in 250 ml of liquid, sipped slowly over 90 minutes and repeated one time, usually caused complete disintegration of the bezoar.[10,11] Rarely, gastroscopic mechanical fragmentation with grasping-forceps was necessary. Some patients were maintained on metoclopramide 10 mg per os before each meal and at bedtime, which increased the motor activity of the pouch.[13]

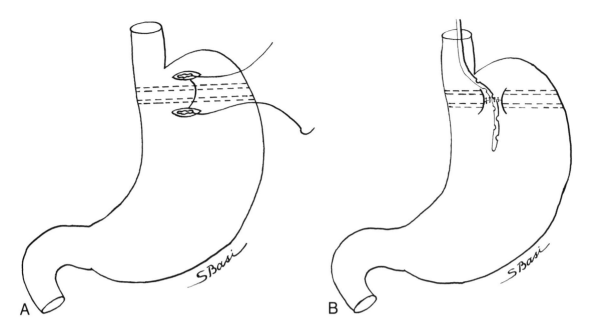

FIGURE 13.2 A and B. Two applications of linear stapling instrument loaded with 4.8-mm-staple cartridge produce two double rows of staggered staples for a secure, complete gastric partition. Then the upper 25–50 ml gastric pouch is anastomosed to stomach immediately below the staple-lines with first an inner layer; the outer anterior layer is continuous seromuscular 3–0 monofilament nonabsorbable suture, in an attempt to prevent stomal dilatation. The anastomosis is performed about a no. 18 nasogastric tube, creating a 0.8-mm diameter stoma.

GOMEZ GASTROPLASTY

Gomez performed horizontal gastric partitioning with two closely placed applications of the re-usable TA-90 or PI-90 stapler, with the opening at the greater curvature (Fig. 13.3).[14] He made a pouch of measured size of ≤50 ml under 70 cm of H_2O pressure (see Chapter 16). Without reinforcement, the outlet would expand over a period of months.[15] Gomez reinforced the outlet by a continuous, totally circumferential, Lembert seromuscular, imbricating 2–0 polypropylene suture over a 12 mm-diameter Maloney bougie, in an attempt to prevent enlargement of the outlet.[16,17] This operation had a 0.5% mortality rate and was performed widely. Many surgeons produced the outlet by removal of 3 or 4 staples from the greater curvature side of the cartridge.[10,15] However, crushing by the stapler fractured the mucosa and traumatized the wall, which occasionally resulted in postoperative outlet edema and obstruction.[5,10,18–20] Gomez used a C-clamp (Behlke Precision Instruments, St. Louis, MO 63116) which was specially constructed to stabilize the TA-90 stapler without using the pin, so that there was no crush to the greater curvature channel.[17]

The left triangular ligament of these often-fatty livers was not divided. A penrose drain about the esophagus identified the cardia. Many surgeons used a TA-55 stapler to construct the tiny pouch, and divided no short gastric vessels. It was found that closely adjacent staple-lines gave less chance of disruption.[21] A no. 18 F nasogastric tube was placed through the outlet at the end of the operation to decompress both sides of the partition.

Buckwalter and Herbst preferred the anterior gastrogastrostomy to the Gomez horizontal partitioning, because they found an incidence of outlet stenosis and obstruction requiring reoperation in only 1.4% after gastrogastrostomy compared to 14.9% after Gomez gastroplasty.[10] Obstructions after Gomez gastroplasty were easily relieved by an anterior gastrogastrostomy operation[22] (Fig. 13.2).

Gomez and others were encouraged by the good early results, with a mean loss of excess body weight of 70% at 1 and 2 years.[15–17] Series comparing the Gomez gastroplasty with the gastric bypass found more successful weight loss with the gastric bypass, although the horizontal gastroplasty was acknowledged to be a simpler procedure.[3,19,20,23] Unfortunately, follow-up of the Gomez horizontal gastro-

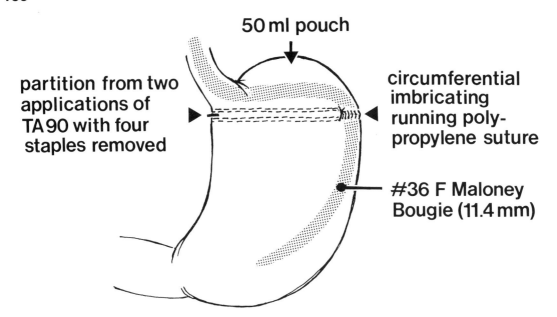

FIGURE 13.3. Gastric partitioning with reinforcement of the outlet by a cirumferential nonexpandable imbricating polypropylene suture, which is placed around the staple-line at the medial side of the outlet. Diameter d of bougies is calculated from the circumference c, by the formula $c = \pi d$, where $\pi = 3.14$. Thus, 38 French (i.e. circumference 38 mm) has diameter 12.1 mm, 36 F has diameter 11.4 mm, 34 F has diameter 10.8 mm, and 32 F has diameter 10.2 mm.

plasty at 5 years found a failure to sustain a loss of 50% or more of excess body weight in 40–70% of patients.[19,20,24,25] Weight gain occurred due to erosion and migration of the circumferential polypropylene suture into the lumen, with stomal enlargement and partial disruption of the doubly applied staple-line[3,9,19,20,25] (Fig. 13.4). Pouch enlargement was also a frequent long-term sequela.

Sugerman and Wolper reinforced the entire staple-line with a running through-and-through 2–0 polypropylene suture.[3] MacLean and co-workers[5] reinforced the greater curvature orifice of the Gomez gastroplasty by two Teflon pledgets at the end of the staple-lines. However, disruption and weight gains still occurred.

Grace attempted to stabilize the greater curvature outlet by wrapping it with a 6 × 2-cm strip of polypropylene (Marlex) mesh in 162 patients.[26,27] The mesh was held in place by a 2–0 polypropylene suture passed through the mesh 5 mm from each end and through the stomach just above and below the greater curvature end of the staple-line, where the band was fixed to the stomach. Omentum was placed over the mesh, so that adherence and kinking obstruction would not occur. Grace reported that both early and late stenosis with obstruction occurred in 12 patents, due to fibrosis under the mesh, erosion of the mesh

into the lumen, and adherence of the mesh to the liver, spleen or diaphragm. At 2 years, an average of 33% of initial body weight was lost (with 30% of patients losing less than 25% of body weight), but subsequent pouch enlargement and late weight gain occurred. When obstruction of the Marlex-covered channel was treated by simple gastrogastrostomy, weight gain resulted, whereas reconstruction by vertical banded gastroplasty or Roux-en-Y gastric bypass allowed continued weight loss.

COMPLICATIONS OF THE GOMEZ GASTROPLASTY

With the dissection at the upper part of the greater curvature, splenic injury was a hazard.[4,19] Early postoperative complications included leaks and subphrenic abscesses, with re-operation difficult in the area between fundus of stomach, diaphragm and spleen. A leak was heralded by unexplained tachypnea, tachycardia, fever, high epigastric pain radiating to the back and pleuritic left lower chest and left shoulder pain, and must be differentiated from pulmonary embolism and atelectasis. Re-operation for a leak was usually a surgical emergency, before adult respiratory distress syndrome and acute renal failure supervened. The emergency re-operation in-

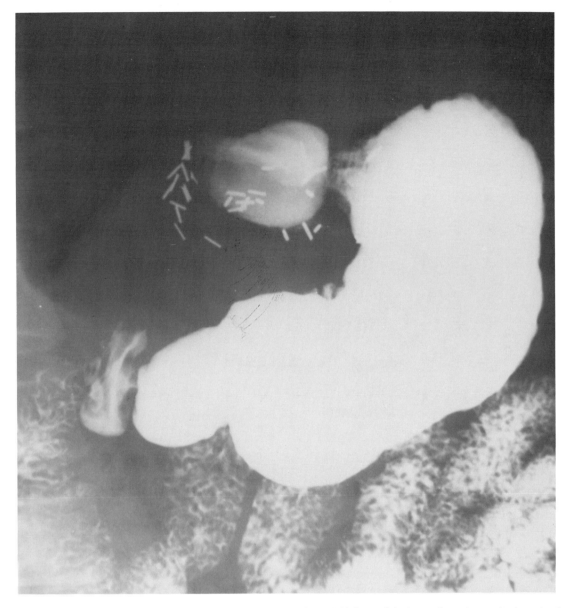

FIGURE 13.4. Upper GI series of a horizontal gastroplasty, which was initially too tight, in a patient who now had regained the weight. Oblique view shows rapid emptying of the pouch through the dilated stoma. This can progress to disruption of the entire staple-line.

cluded drainage of the leak, decompression gastrostomy and frequently a feeding jejunostomy. A subphrenic abscess required CT-guided drainage or open drainage. A sympathetic left pleural effusion was an occasional finding after the Gomez gastroplasty, and was usually of no significance.

After gastric operations in the morbidly obese, 32% of patients have been observed to have amber urine with a pink coating on the plastic urinary collection tubing for up to 48 hours postoperatively.[28] This pink urine is due to a transiently high postoperative urinary level of uric acid dihydrate crystals.

Reflux esophagitis has not been a sequela if the proximal gastric pouch was small. Simonowitz and co-workers[29] studied patients who had had symptoms of reflux esophagitis before Gomez gastroplasty, and were followed for more than 1 year postoperatively. In all 15 patients there was an immediate decrease in acid reflux and symptoms. If the proximal gastric pouch was small enough (<50 ml), it contained few parietal cells, and

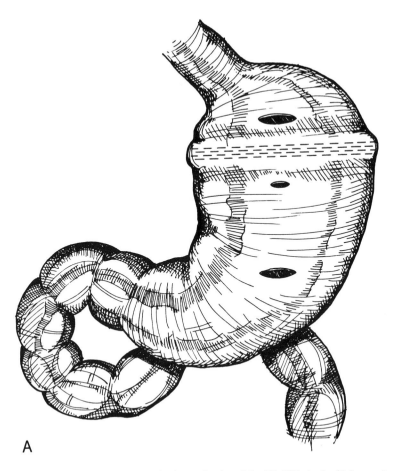

A

FIGURE 13.5A. Complete gastric partitioning by a single application of the TA-90B stapler (4.8-mm staples) high across the stomach, providing four equidistant staggered rows of staples and a ≤50-ml pouch. Sites of the anterior gastrotomies of proper size are shown.

no acid was produced in the pouch. The 12-mm diameter outlet acted as a barrier to the migration of gastric acid to the distal esophagus. Thus, there was a significant increase in proximal pouch pH. Heartburn, of course, can occur from ingested material (e.g. aspirin) above the partition.

A drawback of the outlet on the greater curvature was the difficulty in visualizing or dilating it gastroscopically. The greater curvature channel was frequently best visualized in the right lateral recumbent position (left side up).[30] Gruntzig balloon dilatation was often effective. The surgical treatment of stomal obstructions has already been mentioned. The gastrogastrostomy shown in Figure 13.2 can be simplified by using the GIA (3M anastomotic stapler or ILA) with the forks inserted on either side of the staple-line. If prolonged vomiting is permitted to continue, peripheral neuropathy and Wernicke's disease may occur, due to thiamine deficiency[31] (see Chapter 28).

RE-OPERATIONS FOR INADEQUATE WEIGHT LOSS FOLLOWING HORIZONTAL GASTROPLASTY

Revisions of a horizontal gastroplasty for inadequate weight loss to another horizontal gastroplasty of smaller dimensions is frequently followed again by failure to lose adequate weight. Conversion to a Roux-en-Y gastric bypass has achieved the best weight loss.[3,20,27] Conversion of a horizontal gastroplasty to a vertical banded gastroplasty often requires a gastrogastrostomy over the re-

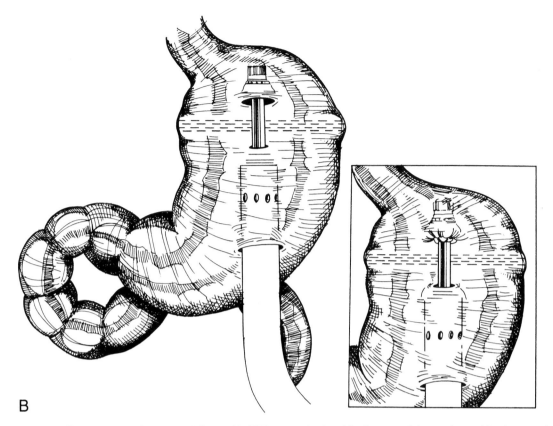

B

FIGURE 13.5B. Placement of the angled disposable EEA-21 stapler (outside diameter of the staple cartridge is 21 mm). The instrument, without the anvil, is passed into the stomach through a mid-anterior gastrotomy. The center rod is then brought out the stab-wound just below the staple-lines. The anvil is attached and advanced into the proximal pouch. A pursestring suture, which was previously placed about the proximal gastrotomy, is tied about the center rod adjacent to the anvil (see inset), so that two complete gastric rings will be cut.

maining partition at the lesser curvature; although a weight loss of 34.4% of initial weight has been reported at 1 year, a 28% incidence of leaks from poor blood supply where the staple-lines intersected and an 11% incidence of postoperative gastric obstruction makes this revision somewhat hazardous.[32] A decompressive gastrostomy in the body of the stomach near the greater curvature and away from the operative area may be beneficial after revisions.[15] Leaks are more common after revision operations.[33]

GASTRIC PARTITIONING WITH STAPLED GASTROGASTROSTOMY

Recently, Clark and colleagues[34] have revived the anterior gastrogastrostomy, by constructing a stapled stoma which they believe will not dilate (Fig. 13.5 A–C). In the 54 patients who have been followed from 1 to 3 years, the mean loss of excess body weight was 53% at 1 year, 52% at 2 years and 51% at 3 years (19 patients followed >3 years). Stapled gastrogastrostomy is a simple and apparently effective operation for providing sustained weight loss. However, it is known that after Roux-en-Y gastric bypass operations, EEA-stapled gastrojejunal anastomoses have enlarged in the long-term.[35] Thus, further follow-up is needed to evaluate whether the weight loss with the stapled gastrogastrostomy will be sustained.

SUMMARY AND CONCLUSION

The horizontal gastric partitionings were followed by a significant incidence of stomal stenosis, stomal enlargement and staple-line breakdown. The procedures were mechani-

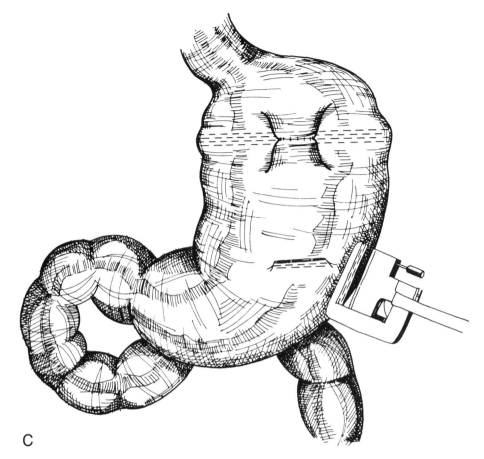

C

FIGURE 13.5C. The 11.4 mm diameter anterior gastrogastrostomy completed. The distal gastrotomy is closed by a linear (TA, PI or RL) stapler. (Figures 13.5 A–C courtesy of J.R. Clark, P.A. Conarro, G.R. Culbertson, T.L. Hovenga, L. Schoelkopf, General Surgery Service, Fitzsimmons Army Medical Center, Aurora, Colorado.[34])

cally unreliable and long-term weight loss was generally inadequate and not maintained. After the operations, tiny liquid meals were advised for 8 weeks from a 30-ml plastic medicine glass, followed by a very soft, small diet. However, continual high caloric junk foods can circumvent the gastric restriction.[36] It was soon found that the Roux-en-Y gastric bypass, although technically more difficult, gave better results.[8,9,12,19,20,23,25]

The results of a questionnaire filled out at the Annual Meeting of the American Society for Bariatric Surgery in 1987 showed that, whereas in 1981 45% of surgeons performed the horizontal gastric partitioning as their bariatric operation of choice, in 1986 0.6% of surgeons performed this procedure. However, many principles were learned from this experience. Good weight-loss results can be deceptive in the short-term. Long-term follow-up is mandatory. The thin-walled fundal pouch can dilate. Mechanically, the highest stress-point in the horizontal gastroplasty is at the end of the staple-line adjacent to the stoma. The stoma should be placed away from the staple-line; this led to a switch to the gastric bypass and the development of vertical banded gastroplasty. Use of polypropylene mesh and silastic tubing to reinforce the outlet has been an extension of this experience. The recent stapled gastrogastrostomy awaits further observation.

ACKNOWLEDGEMENT

The authors thank Dr. Bernard Perey, Professor and Chairman, Department of Surgery, Dalhousie University, Halifax, for suggestions in preparing this material.

REFERENCES

1. Pace WG, Martin EW Jr, Tetirick CE, et al: Gastric partitioning for morbid obesity. Ann Surg 190:392–400, 1979.

2. Cohn R, Merrell RC, Koslow A: Gastric stapling for morbid obesity. Am J Surg 142:67–72, 1981.

3. Sugerman HJ, Wolper JL: Failed gastroplasty for morbid obesity: revised gastroplasty versus Roux-Y gastric bypass. Am J Surg 148:331–339, 1984.

4. Smih LB: Modification of the gastric partitioning operation for morbid obesity. Am J Surg 142:725–730, 1981.

5. MacLean LD, Rhode BM, Shizgal HM: Gastroplasty for obesity. Surg Gynecol Obstet 153:200–208, 1981.

6. Ellison EC, Martin EW Jr, Laschinger J, et al: Preventing early failure of stapled gastric partitions in treatment of morbid obesity. Arch Surg 115:528–533, 1980.

7. Carey LC, Martin EW Jr: Treatment of morbid obesity by gastric partitioning. World J Surg 5:829–831, 1981.

8. LaFave JW, Alden JF: Gastric bypass in the operative revision of failed jejunoileal bypass. Arch Surg 114:438–444, 1979.

9. Pories WJ, Flickinger EG, Meelheim D, et al: The effectiveness of gastric bypass over gastric partition in morbid obesity. Ann Surg 196:389–399, 1982.

10. Buckwalter JA, Herbst CA Jr: Gastric partition for morbid obesity: greater curvature gastroplasty or gastrogastrostomy. World J Surg 6:403–411, 1982.

11. Buckwalter JA, Herbst CA Jr: Perioperative complications of gastric restrictive operations. Am J Surg 146:613–618, 1983.

12. Naslund I, Wickborn G, Christoffersson E, et al: A prospective randomized comparison of gastric bypass and gastroplasty. Acta Chir Scand 152:681–689, 1986.

13. Winkler WP, Saleh J: Metoclopramide in the treatment of gastric bezoars. Am J Gastroenterol 78:403–405, 1983.

14. Gomez CA: Gastroplasty in morbid obesity. Surg Clin North Am 59:1113–1120, 1979.

15. Deitel M, Bojm MA, Atin MD, et al: Intestinal bypass and gastric partitioning for morbid obesity: a comparison. Can J Surg 25:283–289, 1982.

16. Gomez CA: Gastroplasty in the surgical treatment of morbid obesity. Am J Clin Nutr 33:406–415, 1980.

17. Gomez CA: Gastroplasty in the surgical treatment of morbid obesity. World J Surg 5:823–828, 1981.

18. Deitel M: 27. Horizontal gastric partitioning for morbid obesity. Can J Surg 27:237, 1984.

19. Freeman JB, Burchett H: Failure rate with gastric partitioning for morbid obesity. Am J Surg 145:113–119, 1983.

20. Linner JH: Comparative effectiveness of gastric bypass and gastroplasty. Arch Surg 117:695–700, 1982.

21. Eskind SJ, Massie JD, Born ML, et al: Experimental study of double staple lines in gastric partitions. Surg Gynecol Obstet 152:751–756, 1981.

22. Cogbill TH, Moore EE: A simple method for reversal of gastric partitioning. Surg Gynecol Obstet 156:505–506, 1983.

23. Lechner G, Elliott DW: Comparison of weight loss after gastric exclusion and partitioning. Arch Surg 118:685–692, 1983.

24. Martin MB, Kon ND, Meredith JH: Greater curvature gastroplasty: follow-up at 34 months. Am Surg 51:197–200, 1985.

25. Knol JA, Strodel WE, Eckhauser FE: Critical appraisal of horizontal gastroplasty. Am J Surg 153:256–261, 1987.

26. Grace DM: 18. Use of Marlex in horizontal gastroplasty. Can J Surg 27:231, 1984.

27. Grace DM: Recognition and management of Marlex erosion after horizontal gastroplasty for morbid obesity. Can J Surg 30:282–285, 1987.

28. Deitel M, Thompson DA, Saldanha CF, et al: "Pink urine" in morbidly obese patients following gastric partitioning. Can Med Assoc J 130:1007–1011, 1984.

29. Simonowitz DA, Dellinger EP, Stothert JS Jr, et al: Gastroplasty in patients with symptoms of reflux esophagitis. Surg Gynecol Obstet 154:235–237, 1982.

30. Paulk SC: Formal dilation after gastric partitioning. Surg Gynecol Obstet 156:502–504, 1983.

31. Villar HV, Ranne RD: Neurologic deficit following gastric partitioning: possible role of thiamine. JPEN 8:575–578, 1984.

32. Forse RA, Deitel M, MacLean LD: Revision of failed horizontal gastroplasty by vertical banded gastroplasty. Can J Surg 31:118–120, 1988.

33. Buckwalter JA, Herbst CA Jr: Leaks occurring after gastric bariatric operations. Surgery 103:156–160, 1988.

34. Clark JR, Conarro PA, Culbertson GR, et al: Gastric partitioning with stapled gastrogastrostomy for morbid obesity. Scientific Exhibit, 73rd Annual Clinical Congress, American College of Surgeons, Chicago, Oct. 19–23, 1987.

35. Torres J, Oca C: Gastric bypass lesser curvature with distal Roux-en-Y. Bariatric Surgery 5:10–15, 1987.

36. Halverson JD, Koehler RE: Assessment of patients with failed gastric operations for morbid obesity. Am J Surg 145:357–363, 1983.

14

Vertical Banded Gastroplasty

MERVYN DEITEL
BEVERLY A. JONES

The horizontal gastric partitionings had a high failure-rate because of dilation of the thin-walled fundal pouch, enlargement of the outlet, and "unzipping" of the partition. It has been realized that the thicker muscular wall of the stomach with less distensibility is along the lesser curvature.[1] The concept of a lesser curvature channel for treatment of morbid obesity was first published by Laws.[2] The outlet of the vertical pouch was restricted by a silastic ring containing a polypropylene suture.

In 1980, Dr. Edward E. Mason introduced a technique using the end-to-end anastomosis (EEA) stapler to cut a window through the stomach. The window facilitated the placement of a vertical partition, by two applications of a linear stapler from the window to the angle of His[3] (Fig. 14.1). An added benefit was the separation of the outlet of the pouch from the staple-lines, unlike the previous horizontal gastroplasties where the outlet enlarged and the adjacent staple-lines disrupted. Mason banded the outlet with a strip of Marlex (polypropylene) mesh. Initially he used a 5.0-cm circumference collar, but then changed to a 5.5-cm collar, suggesting that the larger size may produce the same ultimate weight loss but over a longer period of time.[3] Because inadequate weight loss occurred with the greater cross-sectional area of the outlet provided by the larger collar, the 5.0-cm collar was resumed.[4]

This technically simple operation carries a low risk, produces minimal disturbance of digestion and absorption, and has a fairly secure non-distensible calibrated lesser curvature stoma. Mean loss of excess weight in the long term is 54–70%, and is largely maintained if the proper dimensions and techniques have been employed.[5-9] Whereas in 1981 only 18% of bariatric operations were forms of vertical gastroplasty, by June 1988, 69% of the bariatric operations in the U.S.A. were vertical gastroplasties.[10,11]

TECHNIQUE OF VERTICAL BANDED GASTROPLASTY (VBG)

PRELIMINARY DISSECTION

The abdomen is entered through a high midline incision. We start to the left, right or through the xyphoid, but almost never find it necessary to remove the xyphoid. The incision ends about 3 fingers' breadth above the umbilicus. In males, who generally have less midepigastric subcutaneous adipose tissue, care is taken in the depth of the skin incision. The subcutaneous tissue is pulled laterally to

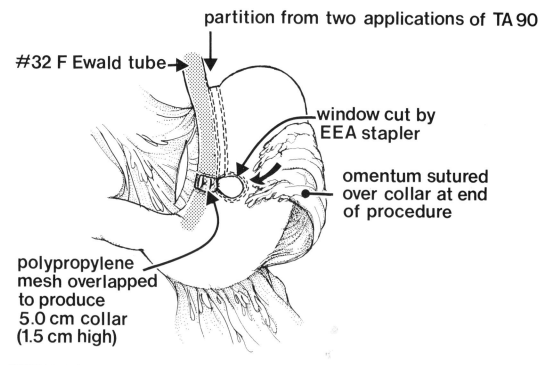

partition from two applications of TA 90

#32 F Ewald tube

window cut by EEA stapler

omentum sutured over collar at end of procedure

polypropylene mesh overlapped to produce 5.0 cm collar (1.5 cm high)

FIGURE 14.1. Vertical band gastroplasty.

find the decussating fibers of the linea alba. Exploration of the pelvis (uterus and ovaries) and abdomen (gallbladder) is done. We routinely take a baseline liver biopsy with a Tru-Cut needle (Travenol Laboratories) along the margin of the left lobe of the liver. A proper retractor is inserted (see Chapters 15 and 25). We use the upper part of the Polytract retractor with the Gomez hand over the padded left lobe of the liver. A great deal of the operation is done quickly by palpation, which comes with experience.

We do not use the reverse Trendelenberg position, as a single high left-upper-quadrant pack holds the splenic flexure of the colon to the left and the greater omentum inferiorly. Our incision ends about 6 cm above the umbilicus, so that the abdominal wall holds the abdominal contents inferiorly.

The 32F Ewald tube (Ewald Stomach Evacuator, InMed Corporation, 2950 Pacific Drive, Norcross, GA 30071) is passed into the stomach by the anesthesiologist, and the blunt tip of the tube is guided through the cardia into the stomach by the surgeon's right hand, to prevent perforation of the distal esophagus. The left triangular ligament of the liver is not divided; indeed its division can be hazardous with a fatty liver where the liver enlarges into the left triangular ligament towards the spleen. Furthermore, the frequently fatty liver cannot be folded on itself without tearing. By blunt finger dissection high up around the esophagus with the hand against the diaphragm, making sure that the stomach is reduced into the abdomen to avoid any perforation, the fingers and the thumb of the right hand are placed carefully about the abdominal esophagus to free a space around it. We do this mainly blindly, because of the difficulty in exposing this area in the massively obese. Next a long ½-inch-wide Penrose drain is looped about the esophagus, by being passed with the left hand behind the esophagus where it is grasped between the second and third fingers of the right hand and withdrawn, and the drain is clamped. This identifies the angle of His.

The left index and middle fingers are then placed in an avascular area of the gastrohepatic omentum, just above the level of the crow's foot, and they open into the lesser sac and retrogastric space superficial to the pancreas. There are no vessels to divide. The smooth posterior surface of the stomach is palpated, and the fingers are then directed towards the angle of His. The second and

third fingers of the right hand are also directed downward from the angle of His to this same space from above and are spread, opening up the portion of the gastrophrenic ligament immediately lateral to the esophagus for the later portion of the procedure (Fig. 14.2A to F).

CREATION OF THE WINDOW

The anvil of the EEA-28 mm (i.e., the outside diameter of the circular staggered double row of staples is 28 mm) is placed with the second and third fingers of the left hand into the opening into the lesser sac, and placed retrogastrically above the crow's foot and against the Ewald tube which is against the lesser curvature of the stomach. The Hearn needle (available from Richard F. Hearn, MD, 915 East Summit Avenue, Oconomowoc, WI 53066), which is the same diameter as the EEA shaft, is attached to the end of the fully open shaft of the EEA stapler. The Hearn needle is then thrust against the center of the anvil and brought through the anterior and posterior walls of the stomach. The 2-cm rubber tip cut off the end of the 18F red rubber catheter is now placed over the sharp tip of the Hearn needle to prevent puncture of the liver. The Hearn needle is then removed by 2½ turns of the needle clockwise. Dr. Hearn suggests holding the needle stationary by a long hemostat and removing the EEA shaft by rotating the stapler 2½ turns counterclockwise, but this will make a larger hole in the stomach. The reusable Hearn needle is also available with a different sized thread to fit the ILS circular stapler.

The anvil is then attached to the EEA stapler, which is screwed down to its maximum, while the left hand about the anvil makes sure that no extraneous tissue is caught. The EEA stapler is fired. In early operations when we used a large hemovac needle with a rubber tube tied to its end, with the rubber tube attached to the shaft of the EEA, on occasion the tube came off the trocar, leaving a hole in the posterior wall of the stomach (see Chapter 15). This does not occur with the Hearn needle. Furthermore, we have always had two complete gastric rings when using the Hearn needle.

Rather than suturing occasional bleeding vessels at the window, we routinely run a 2–0 chromic catgut suture around the entire window, just beyond the circular double row of staggered staples. We have never had a leak

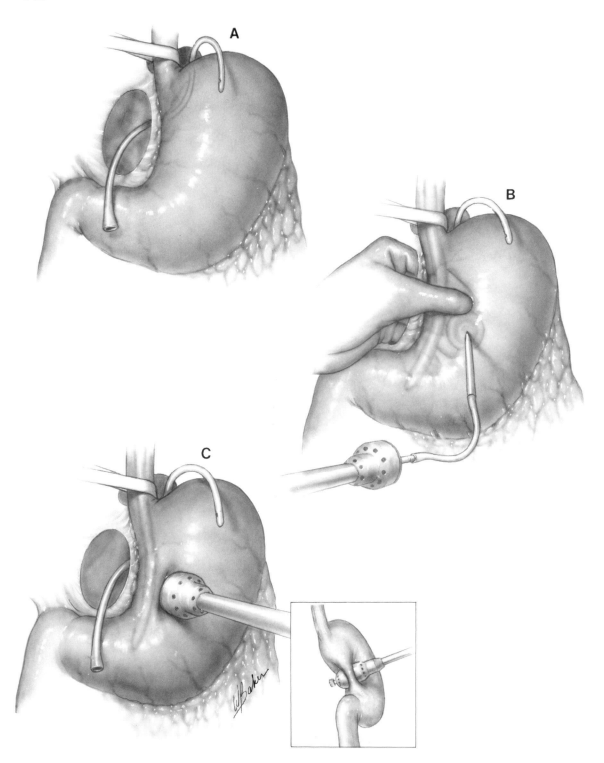

FIGURE 14.2. *A,* A 32F Ewald tube is passed into stomach. A Penrose drain is passed about the mobilized esophagus. The hand opens up an avascular area of the lesser omentum and the lesser sac. We do not pass the rubber catheter retrogastrically to the angle of His until after the window is cut. *B,* Anvil is placed against posterior gastric wall adjacent to Ewald tube, above crow's foot. Trocar is shown being passed through anterior and posterior gastric walls against center of anvil, to introduce attached tubing and EEA center rod. Instead, we use the Hearn needle attached directly to the EEA rod. *C,* Anvil is secured to EEA shaft. Instrument is closed and fired, taking care that a portion of lesser omentum is not included. Stapler is opened 3 turns and anvil is removed through the window.

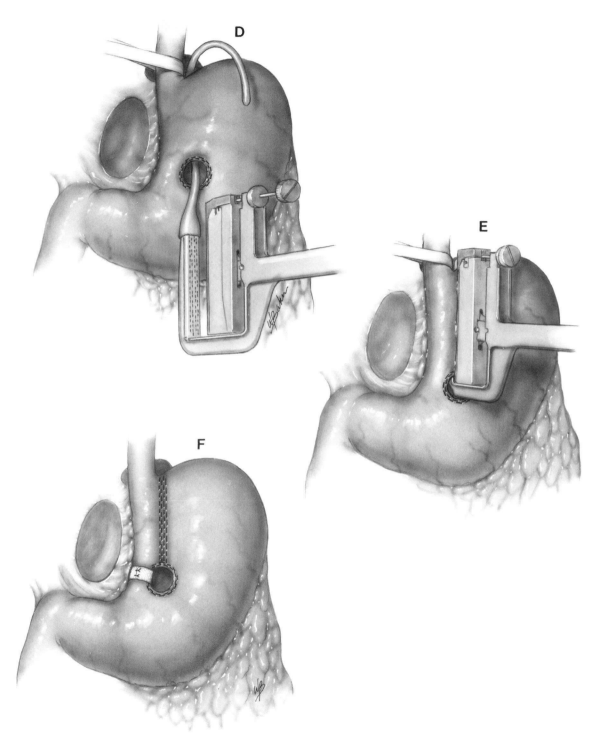

FIGURE 14.2 *Continued.* *D,* Upper end of catheter has been retrieved at angle of His. Wide end of catheter is brought through window and attached to lower jaw of linear stapler. Catheter guides stapler vertically. *E,* Retaining pin is screwed. Sponge-sticks hold fundus to left, aligning staple-lines (evenly distributed to avoid tissue bunching) from angle of His to lesser curvature side of window, as instrument is closed. Pouch volume is measured. Instrument is fired. *F,* TA90B delivers 4 equidistant rows of staples. Premarked mesh strip (1.5 cm wide) is wrapped flat around the channel between lesser curvature and window, and sutured to itself with 3 polypropylene sutures so that its circumference is 5.0-cm. Unlike the diagram, we apply these sutures through small vertical bites of mesh. Window and mesh are covered with anchored omentum. (Figs. 14.2A to F: copyright United States Surgical Corporation, 1986. Used by permission.)

from the window since we started oversewing it circumferentially in the last 675 VBG operations. Before we started oversewing, in one patient a leak occurred at the window where a staple had fallen out of the EEA cartridge. We find that the time to run a suture around the window is not much longer than oversewing the occasional bleeding vessels instead. We prefer to insert this absorbable suture *after* applying the vertical staple-lines. However, if there is significant bleeding from the window when it is cut, we insert this suture at that time.

CONSTRUCTION OF THE TUBULAR POUCH

The red rubber catheter is placed upward retrogastrically through the opening in the lesser omentum with the left hand, and the tip is hooked by the right index finger from the opening at the angle of His where the catheter is retrieved and advanced. The lower wide end of the catheter is brought out the window. The surgeon makes sure that the catheter moves readily up and down retrogastrically, and that its course is not instead around the esophagus, to the right of the lesser curvature, and through the window, which could result in dangerous stapling off of the left gastric artery.

The footpiece of the TA90B (with staple leg length 4.8 mm before closure) is then attached to the wide end of the catheter and brought retrogastrically (Fig. 14.2 D). With a posterior and cephalad direction initially and then an anterior and cephalad direction, the stapler presents at the angle of His, where the catheter is disconnected from the footpiece with a Mixter clamp. The hooked right index finger keeps the proximal stomach in the stapler until the pin, which is inserted with the left hand, is in place. The pin (wing-nut) is then screwed into place in order to stabilize the instrument (Fig. 14.2 E).

The Penrose drain holds the esophagus to the right. Two sponge-sticks cephalad to the window hold the fundus taut to the left, creating as small a pouch as possible. The TA90B is then closed but not fired, checking that there is a straight application from the angle of His to the lesser curvature side of the window without puckering, and making sure that the Penrose drain is not caught in the jaws of the stapler. If the top of the stomach is immediately against the pin, a tiny space can be left unstapled between the pin and the cephalad staples; the surgeon must view that the portion of the cartridge with cephalad staples extends beyond the top of the stomach.

The technique for measuring the volume of the pouch is presented in Chapter 16. We performed this measurement in more than 50 patients, and uniformly found a pouch volume ≤25 ml under 70 cm of water gravity pressure. Accordingly, we do not measure the volume of the pouch, but believe that this should be done initially by surgeons doing the VBG, until they are sure that their technique produces a pouch of less than 30 ml.

The TA90B is then fired, delivering four equidistant rows of staples 2 mm apart. We inspect to confirm that the staples have made the configuration of a letter "B."

Alternatively, two applications of a PI-90 stapler (3M) may be made. The 90-mm staplers appear to be too long for the partition, but the 55-mm instruments are too short to construct the partition without puckering. The length of the vertical partition ranges from 50–70 mm. Mathias A.L. Fobi used two PLS-60 mm staplers (Ethicon) to place the four rows of staples.[12] William M. Headley creates a shorter channel by two applications of the TA55.[12] Michael B. Butler of Florida creates the channel with the GIA stapler.[13] The ILA (3M) may likewise be used.

If two stapler applications, each having a double row of staggered staples, are used, the two staple-lines should be placed immediately adjacent with perfect alignment.[14] Separated staple-lines leave islands of viable epithelium between the staple-lines, which coalesce to form mucous cysts and breakdown of the partition. Dr. Lloyd D. MacLean used to insert two TA90 staplers at once before firing, which left considerable distance between the stapler applications and was followed by dehiscence of the partition in 23% of patients, with regain in weight. However, MacLean used a tighter collar (41–45 mm), which would cause obstruction of the pouch and stress on the staple-lines.[15] MacLean now divides the partition after applying a double cartridge PI-90 (3M), which applies two sets of double staggered rows with a 5-mm space between the two double rows. He incises between the 4 rows of staples, and oversews each side with a running silk Lembert suture. Douglas S. Hess uses a similar technique to divide the partition.[16] Whether division of the partition results in increased leaks and infection has not been determined yet. There is a risk in placing inverting sutures over a staple-line when the underlying lumen is small.

BANDING THE OUTLET

A pair of long Metzenbaum scissors is used to incise the peritoneum in an avascular area on the lesser curvature side of the gastric channel at the level of the window. Rarely, a vessel has to be divided here, between fine silk ties; hemostatic clips are to be avoided under the collar. A small curved clamp is passed under the peritoneum, nerves of Latarjet and adipose tissue at the channel, with its concavity facing the stomach. When the clamp reaches the end of the adipose tissue, it is rotated so that the curve faces outward to the right, is moved up and down to enlarge the tunnel, and then grasps the Marlex band.

We cut the Marlex (knitted polypropylene) mesh band preoperatively from a sheet of Marlex, oriented so that the stretch in the collar is vertical and not horizontal. The bands are marked out with a magic marker so that they are 7 cm long, 1.5 cm wide, and have black lines at 0.5 and 5.5 cm from one end (i.e. the distance between the two lines is 5.0 cm). We do not leave the raised border of the Marlex sheet, which could erode through the gastric channel outlet. About 69 collars are cut from one sheet. These are then individually packaged and sterilized by ethylene oxide gas sterilization. If steam autoclaving were used, polypropylene would not liquify but would fray readily.

The collar is brought through flat (not twisted or folded), and is looped about the outlet and overlapped so that the two previously placed black lines coincide. It is sutured to itself (and not to the stomach) with three 3–0 polypropylene sutures, with small needles. The first of these sutures is placed through the black lines and the Ewald tube is removed by the anesthesiologist before the suture is tied. We have found that the presence of the Ewald tube and gastric thickness may prevent a 5.0-cm collar. A Mixter clamp is then inserted under the collar, so that the collar can be easily sutured to itself with the two further sutures without entering the gastric wall. A total of three vertical sutures are used, with short bites to prevent puckering of the collar (Fig. 14.2 F). We apply a tiny metal hemoclip to the lower margin of the overlap of the collar as a potential radiological marker.

The anesthesiologist passes a 16F nasogastric tube which is negotiated to just beyond the outlet, so that its holes are on both sides of the outlet. As gastric ileus has been found to last up to 48 hours, we remove the nasogastric tube at about 36 hours postoperatively. However, many surgeons, including Mason and Doherty,[4] use no nasogastric tube following routine VBG operations.

At this point, if one has any suspicion regarding a leak, this should be tested by filling the wound with warmed sterile saline and having the anesthesiologist introduce air down the nasogastric tube. No bubbles should be produced. The anesthesiologist then aspirates the air from the distended stomach. Methylene blue may also be instilled down the nasogastric tube in the channel, after occluding the esophagus and distal end of the outlet, to identify a leak. Surgeons who do not use a nasogastric tube test for a leak by instilling air or methylene blue down the Ewald tube, before it is removed.

The greater omentum on the greater curvature of the stomach is brought loosely over the window and collar, and sutured to the lesser omentum with a few fine catgut sutures. This prevents adherence of the collar to the undersurface of the left lobe of the liver and kinking obstruction of the outlet.

Microporous expanded polytetrafluoroethylene (PTFE, Gor-tex) is also malleable and resists stretching. We have not used Gor-tex for the restraining collar, but a preliminary report by Owen has found that a Gor-tex band is suitable.[17]

CLOSURE

The periesophageal Penrose drain is removed and then inserted to the angle of His, from which it is brought out directly through the upper end of the incision. The need to drain after VBG is controversial, and most surgeons do not drain the VBG. We believe that a drain at this site will drain a potential leak or hematoma. Although it is a surgical principle not to bring drains through an incision, the principle of direct drainage takes precedence. We have never had a ventral hernia at the upper end of the incision.

The abdominal fascia is then closed in a standard secure fashion. We do not approximate the peritoneum in these patients. No sutures or drains are placed in the subcutaneous tissue. Skin is closed with staples.

The techniques of VBG described above have worked well in our hands, with a skin-to-skin operating time averaging about 35 minutes. There are many other technical variations for performing VBG. Techniques that can get the surgeon out of trouble are detailed in Chapter 15.

PROBLEMS DURING THE PROCEDURE

If a hole is incurred in the outlet when bringing through the collar, the collar is removed and the hole is closed transversely with interrupted chromic catgut sutures, which are tied and clamped long. The collar is inserted more proximally through the window and about the channel. The ends of the catgut sutures are then individually grasped with clamps through the portion of the greater omentum brought over to cover the collar, and are tied to their partner, producing a secure omental seal.

If the operation has not gone smoothly, a gastrostomy tube is brought out from the greater curvature side of the antrum, away from the operative area,[18] and placed to a straight drainage bag to the floor, to ensure decompression. A feeding jejunostomy may also be considered.

GALLSTONES

In our experience, 26% of patients have had prior cholecystectomy before VBG.[19] Ultrasonography is done preoperatively on the remainder, and a further 12% of patients are found to have gallstones. We have found that palpation of a distended gallbladder at operation frequently misses small gallstones. We do not have intraoperative ultrasonography available. In patients with gallstones, cholecystectomy is done at the time of VBG, following completion of the VBG part of the operation.

Willbanks'[20] and Woodward's[21] groups remove the gallbladder routinely, with pathologic evidence of gallbladder disease found in 95%. Still other surgeons aspirate gallbladder bile which is spun down during the operation, and if crystals are observed microscopically, the gallbladder is removed.[22,23] However, the presence of biliary crystals at the time of VBG does not necessarily indicate future formation of gallstones.[24,25]

Our incidence of postoperative symptomatic cholelithiasis is 5% per year for the first 2 years, with a peak incidence at 15.7 months (Fig. 14.3). The incidence then falls to the 0.3% per year of the general population. This overall postoperative incidence of patients undergoing cholecystectomy is 11.5%.[19] We do not believe that this incidence warrants routine cholecystectomy at the time of VBG.

There is evidence that postoperative small asymptomatic gallstones form more frequently, but disappear with time.[24] Postoperative rapid weight loss is accompanied by the formation of gallstones, as cholesterol is liberated from mobilized adipose tissue, with saturation of bile with cholesterol during the period of rapid weight loss. After weight reduction has stabilized, the lithogenic state reverses.[25] Unfortunately, ursodeoxycholic acid cannot be given postoperatively for prevention or dissolution of gallstones in these patients, because the large 1.5×0.5 cm capsule would halt and irritate the gastric pouch and outlet. If the capsule is opened and consumed, the very bitter bile acid would interfere with long-term acceptance.[24,26] Increased glycoprotein secretion by the biliary mucosa which occurs during rapid weight loss and promotes nucleation of cholesterol crystals has been prevented by daily acetylsalicylic acid.[26] The latter would ulcerate the gastric channel. The incidence of gallstones developing after a VBG differs from the biliopancreatic bypass operation where the majority of patients will eventually develop gallstones, so that the gallbladder should be removed with that operation.

Cholecystectomy, when necessary after a VBG, is a relatively simple procedure in a much thinner patient through a virgin right subcostal hockey-stick incision, which avoids an acute angle with skin necrosis medially.

DIFFERENCES IN TECHNIQUE OF DR. EDWARD E. MASON

Mason recommends that the right-handed surgeon do the VBG operation from the left side of the operating-table (i.e., the patient's left side), because much of the later dissection is done with the left hand. He uses 10–15° reverse Trendelenberg position during the operation, with an upright footboard to prevent the patient from sliding, so that gravity does much of the retraction of the abdominal viscera. To pass the Penrose drain about the esophagus, he inserts it into the jaws of a long right-angled clamp behind the esophagus. Mason encircles the lesser omentum and the neurovascular bundles, adjacent to the stomach, at the level just proximal to the crow's

INCIDENCE OF SYMPTOMATIC GALLSTONES / YR
General Population VS Morbidly Obese Population Before and After Weight-Loss Surgery

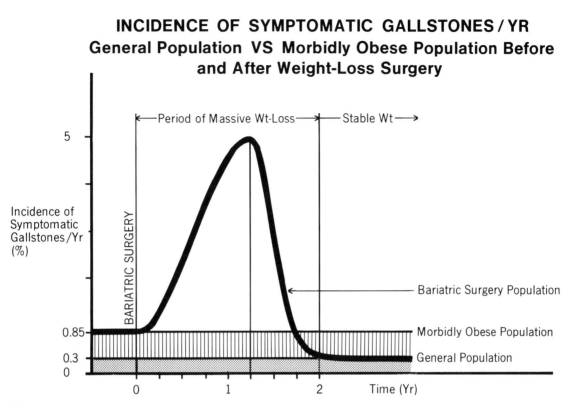

FIGURE 14.3. Yearly incidence of symptomatic cholelithiasis in the general population from age 15 to 60 years is 0.3%. Incidence of gallstones of 38.5% in our morbidly obese patients before weight loss, from age 16 to 61 years, corresponds to a yearly incidence of 0.85% over the 45 year period. Postoperative peak incidence is at 15.7 months. The incidence then falls to 3% during a 2 to 12 year period (10 years), which corresponds to the 0.3% yearly incidence of the general population. (Reproduced with permission from Deitel M, Petrov I: Surg Gynecol Obstet 164:549–552, 1987.[19])

foot with a Penrose drain, which is thus through the tunnel through which the Marlex collar will be threaded (Fig. 14.4 A and B). To find this site, he pinches the stomach edge and omentum and vessels, which pushes the stomach out of the way.

Mason uses a large hemovac needle as a trocar. The needle is attached to tubing which is then attached to the shaft of a 25-mm circular stapler, to guide the stapler through the stomach (Fig. 14.4 C to E). A Mixter clamp through the window grasps the end of the Penrose drain at the lesser sac opening, so that the drain is brought to encircle the outlet, so that it can be occluded for testing of pouch volume (Fig. 14.4 F to J). Dr. Mason makes a pouch with volume 9 to 20 ml at 70 cm of saline gravity pressure (with average pouch volume 15 ml). He inserts the mesh collar through the opening between the lesser curvature of stomach and the lesser omentum by carrying it on a long angled clamp placed through the window and behind the channel from right to left (Fig. 14.4 K to M).

For the super-obese patient (>225% above ideal body weight), Mason utilized a 4.5-cm circumference collar, but he found that this occasionally produced too much obstruction and back-pressure with breakdown of the partition. Weight loss was equivalent with the 5.0-cm collar, and he now uses a collar of 5.0-cm circumference in all patients.[4,9] A trial with the 4.5-cm collar by Doherty[12] did not improve weight loss; instead, an increased incidence of maladaptive eating behavior (liquids and junk food) and staple-line disruption occurred. With the 5.0-cm collar, the incidence of staple-line disruption during the first 3 years following two applications of a two-row stapler has been 0.9%/year.[4]

REFLUX ESOPHAGITIS AND HIATAL HERNIA

In morbidly obese individuals, gastroesophageal reflux symptoms have been found in 73% of patients, subnormal lower esophageal sphincter pressure in 47%, and hiatal

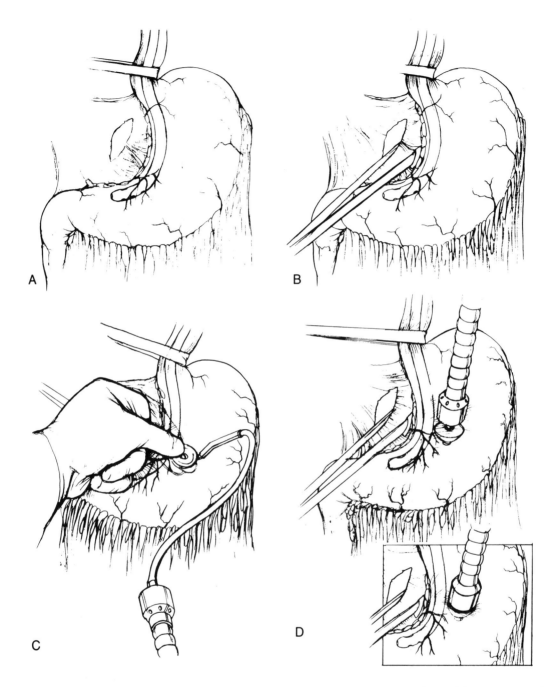

FIGURE 14.4. *A* and *B,* By pinching the omentum and stomach edge to move the stomach out of the way, an opening is made to place a Penrose drain around the lesser omentum. *C to E,* Anvil held in lesser sac at the previously selected site for the window. An angled trocar needle attached to tubing brings through the rod of the circular stapler. Window is cut, instrument is opened partially and withdrawn, and any bleeding controlled. The closed end of the rubber catheter is grasped with a Mixter clamp and brought through the lesser sac to the angle of His. *F to J,* The Penrose drain now surrounds the outlet. Back end of rubber catheter is brought out window, and the lower jaw of a linear stapler, here the PI-90, is attached. The stapler is brought through and pulled against the Ewald tube and the jaws approximated. The anesthesiologist pulls the Ewald tube back into the pouch, and volume is measured. Once pouch size is satisfactory, the stapler is fired. A second parallel line of staples is applied 1–3 mm to the left of the first. *K to M,* Collar passed, secured, and covered by greater omentum. (Figs. 14.4 A to M courtesy of 3M).

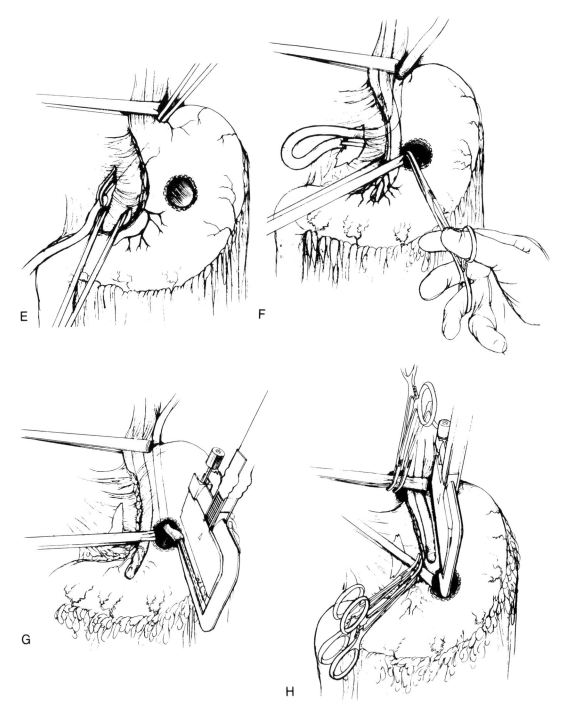

FIGURE 14.4.

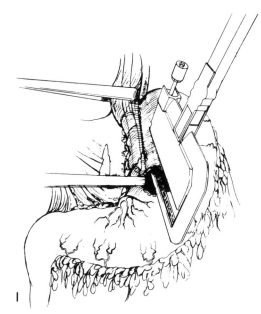

I

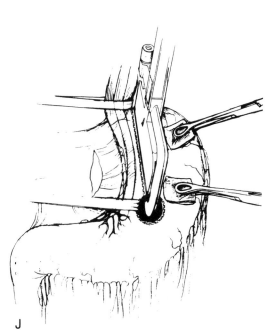

J

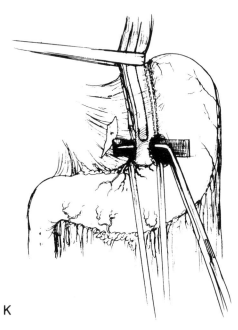

K

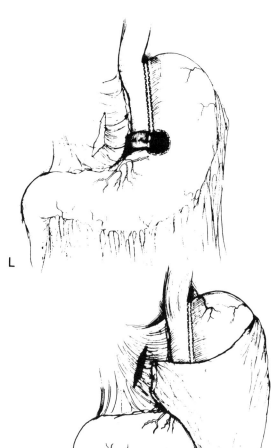

L

M

FIGURE 14.4.

hernia in 29%.[27] A Nissen fundoplication or a Hill stitch could be added to the VBG. However, we add no further procedure, as our studies have demonstrated that the VBG is an excellent antireflux procedure if the vertical staple-line is in line with the angle of His.[1] The operation results in a high pressure under the collar and a high pressure gastroplasty tube (compared to baseline gastric pressure), which inhibit reflux of gastric contents distal to the Marlex mesh collar (Fig. 14.5). The lesser curvature gastroplasty tube itself is an achlorhydric mucous tube.[28,29] The lower esophageal sphincter pressure is also elevated by the VBG operation.

IMMEDIATE POSTOPERATIVE FEATURES

For 4 to 48 hours postoperatively, one-third of patients have an amber urine which coats the plastic urinary collection apparatus as a pink or even red precipitate.[30] The "pink urine" is due to precipitation of uric acid dihydrate crystals, and correlates with increased urine concentration and decreased urine pH and volume. Crushed gastric tissue with release of nucleotides may be a contributing factor. The pink urine is transient and has no clinical importance.[31] We do not insert a Foley catheter routinely except in very poor-risk patients for monitoring.

Patients frequently have a very high white count postoperatively, reaching as high as 25,000 at 24 hours after the operation and falling into the normal range within 5 days. There may be elevated temperatures in the first 2 days, with a mild tachycardia and facial flushing. The head of the bed is maintained elevated at 30°. Patients receive chest physiotherapy and incentive spirometry, having been instructed preoperatively.

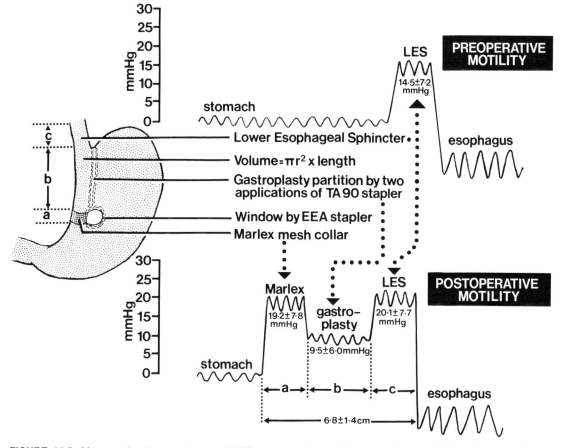

FIGURE 14.5. Manometric characterization of VBG, using station pullthrough technique. LES = lower esophageal sphincter. Using gastric baseline as 0, mean preoperative LES pressure was 14.5 mm Hg (normal ≥15). After VBG, mean pressure in the orifice (under the collar) was 19.2, in the gastroplasty tube 9.5, and at the LES 20.1 mm Hg. Mean channel length was 6.8 cm. (Reproduced with permission from Deitel M, Khanna RK, Hagen J, et al: Am J Surg 155:512–516, 1988.[1])

Patients receive one dose of a cephalosporin intravenously (cefazolin 2 g) at induction of anesthesia and one repeat dose 8 hours later. Ranitidine 75 mg is added to each litre of intravenous fluids postoperatively, while the I.V. is in place.[6,32] Legs are wrapped in tensor bandages or antiembolism stockings before surgery and these are maintained for 48 hours postoperatively, when the patients are adequately ambulatory. Other surgeons use intermittent venous compression pneumatic pressure-gradient boots. We do not give prophylactic subcutaneous mini-dose heparin routinely preoperatively, as some of our patients have a thoracic epidural catheter inserted in the operating-room (see Chapter 25) and potential hemorrhagic complications could ensue. Patients who have a past history of deep vein thrombosis receive mini-dose heparin. In more than 1,400 bariatric operations since 1973, we have had only four known deep vein thromboses and two pulmonary emboli, both patients surviving. Our operating time is short, and we suspect that deep vein thrombosis commencing intraoperatively is time-related.

If the course is smooth, the Penrose drain is shortened on the third postoperative day, if the patient is afebrile, and removed on the fourth postoperative day. Clear fluids are started on the third postoperative day, advanced to full fluids wihout cereals on the following day, taken from a 30-ml plastic medicine glass (up to five per hour). Patients are discharged home on the fifth to sixth postoperative day if they live nearby, and the seventh to tenth day if they live >100 miles away. The skin staples can be removed in the office. There is gastric pouch and stomal edema during the first 4 to 6 weeks postoperatively[33] (Fig. 14.6). The diabetic patient is allowed to show occasional elevated blood glucose; this is because the caloric intake may vary daily, and cannot be guaranteed during the postoperative period. Adult-onset insulin-dependent diabetes resolves as the weight is lost.

Further discussion regarding postoperative care is in Chapters 7 and 26.

LATER POSTOPERATIVE CARE

Patients take a full liquid diet for the first 4 weeks postoperatively. Nothing is taken that is too cold or too hot, and if pop is taken, it is permitted to become flat first. For the second 4 weeks, patients take tiny pureed or blended meals.[34] After 8 weeks, they are advanced to tiny meals, chewed well and taken slowly. Overloading the pouch will produce distress. Patients take low calorie beverages, avoid snacking, and are advised to exercise. A multiple vitamin is taken. Medications must be liquid, chewable, tiny or crushed. Irritating medications which damage the mucosa in the gastric channel such as non-steroidal anti-inflammatory drugs, iron, potassium or tetracycline are prohibited or taken as liquids, preferably with 2% milk. Because the patients cannot manage beef or steak, thus 2% or skim milk, cheese, yogurt, eggs, and fish are encouraged for protein. On occasion, a liquid nutritional supplement may be temporarily necessary.[35]

POSTOPERATIVE COMPLICATIONS

We have had no operative deaths thus far in more than 750 VBG operations. An operative mortality of 0.29 to 0.4% is reported.[4,8,11] The annual revision rate for the VBG with the 5.0-cm collar has been 1.9%.[4,6,8]

EARLY COMPLICATIONS

Leak

The most dreaded complication is a leak, which is fortunately very rare (0.79% of first operations).[6,11,36] This is heralded by unexplained tachycardia, tachypnea, and left chest and shoulder pain. Gastrografin and thin barium in small amounts may be used if the diagnosis is in question, but may not reveal the leak. Unless there is a controlled fistula, a leak requires prompt re-operation and adequate drainage (including soft sump drains), removal of the collar, decompressive gastrostomy, and feeding jejunostomy. The leak is closed if it can be found, and is covered with omentum; however, closure of the leak in this inflamed field is usually impossible. The patient requires I.V. fluids and antibiotics, ventilatory support and nutritional support as necessary. We have had only one leak in a primary VBG[6] but two leaks in revision operations (from a Gomez gastroplasty to a VBG),[37] and the three patients survived stormy postoperative courses.

Subphrenic Abscess

A subphrenic abscess is a rare complication (0.29 to 0.48% of primary operations).[8,11] It generally indicates a walled-off leak and re-

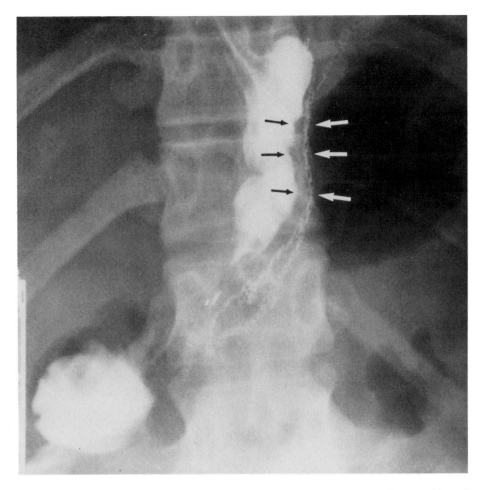

FIGURE 14.6 Postoperative edema is present in the gastric wall, resolving in 4–6 weeks. This is evidenced as a wide distance (arrows) between contrast medium in the pouch and the staple-lines, where it is most marked. GI series above is on 16th postoperative day.

quires drainage. A localized collection may be managed by CT-guided percutaneous drainage. A sympathetic left pleural effusion is an accompaniment.

LATE SEQUELAE

Menstrual periods may be irregular postoperatively, as occurs following any major abdominal operation, but usually revert to cycles which are more normal than preoperatively as weight is lost.[38–40] Pregnancy is usually deferred for one year, to the period beyond massive loss of weight and when lean tissue (protein) is no longer lost.[41] Pregnancy may be a cause of sudden onset of nausea and vomiting episodes, especially in the morning.

The first winter following the surgery is frequently a cold one, as the patient gets ad-

justed to the loss in subcutaneous adipose tissue with its insulation effect.

Vomiting

The patient requires adequate dentition and mastication to create the tiny minced meals. If the patient eats quickly or eats hard fibrous foods or is upset, regurgitation will occur. Bezoars are uncommon, and are treated with meat tenderizer or papain dissolution, endoscopic fragmentation and removal, or metoclopramide.[42] A large pouch can result in vomiting without adequate weight loss. Excess vomiting, midepigastrc pain, and bloating can be related to the development of postoperative cholecystitis, and will require cholecystectomy. If the EEA window was not made immediately adjacent to the Ewald tube, the 5.0-cm Marlex band could infold too much stomach at the outlet, resulting in obstruction.

Edematous narrowing of the stoma may be related to stasis of irritating pills or food. If the orifice is made too small, vomiting and malnutrition can develop.[15] Constant vomiting in the obese may result in starvation with polyneuropathy and ataxia as early as 3 months postoperatively.[43] Rapid excess weight loss may be accompanied by Wernicke's disease, requiring thiamine replacement (see Chapter 28). With a narrowed outlet, thiamine which is a small pill may be given as 25 mg (one-half tablet) twice daily, but when the patient is symptomatic, thiamine is given I.M. All patients are placed on vitamins, e.g., two chewable Centrum vitamin/mineral supplements daily.

Stenosis may require dilatation, which may require repeated sessions. Dilatations may be performed under fluoroscopic control over a soft spring-tipped flexible guidewire with the Eder-Puestow metal-olive dilators or, more safely, with the Savary-Celestin tapered semiflexible polyvinyl dilators which give better tactile sensation of stenosis resistance. There is some danger that the axial (longitudinal) force of these dilators against the stenosis can cause a tear (Fig. 14.7). Thus, the Rigiflex Through-the-Scope Balloon Dilators (MicroVasive, 31 Maple Street, Milford, MA 01757) provide safer radial force against the stenosis, with a 12-mm diameter inelastic

non-distensible balloon filled with fluid to 50 lb per square inch pressure, maintained for 30 seconds to 5 minutes.[44] Larger diameter balloon dilators have the danger of eroding to the mesh collar. Dilatations will be effective in providing a lasting adequate stoma in less than 50% of stenoses.[42]

Post-VBG Endoscopic Appearance

Endoscopy normally observes the cardia at 36 to 42 cm and the outlet (rosette or pseudopylorus) at 46.6 ± 2.1 cm from the incisor teeth. The 11-mm diameter gastroscope passes through the outlet snugly and the 9-mm scope easily.[42]

Erosion of the collar may be caused by chronic overstuffing of the outlet by food and is frequently associated with obstruction. However, this is usually followed shortly by an increase in eating capacity and regain in weight, as part of the collar migrates completely into the lumen. Breakdown across the partition may also result from chronic gorging and be followed by a sudden increase in eating ability and loss of sensation of satiety.

Re-operation for a Stenotic Outlet

Re-operations for a recurring and non-responding stenotic outlet are generally easy in a thin patient. The Marlex mesh collar is found easily by palpation of a small "nut" under the liver, and a Maloney bougie passed by the anesthesiologist is negotiated through this. The collar may be severed, following which a bridge of Marlex mesh is sutured to each end over a 36F Maloney bougie in order to enlarge the collar. Another method of enlarging the collar is to cut the polypropylene sutures, free the overlapped anterior portion of the collar, and suture the ends of the collar together over a 36F Maloney bougie. Merely excising the anterior portion of the collar generally results in regain of lost weight. A vertical gastrogastrostomy anterior to the vertical staple-lines[45] (which can be performed rapidly with a GIA, ILA or PLC stapler) will frequently result in regain of all lost weight. Re-operations are protected when indicated by a decompressive gastrostomy on the antrum near the greater curvature. A gastroscopic examination should not be done immediately before re-operations, because resultant gas-distended bowel makes surgery difficult.

Ventral Hernias

We have had a 5% incidence of known ventral hernias, with an additional unsuspected

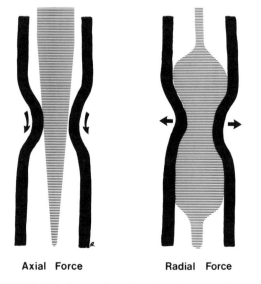

Conventional Dilatation   Hydrostatic Dilatation

Axial Force   Radial Force

FIGURE 14.7. Comparison of action of tapered dilators with longitudinal pushing stresses (left) to the newer balloon dilators with radial force (right).

3% found during abdominal lipectomy. Hernia at the umbilicus has not been a sequela of our VBG, since the incision ends well above the umbilicus.

POSTOPERATIVE WEIGHT LOSS

With the 5.0-cm collar, the maximum weight loss is in the first 12 months. The mean loss of excess weight at 3 years has been 54–70%, with 70% of patients losing more than 50% of excess weight. This weight loss has been maintained in 80% of patients at 5 years.[5,6,8,15] Using the 5.0-cm band, Doherty found that 70% of 180 consecutive patients at 5 years maintained an excess weight loss of >40%.[12]

Sugerman and co-workers[46] have noted a correlation between patients addicted to sweets (nondietetic colas, cakes, candy, cookies) and failures after VBG. In a small prospective study, they found better weight loss in the "sweets-eater" group with a Roux-en-Y gastric bypass, because the patients restricted sweets to avoid the dumping syndrome (flushing, sweating, nausea, lightheadedness and diarrhea). Sugerman's original VBG collars were slightly larger than 5.0-cm.[12] Sweets-eating was determined by a dietitian on an intensive dietary history, including 24-hour recall and a 2-day diary food frequency check. Non-sweets-eaters take <10% of their calories from refined, simple sugars. Severe sweets-eaters take >25% of their total caloric intake from simple sugars.

In a further study, Sugerman and co-workers[47] selectively assigned sweets-eaters to Roux-en-y gastric bypass and non-sweets-eaters to VBG. This significantly improved the VBG results. Weight loss with gastric bypass was still superior to VBG, but at the expense of more complications.

Sugerman acknowledges that this may depend on patient populations. Patients in Richmond may eat more sweets, whereas patients in Iowa or Toronto may eat more meat, potatoes, and vegetables. However, there is no question that some patients after VBG, despite dietary counselling, will gorge and vomit or will ingest high caloric liquids to their limit through the channel. Furthermore, the VBG does turn some patients towards easily consumed junk foods, although the intake of even these foods down the narrow channel is limited. Use of a 4.5-cm collar leads to increased intake of junk foods as well as an increased incidence of breakdown of the par-

tition; with the 5.0-cm collar, masticated fibrous foods taken in small amounts slowly pass through the outlet. As important as the preoperative sweets-eating history in the determination of outcome may be adequate dentition to enable mastication of foods to a fine consistency. Otherwise, the patient may only be able to take junk foods. Furthermore, the internal diameter of the VBG orifice under the 5.0-cm collar varies with the inherent thickness of the contained gastric wall and a possible loss of fat in the gastric wall. With respect to the gastric bypass operation, not all patients dump postoperatively and indeed the dumping syndrome ultimately disappears in many patients.

Loss of excess weight following VBG is about 10% less than following gastric bypass. However, the VBG is preferred by many surgeons because of its simplicity, safety, less serious complications, shorter operating time, ease of gastroscopic examination, and lack of marginal ulcer, stomal enlargement, and iron and B_{12} deficiencies.[48]

REVISION OF A FAILED HORIZONTAL GASTROPLASTY TO A VBG

This conversion will require an anterior gastrogastrostomy over the lesser curvature part of the horizontal partition, if it is still intact. Mason has had considerable success with this revision. The most common long-term complication after this revision is stenosis of the gastrogastrostomy in the pouch.[49] Mason has occasionally required balloon dilatation for later scarring of the gastrogastrostomy. The pouch cannot be made as small as in the virgin VBG, because the middle of the pouch where the gastrogastrostomy is located must be left patulous, so that his pouch volume is 20–25 ml at 70 cm saline gravity pressure.

There is a hazard to the blood supply by the crossing horizontal and vertical staplelines. Our combined experience, with occasional leaks and stenoses after this revision, has led us to conclude that a failed horizontal gastroplasty should not be converted to a VBG.[37] Each surgeon must make the decision regarding revisions on the basis of his or her experience. If the conversion is made to a VBG, a concomitant greater-curvature antral gastrostomy and occasionally a feeding jejunostomy should be included. Revisions are long and difficult operations, and carry the risk of infection, leak, and other complications.

REVISION OF A FAILED ROUX-EN-Y GASTRIC BYPASS TO A VBG

Mason has revised the failed Roux-en-Y gastric bypass to a VBG.[50] He disconnects the Roux-limb from the stomach to avoid stomal ulcer, since gastrin in the antrum will now be stimulated and the fundus will be empty of food. Two gastrogastrostomies are done and are separate (Fig. 14.8).

The steps used by Mason are as follows: 1. A gastrogastrostomy is made on the lesser curvature as a two-layered anastomosis by hand. 2. The 32F Ewald tube is passed. 3. The window is made with an EEA-28 mm just above the crow's foot. 4. The TA90B partition is made, without encroaching on the gastrogastrostomy. 5. If there is any question regarding viability of the fundus, that part lateral to the vertical partition and above the horizontal staple-line is removed; if the fundus is removed, the surgeon should staple to make sure that there is no leak in the horizontal staple-line. 6. If the fundus appears well vascularized, the gastrojejunostomy is divided, and a gastrogastrostomy is performed to drain the fundus into the lower gastric segment.

REVISION FOR A FAILED VBG

An outlet ≥13 mm is associated with inadequate weight loss. It is visualized as too large when compared to the end of the gastroscope or when the gastroscope passed beyond the outlet is retroverted.[42] The outlet can also be measured by comparing it to the dimensions of the biopsy forceps when open. A Fogarty balloon can also be used for measurement.

In early patients where the outlet collar was made too large (>5.0 cm), we performed revisions by leaving the old collar in situ but inserting a tighter collar cephalad through the same window; in some of these patients, we cut a new window cephalad to the previous window against a 28F Maloney bougie and inserted a 4.8 cm collar. These operations resulted in adequate sustained weight loss in 50% of patients.[6] It appears that failures of one operation have an increased incidence of failing another operation.

Mason of Iowa and E.R.T.C. Owen of Middlesex, England, both create a smaller channel within the previous gastroplasty channel,[13] and have had success at re-doing the VBG (Fig. 14.9). A large and redundant pouch with a proper-sized outlet can cause vomiting without weight loss.[13] The new VBG is thus repeated inside the first VBG. They put a Penrose drain around the esophagus and outlet (i.e., free the window). One can use the old window and re-staple vertically. If the stomach between the old and new staple-lines is of good color, Mason and Owen use a GIA stapler to create a gastrogastrostomy to drain the closed segment into the main stomach.

A breakdown of the partition is identified on a single contrast study as a short-circuit of contrast medium from pouch to fundus. However, if the radiologist looks at the staple-line on a preliminary pre-contrast plain film taken in the right posterior oblique position (or in any position in which the staples in-

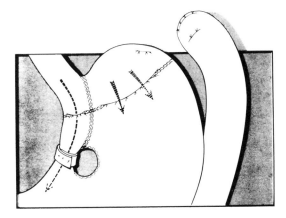

FIGURE 14.8. Conversion of a Roux-en-Y gastric bypass to a VBG.

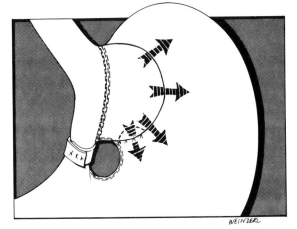

FIGURE 14.9. Revision of a VBG with a large, redundant pouch.

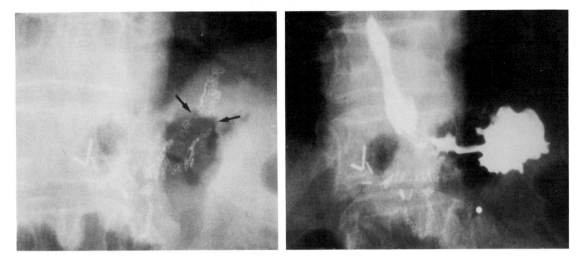

FIGURE 14.10. (Left) With two adjacent applications of a linear stapler (e.g. TA90), the staple-lines are occasionally not uniformly parallel on the plain film. The preliminary precontrast film above shows a defect (arrows) in both staple-lines. (Right) GI series in this patient shows immediate flow of contrast medium from pouch to fundus through this defect. (With the TA90B, the 4 parallel rows of staples cannot be separated on the plain film.)

dicating the partition and window are well seen), a breakdown will be identified by a defect in the staple-lines (Fig. 14–10).[33] Gastroscopy will identify a breakdown as a bifurcation in the channel (carina-like appearance) through which the scope may pass in either direction.[42] Defects in the TA90B staple-lines appear to be virtually non-existent.

A breakdown in the partition is best remedied by re-stapling more medially. Alternatively, the area of the disrupted staple-line may be incised through-and-through and each side oversewn, to reconstitute the partition. There is obviously increased hazard with revisions.

Many surgeons favor revision to some type of malabsorptive operation. Mathias A.L. Fobi of Inglewood, California and George S.M. Cowan Jr. of Memphis, Tennessee favor the distal Roux-en-Y gastric bypass of Oca and Torres (see Chapter 12) for revision of VBG,[12] to produce both restriction and an element of malabsorption. However, Mason does not substitute malabsorption, and points out the risk of bone disease and other long-term complications of malabsorption.[50]

CONCLUSION

The VBG of Mason is an attempt to produce satiety and restrict intake in patients who could not sustain weight loss by exhaustive conservative treatments. It is a relatively safe, rapid, and highly effective operation, which has a normal digestive course, and is generally easily reversible. There are failures for technical reasons and for reasons of extensive liquid high-caloric intake. Follow-up is mandatory for excess vomiting and malnutrition, and must be lifelong for dietary and weight loss support and surveillance. The results are usually very favorable. The treatment of those patients who have failed to have sustained weight loss is a problem area of current investigation for the surgeon. Dr. Mason has pointed out that the ideal treatment of obesity is to reduce intake and not create malabsorption.

ACKNOWLEDGEMENT

The authors are grateful for the recommendations, information and assistance in this work from: Cornelius Doherty, M.D., San Francisco, California; David H. Scott, B.S. and Kathleen Renquist of the National Bariatric Surgery Registry, Iowa City; the Department of Photography of St. Joseph's Health Centre; and Bernard Langer, M.D., Chairman of the Department of Surgery, University of Toronto.

REFERENCES

1. Deitel M, Khanna RK, Hagen J, et al: Vertical banded gastroplasty as an antireflux procedure. Am J Surg 155:512–516, 1988.
2. Laws HL: Standardized gastroplasty orifice. Am J Surg 141:393–394, 1981.

3. Mason EE: Vertical banded gastroplasty. Arch Surg 117:701–706, 1982.

4. Mason EE: Morbid obesity: use of vertical banded gastroplasty. Surg Clin N Am 67:521–537, 1987.

5. Fobi MAL, Fleming AW: Vertical banded gastroplasty vs gastric bypass in the treatment of obesity. J National Med Assoc 78:1091–1096, 1986.

6. Deitel M, Jones BA, Petrov I, et al: Vertical banded gastroplasty: results in 233 patients. Can J Surg 29:322–324, 1986.

7. Mason EE: National Bariatric Surgery Registry Newsletter 2:51, 1987.

8. Mason EE, Maher JW, Scott DH, et al: Vertical banded gastroplasty: a six year review. Scientific exhibit, American College of Surgeons, San Francisco, Oct. 12–15, 1987.

9. Mason EE, Doherty C, Maher JW, et al: Super obesity and gastric reduction procedures. Gastroenterol Clin N Am 16:495–502, 1987.

10. Scott DH, Mason EE, Blommers TJ: Results of the eighth annual bariatric surgery questionnaire. American Society for Bariatric Surgery, 1988.

11. Fourth Pooled Statistical Report, National Bariatric Surgery Registry, Iowa City 52242, Spring 1988.

12. Personal communications.

13. National Bariatric Surgery Registry Newsletter 1:9–11, 1986.

14. Eskind SJ, Massie JD, Born ML, et al: Experimental study of double staple lines in gastric partitions. Surg Gynecol Obstet 152:751–756, 1981.

15. MacLean LD, Rhode B, Shizgal HM: Nutrition after vertical banded gastroplasty. Ann Surg. 206:555–563, 1987.

16. Hess DS: Prevention of staple disruption by complete division and separation of the stomach. Program, Fifth Annual Meeting, American Society for Bariatric Surgery, Iowa City, June 1–3, 1988, p. 98 (poster).

17. Owen ERTC, Kark AE: Assessment and revision of failed vertical banded gastroplasty. Proceedings of the Third Annual Meeting of the American Society for Bariatric Surgery, Iowa City, June 18–20, 1986, pp 77–79.

18. Rice TW, Deitel M: A technique for gastrostomy. Am J Surg 146:397–398, 1982.

19. Deitel M, Petrov I: Incidence of symptomatic gallstones after bariatric operations. Surg Gynecol Obstet 164:549–552, 1987.

20. Calhoun R, Willbanks O: Coexistence of gallbladder disease and morbid obesity. Am J Surg 154:655–658, 1987.

21. Schmidt JH, Hocking MP, Rout WR, et al: The case for prophylactic cholecystectomy concomitant with gastric restriction for morbid obesity. Am Surg 54:269–272, 1988.

22. Howell LM: Intraoperative gallbladder examination with microsopic bile analysis. Proceedings of the Second Annual Meeting, American Society for Bariatric Surgery, Iowa City, June 13–14, 1985.

23. Freeman JB, Meyer PD, Printen KJ, et al: Analysis of gallbladder bile in morbid obesity. Am J Surg 129:163–166, 1975.

24. Wattchow DA, Hall SC, Whiting MJ, et al: Prevalence and treatment of gallstones after gastric bypass surgery for morbid obesity. Br Med J 286:763, 1983.

25. Whiting MJ, Watts J McK: Supersaturated bile from obese patients without gallstones supports cholesterol crystal growth but not nucleation. Gastroenterol 86:243–248, 1984.

26. Chopra R, Sheinbaum R, Marks J, et al: Formation and prevention of gallstones during weight reduction. Gastroenterol 90:1718, 1986.

27. Hagen J, Deitel M, Khanna RK, et al: Gastroesophageal reflux in the massively obese. Int Surg 72:1–3, 1987.

28. Berger EH: Distribution of parietal cells in stomach: histotopographic study. Am J Anat 54:87–114, 1934.

29. Billencamp H: Zur vergleichenden Histologie der Magenstrasse. Beitr Path Anat 82:475–484, 1929.

30. Saldanha CF, Deitel M, Thompson DA, et al: Pink urine in morbidly obese patients following operations. Surg Forum 34:175–178, 1983.

31. Deitel M, Thompson DA, Saldanha CF, et al: "Pink urine" in morbidly obese patients following gastric partitioning. Can Med Assoc J 130:1007–1011, 1984.

32. Abernethy DR, Greenblatt J, Mathis R, et al: Cimetidine disposition in obesity. Am J Gastroenterol 79:91–94, 1984.

33. Deitel M, Leekam R, Shankar L, et al: Radiologic features after vertical banded gastroplasty. Program, Fifth Annual Meeting, American Society for Bariatric Surgery, Iowa City, June 1–3, 1988, p 66 (abstract).

34. Ellison EC, Martin EW Jr, Laschinger J, et al: Preventing early failure of stapled partitions in treatment of morbid obesity. Arch Surg 115:528–533, 1980.

35. Deitel M, McArdle AH, Brown RA, et al: Elemental and liquid diets in surgery. In Deitel M (ed): Nutrition in Clinical Surgery, Second Edition. Baltimore, Williams & Wilkins, 1985, pp 44–59.

36. Buckwalter JA, Herbst Jr CA: Leaks occurring after gastric bariatric operations. Surgery 103:156–160, 1988.

37. Forse RA, Deitel M, MacLean LD: Revision of failed horizontal gastroplasty by vertical banded gastroplasty. Can J Surg 31:118–120, 1988.

38. Deitel M, Stone E, Kassam HA, et al: Gynecologic-obstetric changes after loss of massive excess weight following bariatric surgery. J Am Coll Nutr 7:148–152, 1988.

39. To TB, Deitel M, Stone E, et al: Sex hormonal changes after loss of massive excess weight. Surg Forum 38:465–467, 1987.

40. Deitel M, To TB, Stone E, et al: Sex hormonal changes accompanying loss of massive excess weight. Gastroenterol Clin N Am 16:511–515, 1987.

41. Raymond JL, Schipke CA, Becker JM, et al: Changes in body composition and dietary intake after gastric partitioning for morbid obesity. Surgery 99:15–18, 1986.

42. Deitel M, Bendago M: Endoscopy of vertical banded gastroplasty. Am Surg, in press.

43. Feit H, Glasberg M, Ireton C, et al: Peripheral neuropathy and starvation after gastric partitioning for morbid obesity. Ann Intern Med 96:453–455, 1982.

44. Webb WA: Esophageal dilation: personal experience

with current instruments and techniques. Am J Gastroenterol 83:471–475, 1988.

45. Cogbill TH, Moore EE: A simple method for reversal of gastric partitioning. Surg Gynecol Obstet 156:505–506, 1983.

46. Sugerman HJ, Starkey JV, Birkenhauer R: A randomized prospective trial of gastric bypass vs vertical banded gastroplasty for morbid obesity and their effects on sweets vs non-sweets eaters. Ann Surg 205:613–624, 1987.

47. Sugerman HJ, Londrey G, Kellum JM, et al: Weight loss with vertical banded gastroplasty and Roux-en-Y gastric bypass in sweets and non-sweets eaters: selective vs randomized assignment. Am J Surg, in press.

48. Printen KJ, Halverson JD: Hemic micronutrients following vertical banded gastroplasty. Am Surg 54:267–268, 1988.

49. Faber LA, Maher JW, Mason EE: Balloon dilatation of gastro-gastrostomy strictures in gastroplasty revisions. Am Surg 54:526, 1988 (abstract 13).

50. National Bariatic Surgery Registry Newsletter 1:14–18, 1986.

15

Technical, Stapler and Dissection Related Problems During Gastroplasties: Approaches to Management

GEORGE S.M. COWAN, JR.
THOMAS G. PETERS

EXPOSURE
  A. Incision for Gastroplasty
  B. Resection of Properitoneal Fat
  C. Xiphisternectomy
  D. Retractor Systems
  E. Retractor Maintenance and Familiarity
  F. Splenic Injury
  G. Liver Mobilization
  H. Tilting the Operating-Table
DISSECTION
  A. Encircling the Esophagus
  B. Dissection of the Posterior Stomach
  C. Repairing a High Posterior Gastric Perforation
  D. Clearing the Angle of His for Vertical Stapling

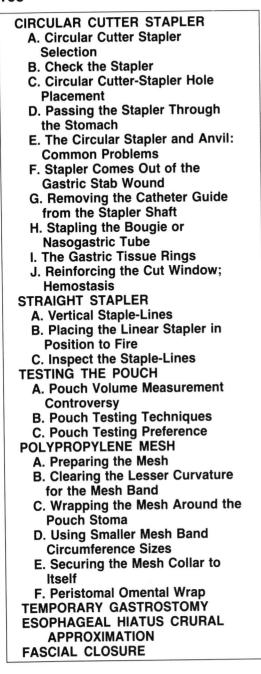

Published step-by-step descriptions of bariatric surgical procedures, postoperative complications and weight loss statistics tend to ignore many of the technical difficulties experienced during surgery.[1–14] Recommended methods for the management of intraoperative problems, or their prevention, are infrequently addressed.[15–18]

Serious morbidity and death may result from staple-line leakage, gastric or esophageal perforation, splenic injury and infection.[2,6–11,16,17,19–28] In addition, staplers are fired within a deep incision in morbidly obese patients who may have received heparin.[16,25,28] Therefore, adequate exposure, careful dissection as well as stapler placement, firing, staple-line reinforcement and coverage are critically important. The following descriptions are largely limited to the authors' preferences for management of a variety of technical, stapler and dissection-related problems experienced while performing Mason's vertical banded gastroplasty.[29] However, certain of the basic and detailed techniques are also applicable to other bariatric surgical procedures.

EXPOSURE

A. INCISION FOR GASTROPLASTY. An adequate upper abdominal midline incision for most gastroplasties extends about 20 cm inferiorly from the xiphisternum to above the umbilicus. After incising the skin, the midline subcutaneous fat is bluntly divided for the length of the incision using the tip of a wide malleable retractor, applying counter-traction with extra large rake retractors. When exactly in the midline, the fat divides readily, there is little bleeding and the linea alba is easily identified. Where the connective tissue does not readily divide, it can be incised while maintaining traction. Gentle handling and minimizing undermining of the subcutaneous fat reduce the risks of seroma, hematoma, fat necrosis and wound infection.

The operative field for gastroplasty lies beneath and slightly superior to the upper abdominal midline incision. The barrel-chested morbidly obese patient, however, may present a considerable challenge in surgical exposure. Great quantities of abdominal wall and visceral fat, a high diaphragm, large spleen or liver and adhesions from any previous surgery pose difficulties in exposure. A good retractor system is essential for the optimum exposure necessary in most bariatric surgery; likewise, liver mobilization and resection of the properitoneal fat pad and xiphisternum should be performed as needed to maximize this exposure.

B. RESECTION OF PROPERITONEAL FAT. In order to improve exposure and wound closure, the properitoneal fat pad, which extends inferiorly from the xiphisternum, is excised.[19] This pad obscures visualization of the deep fascia and may be, in part, responsible for the relatively large percentage of incisional hernias reported in some bariatric surgery series. It is first identified when entering the abdomen and then squeezed medially from posterior to the rectus fascia. It is excised by pushing with partly-opened scissors along each midline fascial edge to the tip of the xiphisternum. In coursing superiorly, the round ligament is divided and ligated. This maneuver exposes the tip of the xiphoid process for dissection and excision as may be required.

C. XIPHISTERNECTOMY. Xiphisternal resection improves exposure. Before or after the properitoneal fat pad resection, the musculofascial insertions on the xiphoid process are incised with the cautery (Fig. 15.1A). The xiphoid is then resected sharply with 45°-angled scissor cuts made from either side and meeting in the midline (Fig. 15.1B). The superior epigastic vessels or their branches are usually divided by these maneuvers, and bleeding can be controlled with the cautery.

D. RETRACTOR SYSTEMS. The ideal retractor system for bariatric surgery should be rigidly based, easily adjusted, placed and replaced in the wound, and have blades and holding power adequate for the largest of patients while remaining immobile after fixation. The retractor may incorporate its own directable light-source[a,b,c] and it should take little time to apply. The retractor system should also allow the operating-table position to change and be easy to maintain. The system should not damage tissue or interfere with the surgeon's operative performance or physical comfort. There are a number of acceptable retractor systems with a selection of interchangeable blades available for bariatric surgery. Retractors currently used include the Iron Intern®,[a] Omni-Tract®,[b] Thompson®,[c] Gomez Poly-Tract® Upper Abdominal System,[d] Upper Hand® and Buckwalter®.[16,17,23,25,30,31] Most surgeons have a preference based upon familiarity and "feel," much like choices of other surgical instruments and suture materials. As long as the retractor system meets the surgeon's needs and preferences for adequate exposure, the particular brand is unimportant.

E. RETRACTOR MAINTENANCE AND FAMILIARITY. Most retractor systems have mechanical parts that may fail or be misplaced; therefore, always have a back-up system available. For any system new to the surgeon or the hospital, a dry-run practice session in the operating-room is time well spent. It is critical that the operating-room nurses understand proper set-up and maintenance procedures for the retractor system.

F. SPLENIC INJURY. Regardless of the specific retractor system, caution must be exercised in placing large retractor blades and performing surgical dissection in the morbidly obese.[18,19,22,28] The spleen has been injured by both deep retractors and laparotomy packs in the left upper quadrant. Anesthesia should be sufficiently deep, with adequate muscle relaxation and absence of bucking, before the deep retractor blades are placed intra-abdominally. Part of the splenic capsule may be avulsed by traction on the omentum, stomach or colon, especially if adhesions are present. Splenectomy should be avoided at all reasonable cost. We have successfully applied double and quadruple strength Thrombostat®-soaked Surgicel® to capsular tear sites and combined this with splenorrhaphy in one case as well. The injured spleen should be removed only after determination that repair cannot be done rapidly without undue blood loss. Hematoma in the left upper quadrant should be assiduously avoided.

G. LIVER MOBILIZATION. Hepatomegaly is common in the morbidly obese patient. It interferes with exposure of the gastroesophageal area and may require mobilization of the lateral segment of the left lobe.[28] Suitable lighting and retraction are essential for this maneuver. With two fingers placed behind the left triangular ligament, it can be incised in its bloodless mid-portion. The most left lateral portion of the ligament may contain a small vein. When present, the lateral portion of the ligament should be divided between large clips or ligatures. More medial extension of the incision in the coronary ligament is lim-

---

[a]Automated Medical Products, 2315 Broadway, New York, NY 10024

[b]Minnesota Scientific, 3839 Chandler Dr, Minneapolis, MN 55421.

[c]Thompson Surgical, P.O. Box 1113, Barrington, IL 60010.

[d]Pilling, 420 Delaware Dr., Fort Washington, PA 19034.

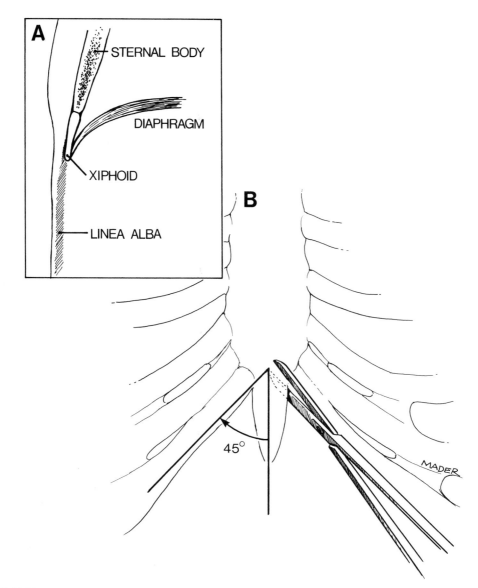

FIGURE 15.1A. Attachments of the diaphragm and linea alba to the xiphisternum are shown in sagittal section. Before resecting xiphisternum, its surface should be completely freed of these attachments and the laterally-attached rectus sheath fibers with an electrocautery. Once freed from its xiphisternal attachment, the diaphragm can be retracted much further upwards than the length of the xiphoid and significantly aid exposure. **B.** After being freed circumferentially, the xiphoid is resected with 45°-angled scissor cuts made from either side and meeting in midline. Bleeding from superior epigastric and other vessels is controlled with cautery.

ited by the hazard of injury to the hepatic veins. It is best to proceed under direct visualization. In this area, dissect no more than is needed to fold the lateral segment of the left lobe upon itself in much the same manner as in exposure for truncal vagotomy. Retractors are then positioned so that the esophagogastric junction and esophageal hiatus are fully exposed.

H. TILTING THE OPERATING-TABLE. We often tilt the operating-table 15 to 45° in reverse Trendelenburg position. By using gravity to pull the adjacent viscera caudally, the esophagogastric junction, the angle of His, the esophageal hiatus and adjacent structures are better visualized. To prevent the patient from sliding off the end of the table, the feet are made to rest securely on a metal footplate, cushioned with foam rubber and taped in place. It is prudent to select a table which tilts sufficiently before the patient is moved into the room for surgery.

DISSECTION

A. ENCIRCLING THE ESOPHAGUS. The esophagus is encircled in a manner similar to distal esophageal mobilization for truncal vagotomy under direct visualization.[17] The entire anterior phrenoesophageal ligament is usually not incised. With an adequate incision in the most left lateral portion of the phrenoesophageal ligament, the index finger frees the posterior esophageal attachments from the anterior aorta. A previously-placed nasogastric bougie helps to clarify the anatomy. With sweeping motions and gentle pressure, the distal posterior esophagus is mobilized. Dissection from each side of the esophagus under direct visualization is indicated when there is resistance to digital pressure, when a hiatal hernia is present or when previous surgery has been performed in this area. A soft rubber (Penrose) drain suffices to retract the esophagus during succeeding stages of the surgery and to later occlude the esophagus when pouch and staple-line testing are carried out (see Chapter 16). The small curved end of a narrow Deaver abdominal retractor may be looped under the esophagus and retracted towards the left to expose the diaphragmatic crura if needed.

B. DISSECTION OF THE POSTERIOR STOMACH. The posterior gastric cardia is difficult to visualize directly and needs to be bluntly separated from its posterior attachments in order to insert staplers and complete the gastroplasty.[17] Blunt dissection should be done gently. Where there is tissue resistance, dissection should be stopped and an attempt made from another direction. The usual starting points for this dissection are from an opening in the gastrohepatic ligament, the angle of His, the circular stapler hole made for a vertical banded gastroplasty or beside or behind the esophagus. Gentle bimanual dissection can be helpful, especially where prior surgery, pancreatitis or other inflammatory processes may have caused posterior gastric adhesions. Direct visualization of the starting point is important to avoid injury to the short gastric or the left gastric vessels and the spleen.

C. REPAIRING A HIGH POSTERIOR GASTRIC PERFORATION. A significant operative complication in obesity surgery is posterior gastric perforation. Repair of a high posterior gastric wall perforation, even in the non-obese patient, can be very difficult due to the inability to mobilize the posterior gastric wall sufficiently to suture the rent under direct visualization. Repair is easier via an anterior gastrotomy.[31]

Locate the gastric wall overlying the posterior perforation and place two stay sutures for a planned anterior gastrotomy. A vertically oriented, anterior gastrotomy is performed using the straight cutter-stapler (Fig. 15.2A). The posterior rent is visualized, and sutures or tissue forceps are placed across the full thickness of the posterior tear at either of its ends. Additional sutures are placed as needed to deliver the posterior tear through the anterior gastrotomy (Fig. 15.2B). Use a 55-mm straight double-row stapler to securely close the perforation, and trim off the small amount of redundant tissue (Fig. 15.2C). Allow the repaired posterior wall to retract to its normal position and inspect for any bleeding. Next, place sutures or tissue forceps across the anterior gastrotomy to approximate its edges, apply a 55 or 90-mm straight, double-row stapler to close the anterior gastrotomy and trim off the redundant tissue (Fig. 15.2D). Depending upon the extent of the posterior tear, spillage of gastric contents and other concerns, the gastroplasty may have to be postponed.

D. CLEARING THE ANGLE OF HIS FOR VERTICAL STAPLING. Approximately 2 to 3 cm of the greater curvature from the angle of His needs to be cleared in order to place four vertical staple rows through this area. It often contains fat which may be carefully divided with a long-handled dissecting scissors. If any blood vessels are seen or if the spleen is closely adjacent on the greater curvature, tissue should be divided between silk ligatures. It is best not to use metal tissue clips in this area, as they may interfere with the staples to be placed there when constructing the pouch.

CIRCULAR CUTTER-STAPLER

A. CIRCULAR CUTTER-STAPLER SELECTION. Any stapler size may be selected, but the larger sizes are recommended. A size 28 or 31 allows easier subsequent placement of the straight stapler and omental coverage. Figure 15.3 illustrates a buttonhole-like tear

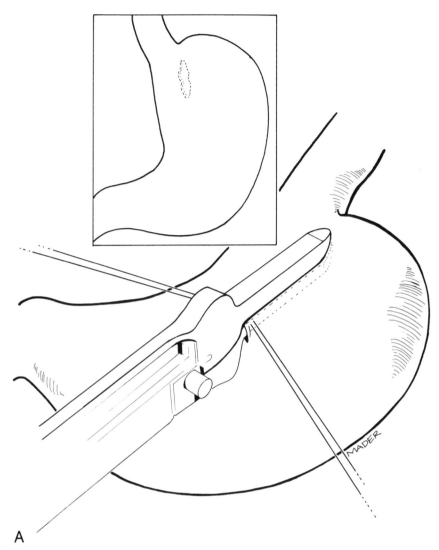

A

FIGURE 15.2A. As the technically easiest means of approach, an anterior gastrotomy is made over the posterior high gastric perforation using a straight cutter-stapler. The gastrotomy should be vertical towards the angle of His.

made by the circular cutter-stapler shaft, which could be a source of gastric leakage.

B. CHECK THE STAPLER. On rare occasions, the staples or the plastic washer in the anvil (stapler cap) of the instrument may be missing. The stapler may have been accidentally fired while being arranged on the back table or a reusable instrument containing a used cartridge may be handed to the surgeon. Therefore, it is important to confirm that all stapler parts are present before using each instrument.

C. CIRCULAR CUTTER-STAPLER HOLE PLACEMENT. Gastroplasty pouch size depends, among other things, upon the distance from the angle of His and the lesser curvature at which the circular cutter-stapler

is fired. A 30 Fr bougie or Ewald tube and an anvil from a previously fired, same-diameter circular cutter-stapler (anvil-spacer) are used to position the stapler an acceptable distance from the lesser curvature of the stomach (Fig. 15.4). The anvil-spacer, tagged with umbilical tape, is passed through an opening in the gastrohepatic ligament and held against the posterior gastric wall, lightly pressing against the more medial bougie. Care must be taken not to trap any lesser omentum under the anvil-spacer. The most craniad point on the anvil-spacer is adjusted to lie about 5 cm from the angle of His (Fig. 15.4—insert).

D. PASSING THE STAPLER THROUGH THE STOMACH. Using the indwelling tube, all air and fluid should be aspirated from within the

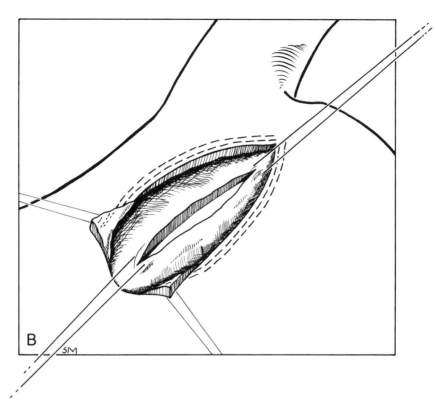

FIGURE 15.2B. Sutures/tissue forceps approximate and deliver the edges of the gastric perforation through the anterior gastrotomy.

stomach. A trochar, connected to the stapler shaft with a piece of tightly-fitting rubber tubing, is used to lead and guide the stapler shaft through the anterior and posterior gastric walls.[29] The trochar is pushed through the gastric walls against the center of the properly-positioned anvil-spacer; the trochar is then grasped by a sturdy clamp as it, the tubing and the stapler shaft are pulled smoothly through the anterior and posterior gastric walls. The trochar is obtained from a medium-sized wound evacuation drainage set; to facilitate manipulation and reduce risks of impalement of the pancreas or liver, it is cut to half its length and the tip reshaped by a machine shop prior to use (Fig. 15.4). It must be emphasized that the trochar should be thrust through the stomach in a single, deliberate, firm movement so that only one passage is made. Multiple thrusts will make multiple holes and, possibly, leaks.

E. THE CIRCULAR STAPLER AND ANVIL: COMMON PROBLEMS. The nut on the anvil must be completely threaded into the shaft of the circular cutter-stapler. If not, the instrument's jaws will be too far apart and the in-

strument cannot fire properly, resulting in inadequately cut gastric rings and staples that form poorly if at all. When properly aligned without tilt, the anvil threads onto the shaft and the shaft tip can be demonstrated to be flush with the anvil nut when the latter is fully tightened.

There may be obstacles to successfully threading the anvil onto the stapler shaft. One is tissue moving down the shaft into the anvil (Fig. 15.5). This interferes with secure threading of the anvil nut. Therefore, it is important to keep the stomach from sliding into the anvil while it is being threaded onto the stapler shaft. There are small metal tines inside the anvil of some models, which orient it relative to the stapler shaft; they may become bent and prevent complete threading of the anvil onto the stapler shaft. If this occurs, the tines should be re-bent to their original orientation parallel with the properly-placed stapler shaft.

F. STAPLER COMES OUT OF THE GASTRIC STAB-WOUND. If the trochar needle inadvertently separates from the rubber tubing or the shaft of the circular cutter-stapler has to be

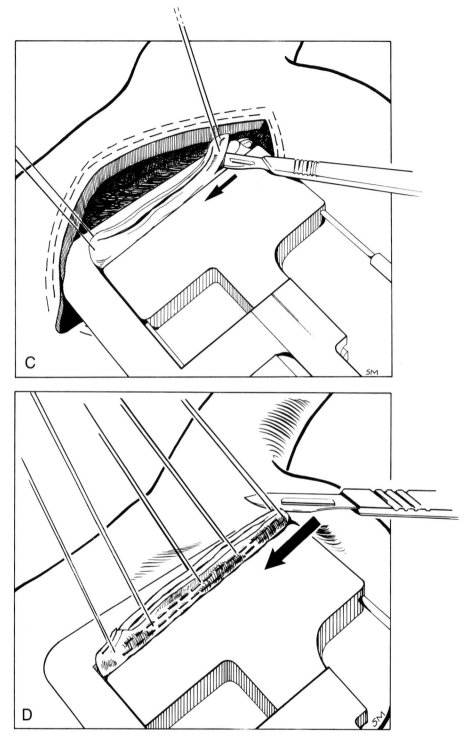

FIGURE 15.2C. A straight 55-mm stapler closes the perforation in the cardia and the redundant tissue is trimmed away. The scalpel cutting angle may be changed relatively to the type of stapler used and other variables. **D.** Sutures are placed across the anterior gastrotomy to approximate its edges, a 90-mm straight stapler applied to close the anterior gastrotomy and the redundant tissue trimmed with a heavy scissors or scalpel. The vertical staple rows for the gastroplasty can be made on each side of these staple-lines if the anterior gastrotomy was well-placed (see legend, Fig. 15.2A).

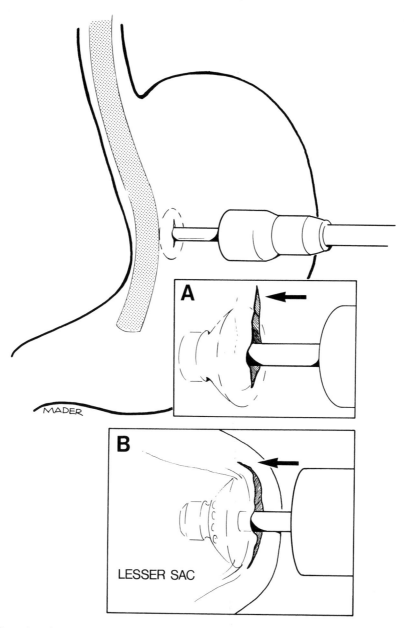

FIGURE 15.3. Central perforation made by stapler shaft may be widened inadvertently by stapler manipulations (Inset A). The central perforations may be widened further, and the final gastric buttons made smaller, by closing the stapler while the stomach walls are stretched by the anvil (Inset B). Extension of the gastric perforation beyond the margins of the stapler cut (arrows) could cause a gastric leak.

removed from the stomach for whatever reason, or it slips out accidentally, the surgeon may have difficulty in re-threading through both of the previously-made transgastric stab-wounds. It is essential to establish the location of the posterior gastric perforation site. The posterior gastric wall with the perforation is usually located by pushing against anterior gastric wall and rotating and everting stomach through the gastrohepatic omentum opening. Babcock clamps may be necessary to grasp posterior gastric wall. Alternatively, the lesser sac may have to be entered beside the greater curvature of the stomach and the greater curve rotated anteriorly and to the right, in order to find the posterior gastric perforation towards the lesser curvature. Place a 2-0 silk suture across the posterior gastric stab-wound (Fig. 15.6A). The ends of the silk suture are threaded through the central

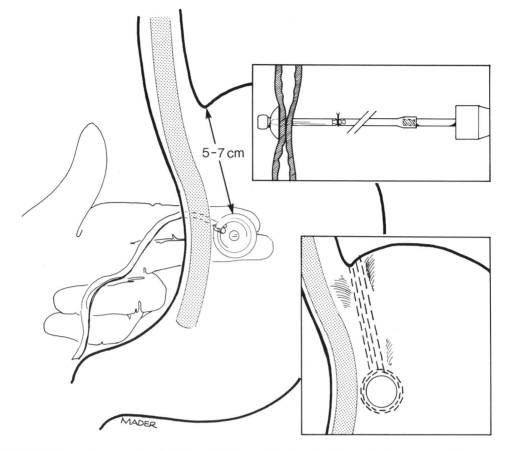

FIGURE 15.4. The anvil-spacer, tagged with umbilical tape, is held against the posterior gastric wall, its upper edge located 5 to 7 cm from the angle of His. It is lightly pressed against a 30 Fr bougie lying along the lesser curvature. The vertical staple-line (lower inset) should intersect with the circular hole at a medial point on its circumference.

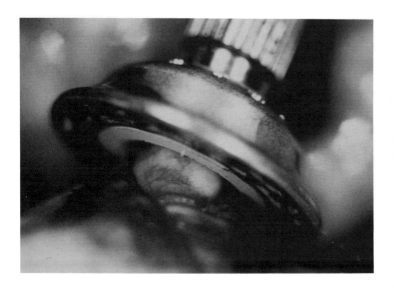

FIGURE 15.5. Gastric tissue tented along the stapler shaft into the anvil.

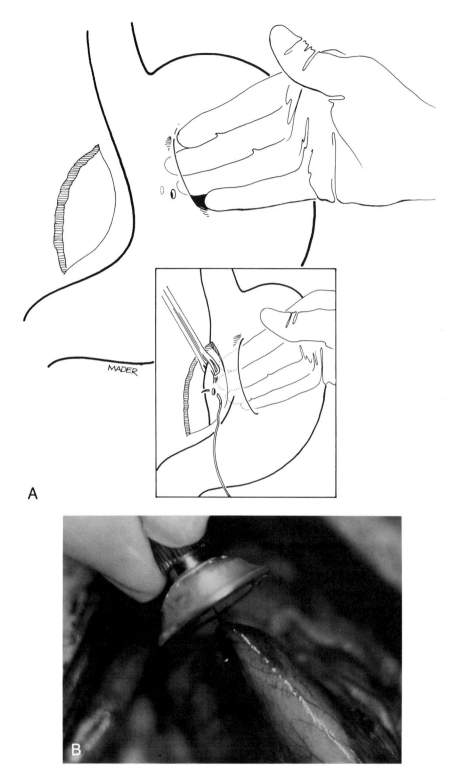

FIGURE 15.6A. The location of the posterior gastric perforation site is established and a 2-0 silk suture is placed across it. **B.** The anvil-spacer should be moved along the silk suture, under direct visualization to the posterior gastric perforation and securely held in place. Thus, the trochar is made to pass through the visible anterior perforation and the anvil-spacer-marked posterior hole without false passages.

hole in the anvil-spacer, with the base of the anvil oriented towards the surface of the stomach. The anvil-spacer should be guided under direct vision to the posterior gastric perforation and securely held in place. This permits the trochar to be properly oriented as it passes through the visible anterior perforation and the anvil-spacer-marked posterior hole and prevents any false passages (Fig. 15.6B).

G. REMOVING THE CATHETER GUIDE FROM THE STAPLER SHAFT. Removing the catheter guide tube from the stapler shaft may be a problem. Pulling the tube off may require such force that the liver or pancreas could be damaged. To prevent this, turn the cutter-stapler so that the flat side of its distal shaft is visible; use a scalpel blade to cut the tube on that flat surface and remove the tube.

H. STAPLING THE BOUGIE OR NASOGASTRIC TUBE. Staplers have been unintentionally fired across a portion of the intragastric nasogastric tube or the bougie. When this occurs, the gastric lumen is entered beside the staple-line (Fig. 17.7A). Babcock tissue forceps grasp the cut edges of the stomach, and the incision is continued parallel to and beside the staple-line (Fig. 15.7B). The tube is eventually visualized and withdrawn. The cut edges may be approximated with an inverting type of Connell stitch around the defect (Fig. 15.7C), reinforced with a row of inverting silk sutures (Fig. 15.7D). This type of defect has also been closed with a continuous over-and-over suture. If the resulting lumen is inadequate, another circular hole could be placed proximally or more laterally with adjustment of the straight stapler-lines and mesh band locations. The Marlex mesh band is next applied as usual. Prior to firing any stapler, we withdraw or assure mobility of any intragastric, perigastric or periesophageal tubes.

I. THE GASTRIC TISSUE RINGS. The gastric rings consist of circles of anterior and posterior gastric wall cut out by the circular cutter-stapler. Each gastric button has a central perforation made by the stapler shaft. These perforations can be torn radially by excessive stapler shaft movement (Fig. 15.3—inset A). The gastric walls adjacent to the stapler shaft can be stretched out over the stapler anvil if the stapler is pulled outwards through the wound (Fig. 15.3—inset B). If this causes a radial tear in the gastric wall to extend beyond the margins of the stapler cut, a gastric leak could result. Therefore, it is important to confirm that the two gastric rings are intact. If one is

incomplete, we suture reinforce the entire cut edge of the circle. Tightening the stapler too securely could cause a gastric leak. Avoidance of traction on the stomach by the stapler anvil or shaft and use of recommended stapler settings are important.

J. REINFORCING THE CUT WINDOW; HEMOSTASIS. The circular staple-line may be reinforced with continuous sutures of 2-0 or 3-0 absorbable or non-absorbable suture material. We place sutures only if the cut edge bleeds or a leak is demonstrated when distending the pouch with fluid. The sutures are placed just deep to the staple-line. Figure-of-8 3-0 chromic or silk sutures are used for hemostasis.

STRAIGHT STAPLER

A. VERTICAL STAPLE-LINES. The vertical staple-lines are placed by a 55-mm or 90-mm straight stapler with large (4.8-mm leg length) staples. If the distance to be stapled could exceed 55 mm, a 90-mm stapler should be used to prevent bunching of the enclosed tissue. A Penrose drain, rubber catheter or straight plastic tubing, tightly adherent to the tip of the anvil, is often used to guide the stapler between the circular stapler hole (window) and the angle of His. When the gastric walls are evenly spread out within the closed stapler-jaws, straight, well-formed staple-lines can be formed.[16] Two, more recently three, applications of a double-row stapler or a single application of a quadruple-row stapler plus one additional double-row stapler are employed. When the double-row stapler is applied and closed the second and third times, the gastric wall is aligned by a sponge-on-a-stick so that the previous staple-line is just visible beside the straight stapler-jaws; this produces four well-spaced (equidistant) rows of staples.

B. PLACING THE LINEAR STAPLER IN POSITION TO FIRE. A posterior gastric tunnel or track is developed from the circular window to the angle of His, wide enough to accommodate two fingers. The anvil end of the linear stapler is passed behind the stomach to the angle of His and the stapler-pin inserted. The stapler is tightened down and then fired after palpating and inspecting the stapler jaws to be sure that they include only the part of the stomach intended for stapling. The vertical staple-line should intersect with the window at a medial point on its circumference

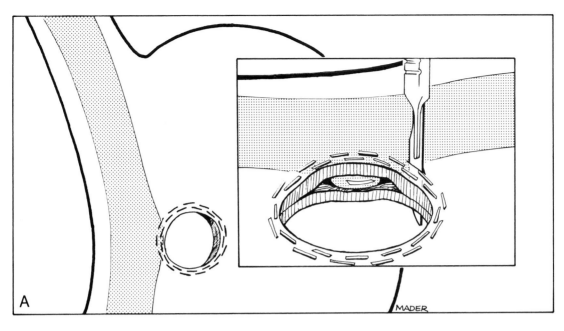

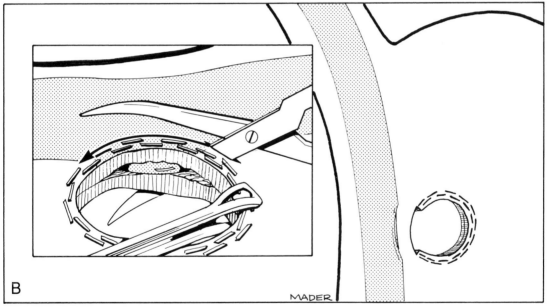

FIGURE 15.7A. When a stapler is fired across a portion of the nasogastric tube or the bougie, the gastric lumen is entered sharply beside the staple-line as shown. **B.** Babcock tissue forceps grasp the cut edges of the stomach, and the incision is continued parallel to and beside the staple-line.

and extend to the angle of His (Fig. 15.4—inset).

C. INSPECT THE STAPLE-LINES. Palpate the staple-line and visually inspect it as well. Staples which were not included in the gastric wall can be inspected to ascertain that they form the letter B. Less than fully secure, evenly placed staple-lines may later become the leading points for staple-line disruption and, if noted during surgery, should be re-

done. Particularly vulnerable locations are the intersections with the angle of His and the circular stapler hole.

TESTING THE POUCH

A. POUCH VOLUME MEASUREMENT CONTROVERSY. One approach to pouch construction is to measure the pouch's volume at a

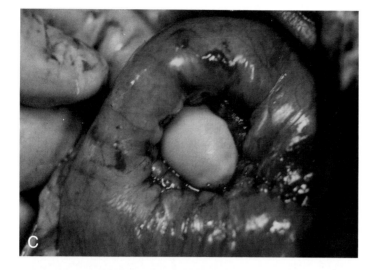

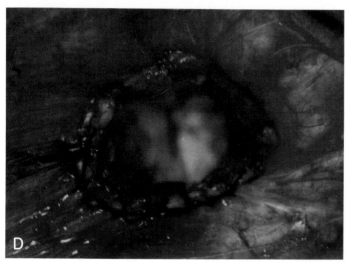

FIGURE 15.7C. The cut edges may be approximated with a Connell suture. **D.** The closure is reinforced with a row of inverting silk sutures.

given pressure, by pouring fluid into a tube elevated 70 cm above the cricoid cartilage, producing a 70 cm H_2O pouch pressure. Since this technique was developed, the trend has been toward smaller pouches; our average pouch volume is 15 mL. Even if a pouch is double the intended 15-mL volume, it still should be an adequately small size. However, some believe that exact knowledge of the pouch volume is essential.[29,32] Practical considerations have led us to simpler maneuvers that test for pouch leakage and provide a rough approximation of the pouch volume; three basic methods are described (see also Chapter 16).

B. POUCH TESTING TECHNIQUES

1. Through a Nasogastric Tube or Hollow Bougie (Fig. 15.8). Only a nasogastric tube or hollow bougie is left within the stomach, its tip placed at the level of the circular gastric window. Pass a Penrose drain through the gastric window around the lesser curvature. Place and close a Silverman or other curved atraumatic clamp over the Penrose drain. This acts as a protective pad for the stomach and leaves as much as possible of the medial half of the staple-line exposed. Have the anesthesiologist gently advance the tube until it reaches the Silverman clamp. Then, pull up on the Penrose drain placed earlier around the distal esophagus. Cross-clamp the stretched Penrose drain with a right-angle clamp as near as possible to the esophagus without entrapping any esophageal tissue in the instrument. Pull the right-angle clamp and Penrose drain anteriorly and apply a second right-angle clamp to the drain stretched between the esophagus and the first clamp (Fig. 15.8). If the tourni-

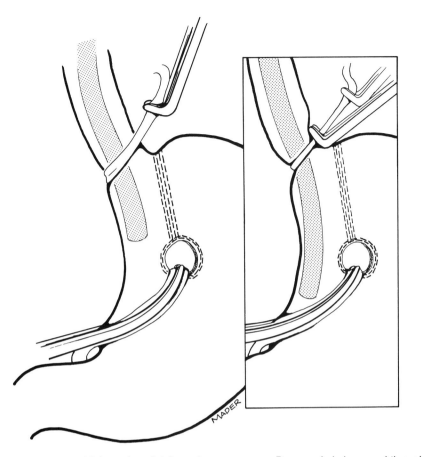

FIGURE 15.8. With the bougie withdrawn into distal esophagus, a narrow Penrose drain is passed through the gastric window and around the lesser curvature. A Silverman clamp is closed over the Penrose drain, allowing the medial half of the circular staple-line to be observed for leakage. The nasogastric tube is inserted to the level of the clamped Penrose drain. Then, a right-angle clamp is applied to the stretched peri-esophageal Penrose drain near the esophagus. A second right-angle clamp, applied onto the tented drain between the esophagus and the first right-angle clamp, produces water-tight seal for testing pouch integrity.

quet effect of the clamped Penrose drain is not tight enough, repeat this maneuver with a third clamp to secure a watertight seal around the tube. Similar gathering of the lower Penrose drain should not be done as it tends to obscure a critical portion of the staple-line when testing for leaks and could damage the staple-line.

The anesthesiologist next injects normal saline-containing antibiotics into the tube (any side-arm or sump tube must be clamped) with a plunger syringe in 5 mL or smaller volume increments until the desired pressure is reached or a leak is identified. If the pouch wall feels tense (like a fully inflated balloon), the pressure is acceptable, and, if no leak is found, pouch testing is complete.

Those who measure the pouch pressure have anesthesia personnel attach an open 60-mL syringe with the barrel removed to a 70-cm tubing. This tubing is connected to the tube which terminates in the gastric pouch. While the system is filled with sterile saline containing antibiotics, the syringe is kept elevated and all air is milked out. The system is filled with fluid to the tip of the syringe. If manual compression of the pouch moves the fluid column, the system is properly connected. The syringe is then elevated to 70 cm above the level of the cricoid and lowered to, or below, cricoid level. The final volume of the pouch is determined by subtracting the fluid in the syringe while it is located at each of these two positions. The tubing in the pouch displaces some of the saline, and some surgeons add a correction volume (e.g. 8 mL) to the final measured pouch volume.

2. Fluid Injected Directly into the Pouch.

Withdraw both the nasogastric tube and bougie into the distal esophagus. Cross-clamp the esophagogastric junction and the gastric window over the Penrose drains in the same locations as in Method 1. Puncture the gastric pouch wall with a 20-gauge plastic angiocatheter or butterfly needle into the pouch lumen. The surgeon may then directly inject the antibiotic-containing fluid into the pouch, observing for leaks.

An objection to this method is that the catheter or butterfly needle may slip partially or completely out of place. Also, solution can inadvertently be injected into the wall of the pouch.[24]

3. Balloon Inflated Inside Pouch. A balloon, mounted on the distal end of an Ewald-type or similar nasogastric tube (extra-length Pingree-Jack Tube®, Wilson-Cook), is passed into the pouch by the anesthesiologist and inflated. The balloon is assumed to conform to the entire pouch dimensions; this may not be true, rendering the measurement inaccurate.

C. POUCH TESTING PREFERENCE. We prefer the first method described and inject antibiotic solution in normal saline through the hollow bougie or nasogastric tube. In the event that a leak is present, only antibiotic solution is leaking into the peritoneal cavity. Some surgeons inject diluted methylene blue or plain sterile saline. We use dye only if we cannot locate the suspected leak. Once the dye is used and a leak persists, or there are multiple leaks, the tissue is so stained that it is difficult to locate any leak with or without the use of dye.

POLYPROPYLENE MESH

A. PREPARING THE MESH. Large sheets of polypropylene mesh can be most economically cut into individually sterilized pieces, each satisfactory for banding a gastroplasty stoma. One entire edge of each mesh sheet has a thickened ridge. The sheet should be cut across (perpendicular to) this thickened edge at 15-mm intervals, extending each cut to 9 cm in length. The mesh stretches less when cut in this direction than when cut parallel to the thickened edge.[31] The mid-length area (4.5 cm) is marked with metal clips so that measurement may be accurate when the mesh is wrapped around the gastroplasty stoma.

B. CLEARING THE LESSER CURVATURE FOR THE MESH BAND. Sufficient gastrohepatic omentum must be cleared from the lesser curvature opposite the gastric window to loosely accommodate the 15-mm-wide mesh band. Although some claim to make an ample opening by blunt dissection, it is safer to divide the tissue between 00-silk ligatures passed on right-angle tissue clamps. Demarcation of the lesser curvature from fat may be made more apparent by bimanually palpating both sides of the stomach and gastrohepatic ligament, with one hand within the lesser sac and the other immediately anteriorly. Injury to the neural or vascular structures along the lesser curvature should be avoided and is best assured if the area of dissection remains near the gastric surface.

C. WRAPPING THE MESH AROUND THE POUCH STOMA. Some Marlex mesh bands do not lie completely flat; they are slightly convex between their long sides. If this occurs, orient the mesh so that the convex surface lies on the tissue to be banded. Pass the mesh around the posterior wall of the stoma between the lesser curvature of the stomach and the gastric window with a right-angled tissue forceps. After wrapping the mesh collar around the stoma, check that the material is not twisted upon itself or wrinkled. It is important to avoid having edges or raised surfaces of the mesh which may erode into or through the gastric wall. The mesh is best wrapped and sutured with the bougie inside the lumen of the stoma. When difficulties arise in reinserting the bougie which was withdrawn into the esophagus during pouch testing, we use no intraluminal stent and later insert the nasogastric tube through the stomal lumen for postoperative suction; we have not had a stomal obstruction in any such cases.

D. USING SMALLER MESH BAND CIRCUMFERENCE SIZES. Most surgeons use the 5.0-cm band circumference. Studies are ongoing concerning the use of a 4.5-cm band circumference. While we are aware of the increased risk of stomal outlet stenosis which may occur with use of this size band, we are now employing it in all our gastroplasties and have not encountered any significant problems yet.

E. SECURING THE MESH COLLAR TO ITSELF. Polypropylene 2-0 is commonly used to suture the non-thickened end of the mesh to each side of the band at the level of the clip marker. It is helpful to overlap the band on itself for another centimeter and use several metal clips to secure the overlapped segment superiorly and inferiorly before trimming off the redundant material. The clips reinforce the sutures and also mark the non-radioopaque band's location in abdominal radiographs.

F. PERISTOMAL OMENTAL WRAP. The largest size of circular-cutter stapler leaves an opening across the stomach >2 cm in diameter. There is adequate room to pass an edge of the mid-portion of greater omentum through the hole, wrap it around the lesser curvature and attach it to itself with 3-0 silk sutures which gently approximate the tissue, thereby covering the mesh band (Fig. 15.9). If a perforation later occurs, the omental covering may seal it off. If later re-stapling of the vertical line becomes necessary, the circular stapler hole may be penetrated easily with gentle, blunt dissection.

The omental fat which lies lateral to the circular hole on the greater curvature of the stomach should not be used to cover or wrap the polypropylene mesh collar. It can cause the collar to be tilted towards the left and distort the stomal outlet resulting in partial or complete obstruction.

TEMPORARY GASTROSTOMY

Where concern for early stomal outlet stenosis due to edema or functionally-induced vomiting is high or there have been significant technical problems during surgery, a Stamm temporary feeding gastrostomy in the distal stomach should be strongly considered.[21] It should also be used as an adjunct to most revisional or gastric bypass procedures. The tube remains in place for at least two weeks postoperatively and until the patient is able to ingest adequate fluids, pureed foods and all prescribed medications orally. Meticulous attention to detail is essential, since death from peritonitis associated with a gastrostomy tube, inserted during a gastroplasty procedure, can occur.[33]

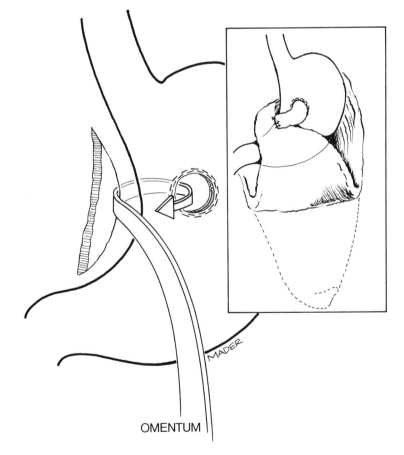

OMENTUM

FIGURE 15.9. A pedicle of the **mid**-portion of greater omentum from the transverse colon, not under tension, is passed into lesser sac through the opening in the gastrohepatic omentum. It is then brought out from behind the stomach through the circular gastric hole, wrapped around the lesser curvature including the left gastric vessels and sutured to itself. It covers the mesh band completely and seals potential leaks which may occur in its area of coverage.

ESOPHAGEAL HIATUS CRURAL APPROXIMATION

Symptomatic gastro-esophagal reflux may not completely resolve after gastroplasty. Our patients who have had esophageal hiatus crural approximation are asymptomatic postoperatively with the exception of a mild, transient dysphagia in some. With adequate exposure and a 30 Fr bougie in place, each crus is identified and held with extra-length Allis tissue clamps. Three or more No. 2 silk, simple, interrupted sutures are placed deeply in the crura and gently approximated. We tag the most craniad suture with a large metal clip to orient the uppermost part of the repair during later upper GI contrast studies. With the bougie in place, the tip of the forefinger should be able to pass along the esophagus above the most superior suture. We prefer to perform this procedure prior to the gastroplasty.

FASCIAL CLOSURE

To close the midline fascia, we use a 1.5 meter long, No. 2, monofilament, polypropylene suture on a large tapered needle, placed as a continuous, running suture from either end of the wound, at least 1.5 cm from the cut edges. The knots are inverted or buried deep to the fascia. Others have used 0 monofilament stainless steel wire, No. 2 Dexon® and other materials, continuous, interrupted or as retention sutures for closure.[18,25,28,30,31,34]

REFERENCES

1. Buckwalter JA: A prospective comparison of the jejunoileal and gastric bypass operations for morbid obesity. World J Surg 1:757–768, 1977.
2. Buchwald H, Schwartz MZ, Varco RL: Surgical treatment of obesity. Adv Surg 7:235–255, 1973.
3. Hallberg, D, Holmgren U: Bilio-intestinal shunt: A method and a pilot study for treatment of obesity. Acta Chir Scand 145:405–408, 1979.
4. Hermreck AS, Jewell WR, Hardin CA: Gastric bypass for morbid obesity: results and complications. Surgery 80:498–505, 1976.
5. Jewell WR, Hermreck AS, Hardin CA: Complications of jejunoileal bypass for morbid obesity. Arch Surg 110:1039–1042, 1975.
6. Linner JH: Comparative effectiveness of gastric bypass and gastroplasty. Arch Surg 117:695–700, 1982.
7. MacLean LD, Rochon G, Munro M, et al: Intestinal bypass for morbid obesity: a consecutive personal series. Can J Surg 23:54–59, 1980.
8. Martin EW, Mojzisik C, Carey LC: Complications of gastric restrictive operations in morbidly obese patients. Surg Clin North Am 63:1181–1190, 1983.
9. Peltier G, Hermreck AS, Moffat RE, et al: Complications following gastric bypass procedures for morbid obesity. Surgery 86:648–654, 1979.
10. Printen KJ, Mason EE: Gastric surgery for relief of morbid obesity. Arch Surg 106:428–431, 1973.
11. Reinhold RB: Critical analysis of long-term weight loss following gastric bypass. Surg Gynecol Obstet 155:385–393, 1982.
12. Rucker RD, Horstmann J, Schneider PD, et al: Comparisons between jejunoileal and gastric bypass operations for morbid obesity. Surgery 92:241–249, 1982.
13. Shamblin JR, Shamblin AE: Gastroplasty in morbid obesity: observations in 300 patients. South Med J 78:1036–1040, 1985.
14. Halverson JD: Obesity surgery in perspective. Surgery 87:119–127, 1980.
15. Brolin RE: Calibrated gastrojejunostomy for gastric bypass using the EEA stapler. Contemp Surg 26:40–44, 1985.
16. Pace WG, Martin JEW Jr, Tetirick T, et al: Gastric partitioning for morbid obesity. Ann Surg 190:392–400, 1979.
17. Pories WJ, Flickinger EG, Meelheim D, et al: Effectiveness of gastric bypass over gastric partition in morbid obesity: consequences of distal gastric and duodenal exclusion. Ann Surg 196:384–393, 1982.
18. Smith LB, Fricke FJ, Graney AS: Results and complications of gastric partitioning: 4 year follow-up of 300 morbidly obese patients. Am J Surg 146:815–819, 1983.
19. Buckwalter JA, Herbst CA Jr: Complications of gastric bypass for morbid obesity. Am J Surg 139:55–60, 1980.
20. Carey LC, Martin EW, Mojzisik C: The surgical treatment of morbid obesity. Current Prob Surg 21:1–78, 1984.
21. Deitel M, Bojm MA, Atin MD, et al: Intestinal bypass and gastric partitioning for morbid obesity: a comparison. Can J Surg 25:283–289, 1982.
22. Freeman JB, Burchett HJ: A comparison of gastric bypass and gastroplasty for morbid obesity. Surgery 88:433–444, 1980.
23. Gomez CA: Gastroplasty in the surgical treatment of morbid obesity. Am J Clin Nutr 33:406–415, 1980.
24. Hartford CE: Near-total gastric bypass for morbid obesity. Arch Surg 119:282–286, 1984.
25. Jones KB: Horizontal gastroplasty: A safe, effective alternative to gastric bypass in the surgical management of morbid obesity. Am J Surg 50:128–131, 1984.
26. Lechner GW, Callender AK: Subtotal gastric exclusion and gastric partitioning: a randomized prospective comparison of 100 patients. Surgery 90:637–644, 1981.
27. Mason EE, Printen KJ, Barron P, et al: Risk reduction in gastric operations for obesity. Ann Surg 190:158–165, 1979.
28. Thompson WR, Amaral JA, Caldwell MD, et al: Complications and weight loss in 150 consecutive gastric exclusion patients. Am J Surg 146:602–612, 1983.

29. Mason EE: Vertical banded gastroplasty for obesity. Arch Surg 117:701–706, 1982.

30. Lechner GW, Elliott DW: Comparison of weight loss after gastric exclusion and partitioning. Arch Surg 118:685–692, 1983.

31. Deitel M, Jones BA, Petrov I, et al: Vertical banded gastroplasty: results in 233 patients. Can J Surg 29:322–324, 1986.

32. Alder LA, Terry BE: Measurement and standardization of the gastric pouch in gastric bypass. Surg Gynecol Obstet 144:762–763, 1977.

33. Mason EE, Printen KJ, Hartford CE, et al: Optimizing results of gastric bypass. Ann Surg 182:405–415, 1975.

34. Holian DK: Biliopancreatic bypass for morbid obesity. Contemp Surg 21:55–62, 1982.

16

Calibration of Pouch or Channel Size

BOYD E. TERRY

In the relatively brief history of gastric restrictive procedures, one sees consistent success only after precise volumetric measurement became standard. To be sure, stabilization of the stoma at a standard diameter of approximately 10 mm was an essential additive for the small pouch to give prolonged success.

Pouch size quickly dropped from 150 to 100 to 50 and 25 mL as weight loss was observed to correlate with the small pouch. Surgeons, careful in observation, now have many special ways to make the pouch small with "uniformity" of execution without actual volumetric measurement. It may be adequate to proceed this way if the pouch is indeed in the 20–50 mL volume range, but an undetected error outside this range may jeopardize good results and lead to a remedial procedure or possibly wrongly place blame on the patient for poor compliance and ofttimes condemn the patient to a hands-off policy regarding remedial procedures. The most secure policy is one that allows the surgeon great confidence in the initial pouch size.

IS THERE AN OPTIMUM POUCH SIZE?

There is a feeling among surgeons who treat obesity that the pouch cannot be made too small, in order to avoid stretching by the adventuresome eater—one who is resistant to satiety signals. Yet it must be admitted that, in order to take solid food in adequate amounts to provide the R.D.A. for protein without snacking continually, there *is* a volume too small. To date, this has not been determined, but I suggest that under 20 mL may be a hazard. This ideal pouch should provide a satiety signal when solid food is ingested after careful chewing so that a minimum of 1.5 to 2.5 ounces of protein can be processed per meal. Three meals per day would provide the R.D.A. for protein. Some additional calories could be accepted plus added vitamins and minerals. Behavior is modified to adapt to this individualized quantity of food chosen for its nutrient composition. The stress on the staple-lines in proportion to the initial volume of the pouch when meal tested has not been studied. Also, esophageal reflux related to small pouch size has not been tested systematically.

Of greatest concern must be to provide a pouch with capacity for adequate nutrition, rather than anticipate later stretching to an acceptable size. To prevent a small pouch from stretching, behavior modification must be the answer. Many construct such a small pouch that food is restricted to liquids or to small frequent meals—not a sound foundation for good nutritional habits based on specific individual needs.

CALIBRATION PRINCIPLES

The following are considered important.
1. Use a simple, precise technique which is controlled as much as possible by the surgeon.
2. Measure volume and pressure *before* firing the final staple-line in pouch construction:
   a. Adjust volume if needed;
   b. Avoid testing the fresh staple-line.
3. Record measurements to correlate with later pouch performance in regard to staple stability and satiety signal.

OPTIONAL TECHNIQUES

1. For vertical gastroplasty, with a 32-Fr hollow esophageal tube defining the lumen of the new gastric pouch, the stapling device is positioned to anticipate a predetermined volume and tightened but not fired. Occlusion of the inlet and outlet allows volumetric filling with saline to a pressure of 70 cm H_2O measured vertically by the anesthesiologist from the level of the pouch (Fig. 16.1). A pressure of 70 cm H_2O was chosen, because this will not disrupt the muscle fibers but will distend the pouch. The volume may be adjusted by repositioning the stapler and repeating the measurement. When the volume is satisfactory, the pressure is released and the stapler is fired. The volume may be 15–20 mL plus the standard volume displaced by the tube.[1]

2. A 30-Fr (1 cm diameter) hollow tube with a balloon cuff mounted on the distal part of the shaft (Pingree-Jack Gastroplasty Calibration Tube, Wilson-Cook, Winston Salem, NC 27105) can be used to measure the volume (Fig. 16.2). However, the shape and compliance of the balloon make the pressure measurement variable. The volume is approximate, as the pressure is undetermined because of balloon tension. Of great concern is to avoid pinching the inflated balloon in the staple-line; the balloon is deflated before the staples are fired. Checking volume *after* stapling would be a distinct hazard to the staple-line. Again, inflation volume is added to the

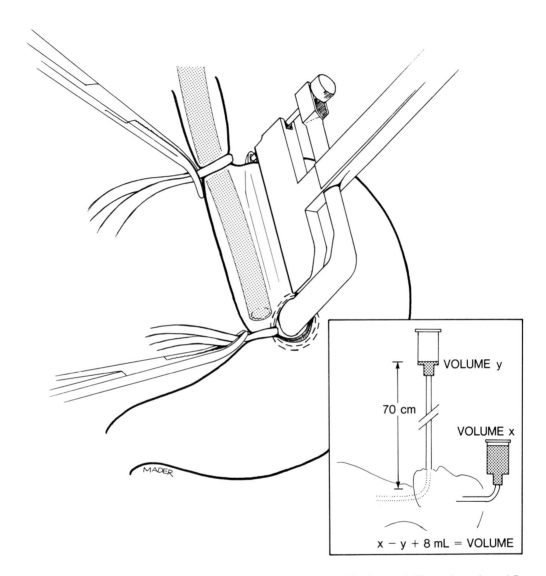

FIGURE 16.1. The 32-Fr Ewald tube is positioned so that all holes are within the pouch. The peri-esophageal Penrose drain is tightened. The lower end of the pouch is occluded by a Penrose drain through the window and through the tunnel developed deep to lesser curve adipose tissue and nerves of Laterjet around the outlet. The surgeon strips all air from the tube and pouch, and directs the anesthesiologist to measure volume of saline in the bulb of a syringe attached to the Ewald tube at 70 cm above the cricoid *and* at cricoid level. The pouch volume equals the difference in volume between the 2 levels plus 8 mL for tube displacement. Stapler is adjusted so that pouch volume is 20–30 mL.

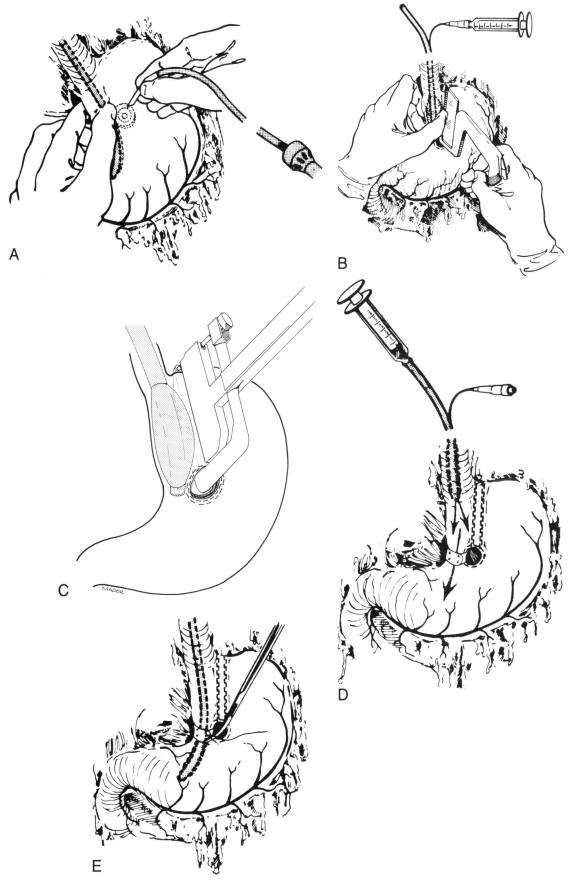

volume displaced by the tube to define the final volume. Lack of a pressure determination may lead to over-stretching the pouch for a given volume.

3. A needle inserted into the pouch with the manometer controlled by the surgeon is the technique I prefer (Fig. 16.3). A 32-Fr bougie is passed, the window cut and the collar applied. The stapler is passed and snugged up against the bougie, forming a taut tube along lesser curve. The stapler is closed (not fired). A 22-gauge butterfly needle is inserted tangentially into the pouch, piercing the outer layer of the bougie. The bougie is removed, thereby placing the needle in the gastric lumen. A Potts clamp is placed carefully at the esophagogastric junction. Thus, esophageal mobilization is avoided. The pouch is stripped of gas. The outlet stoma is occluded by the left forefinger against the heel of the stapler, and the assistant inflates the pouch to the desired volume (20–30 mL). The pressure is measured through the manometer side-arm at 70 cm H_2O above the pouch level. Adjustment of the position of the stapler is done if necessary, before firing the stapleline.

4. For gastric bypass, the stapler is closed across proximal stomach but not fired. The pouch is aspirated of air and fluid by the anesthesiologist, and the esophagus is occluded around the suction catheter by the surgeon's right thumb and index finger. The anesthesiologist then instills saline via an open syringe at 5-mL increments, while volume is measured at 70 cm pressure (70 cm above the cricoid). The volume is usually 12–15 mL, which may be simply injected and visualized or palpated with experience.

Originally for gastric bypass, we used a nasogastric tube marked with arch-bar rubber bands at 5 and 12 cm from the tip. The bands were palpated at the gastroesophageal junction, which enabled marking a site 5 cm on lesser curve and 12 cm on greater curve for transection.[2] This method of pouch measurement lacked precision, resulting in a volume of 50–100 mL; however, this act of measurement led to more optimal pouch volume determinations. Gastric bypass advocates often consider precise pouch measurement to be less important because of the dumping and malabsorptive features of that operation.

CONCLUSION

In conclusion, I continue to measure each pouch volume, aware that initial estimates occasionally require adjustment. Differing methods give reproducible measurements. One must be aware that a given volume may be in addition to tube displacement. Each surgeon must certify to himself a method of achieving reproducible pouch volume, to give predictable patient response. In this way follow-up may eventually define the optimal pouch volume.

SUMMARY

Three available methods for achieving reproducible volume measurement in construction of the gastric restrictive pouch are discussed. The preferred method is the use of a reproducible volume standard at a given pressure. This method makes a valid statement to guide the surgeon and to protect the patient's interest. Subsequent changes in the patient's pouch are influenced by many variables; initial pouch volume should be controlled.

REFERENCES

1. Mason EE: Vertical banded gastroplasty for obesity. Arch Surg 117:701–706, 1982.
2. Alder RL, Terry BE: Measurement and standardization of the gastric pouch in gastric bypass. Surg Gynecol Obstet 144:762–763, 1977.

FIGURE 16.2. A. Pingree-Jack tube is passed by the anesthesiologist through the mouth into stomach and used as a guide for the site of the gastric window. The esophagus is not mobilized. B and C. Jaws of TA stapler are closed. The anesthesiologist then pulls tube up into the intended pouch and inflates the balloon with 10-mL increments of air or saline, while the surgeon palpates the balloon. The pouch should be tense with a volume of <50 mL in the balloon. The balloon is deflated, and the stapler is either moved towards lesser curvature (and the balloon volume rechecked to be <50 mL with the pouch full), or fired. D. The shaft of the deflated balloon tube is passed through the outlet to act as a tube as Marlex mesh or other material is placed around the outlet. E. As the tube is pulled back, dye may be injected by the anesthesiologist through the central lumen to check for leaks.

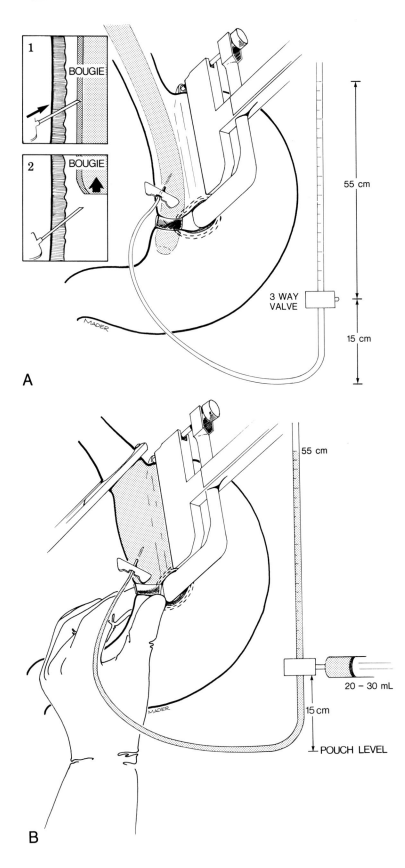

FIGURE 16.3. A and B. Vertical channel occluded between Potts clamp at cardia and left index finger and thumb of surgeon against TA stapler at window. No. 22 needle in channel permits instillation of 20–30 mL of saline, with pressure measured on manometer to 70 cm H_2O (vertical height above stomach).

17

Radiologic Evaluation of the Partitioned Stomach

JOEL B. FREEMAN
ZOHAIR Y. AL-HALEES
RICHARD E. SEPPALA

Gastric operations for morbid obesity which have developed over the past quarter century can be classifed broadly as follows: gastric bypass with loop gastrojejunostomy, gastric bypass with Roux-en-Y gastrojejunostomy, biliopancreatic-enteric bypass, various horizontal gastroplasties, vertical gastroplasties, and gastric wrap. Vertical banded gastroplasty and Roux-en-Y gastric bypass are currently the most utilized operations. Horizontal gastroplasties had an unacceptably high long-term failure-rate.[1]

Gastric partitioning procedures are subject to many potential complications, especially leaks, stenosis and failure to produce the desired weight loss. The radiographic interpretation postoperatively can be difficult. It is important to have full cooperation between surgeon and radiologist. The surgeon should be in the radiology suite during emergency diagnostic procedures and when the radiologist is evaluating pouch and stoma sizes. The surgeon should explain the operation which had been performed. The radiologist should be both interested and knowledgeable in interpreting gastric partitioning films. Prompt, accurate diagnosis of complications is extremely important for proper management. The radiologic procedures that can be used include:

1. Plain radiographs.
2. Contrast examination of the upper GI tract.
3. Ultrasonography.
4. Computerized axial tomography.
5. Gallium scans.
6. Oral isotope studies.

Ultrasound, computerized axial tomography, and gallium scans can be helpful in diagnosing and localizing intra-abdominal abscesses. Oral isotope studies are used to evaluate the emptying time of a fundic remnant and gastroesophageal reflux.[2,3] However, plain radiographs and upper GI contrast studies are most important. The spectrum of complications includes:

1. Leaks with or without intra-abdominal abscesses.
2. Proximal pouch dilatation.
3. Staple-line disruption, early and delayed.
4. Stomal obstruction, early and late.
5. Stomal dilatation.
6. Stomal ulceration.
7. Staple-line ulceration.

PLAIN FILMS

We do not routinely obtain plain roentgenograms of the chest and abdomen in the early postoperative period, unless there is clinical suspicion of a leak or perforation. Chest radiographs may demonstrate atelectasis, pneumonia or pleural effusion. One should be cautious in interpreting such films because, even in the presence of some pulmonary pathology, it is mandatory to rule out an intra-abdominal source. High-quality films in the supine and erect or lateral decubitus positions are obtained. A pleural effusion, localized air bubbles (the "soapsuds" sign), or extra-intestinal air-fluid levels suggest an intra-abdominal abscess (Fig. 17.1). Free air may be seen, posing the difficult distinction between a perforation and air remaining from the operation. Fluoroscopic demonstration of decreased movement or paralysis of a hemidiaphragm, particularly the left, suggests a subphrenic abscess, especially when combined with a subphrenic fluid collection or pleural effusion. Such findings represent leaks until proven otherwise. Pleural effusions should be aspirated with caution, as

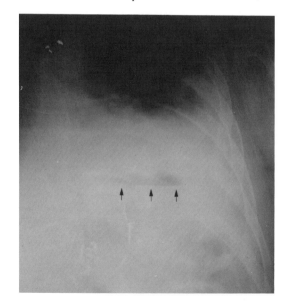

FIGURE 17.1. Patient with fever, tachycardia and left pleural effusion 4 days after gastroplasty. Note the left upper quadrant air-fluid level, supporting the diagnosis of a left subphrenic abscess which was secondary to a leak. Multiple bubbles of air (the "soapsuds" sign") would indicate the same problem.

subdiaphragmatic purulent material may be inadvertently needled, contaminating the chest and leading to empyema.

Routine scout films should be obtained prior to upper GI contrast studies, particularly if a previous leak was studied by barium. Otherwise, barium remaining in the peritoneal cavity will lead the physician to believe that a leak persists.

In gastric bypass, the distal excluded pouch cannot be easily examined radiographically except by abdominal plain films or a distal gastrostomy tube. The outdated loop gastric bypass allowed retrograde endoscopic examination through the afferent limb into the excluded stomach, but this was quite difficult. However, as thinner and longer endoscopes have become available, such examinations are being performed successfully even in those gastric bypass patients with a Roux-en-Y hook-up.[4,5] Routine insertion of a tube gastrostomy into the distal pouch eliminates the problem of distal pouch distention in the postoperative period.

UPPER GI CONTRAST STUDIES

We routinely obtain an upper GI single-contrast barium study on the fifth postoperative day to rule out a leak or obstruction and to provide a baseline comparison for subsequent examinations (Fig. 17.2A, B and C). A double contrast study with effervescent agents is contraindicated, because of the danger of pouch distention and perforation.

Emergency contrast studies are carried out whenever there is a clinical indication. We prefer to be in the radiology suite with the radiologist whenever a postoperative gastroplasty patient is ill. Superior plain films are obtained, and one can proceed immediately with contrast studies. Using this method, a sick patient can be wheeled to the X-ray department and all appropriate films obtained in less than one hour. Conversely, staging the films leads to procrastination. Delays in the diagnosis of a leak are the commonest cause of death. The studies may have to be repeated one to several days later. We have had patients referred with "normal" upper GI studies in whom subsequent re-examinations revealed leaks or abscesses.

If a leak is suspected, a water-soluble contrast medium, such as Hypaque or Gastrografin, is used initially, followed by barium if a leak is not demonstrated. Leaks cannot be ruled out unless a negative water-soluble contrast study is followed by a barium examination (Fig. 17.3A and B). The latter could be eliminated if one has made the clinical decision to re-operate, although we prefer to confirm and note the location of a leak pre-operatively. In one study, 17 of 30 upper GI series were negative despite free perforation.[6] Hence, exploration should be performed based on clinical grounds, even if all the above investigations are negative.

Detection of leaks at re-operation can be difficult.[6,7] Both surgeon and radiologist should remember that while the primary purpose of the study is to locate an anastomotic leak, there is always the possibility that inadvertent damage had occurred to the esophagus or greater curve of the stomach, particularly if the short gastric vessels were divided during mobilization. The distal Roux-en-Y anastomosis must also be visualized. Leaks may occur from displaced gastrostomy or jejunostomy tubes. This may be demonstrated by injecting 20 mL of contrast medium into the tube in question (Fig. 17.4). Pressure necrosis from the tip of a nasogastric tube in the proximal pouch is another potential cause. Finally, there is the possibility that careless use of the electrocautery or a closing suture may have inadvertently damaged the stomach (or intestine). Hence, a number of different sites need to be examined when considering a leak. It is important that such patients also *drink* contrast material, even if a nasogastric tube is in place. Otherwise, high esophageal or gastric leaks may not be detected.

Upper GI contrast examinations must be done in the erect and supine positions. The latter assures filling of the fundus (Fig. 17.2A–1). Oblique views are important to adequately demonstrate the stoma and to accurately distinguish between staple disruption and leaks.[8]

There is a risk of aspiration after contrast studies with water-soluble agents if the throat has been anesthetized (as occurs when the study follows a dilatation) or if the stoma is obstructed. To avoid aspiration in the former case, delay the procedure for 90 minutes if possible. If there is an element of obstruction present, the contrast material should be aspirated via a nasogastric tube after the study is terminated, to prevent aspiration and because water-soluble materials can cause pouch distention or hemorrhage.[9]

A left pleural effusion, left lower lobe pneumonia or atelectasis or unusual air-fluid level in the left upper quadrant suggests a sub-

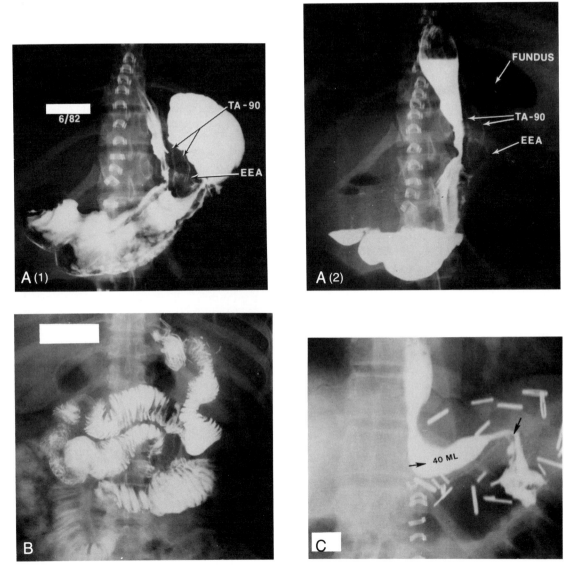

FIGURE 17.2A–1. Normal appearance of a vertical banded gastroplasty 5 days postoperatively. The two rows of parallel staples (TA-90) and the circular row (EEA) are seen creating a long, narrow pouch. The constriction to the viewer's left of the EEA staple-line indicates the position of the Marlex ring. **A–2.** GI series with vertical banded gastroplasty demonstrates air in the fundus—that portion of the stomach to the patient's left of the vertical staple-lines. This area must be filled with barium by proper positioning (as in Fig. 17.2A–1) or it may be confused with an abscess cavity. There is a degree of obstruction at the Marlex collar, and the channel proximally, as well as the distal esophagus, has dilated as a result. This demonstrates the vast capacity of even a very small gastric pouch to dilate. The same can occur with overeating. **B.** Normal appearance of a Roux-en-Y gastric bypass on the fifth postoperative day. One can see the gastroesophageal junction, gastric pouch and gastrojejunal anastomosis. The dilatation in the middle of the figure is the area of Roux-en-Y anastomosis. **C.** Normal appearance of a horizontal gastroplasty. A very small pouch is seen with two rows of horizontally applied staples below the pouch and a narrow greater curve outlet (arrow). The large air cavity represents the distal stomach.

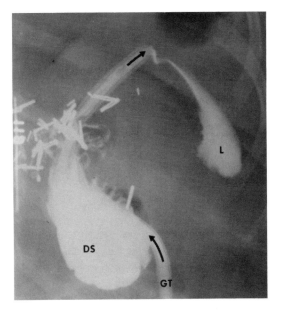

FIGURE 17.4 Demonstration of a leak (L) by the retrograde injection of barium through the gastrostomy tube (GT). DS = distal segment. The operative report of this referred patient indicated that the revisionary operation was extremely difficult. During such operations, the gastroesophageal junction may be damaged or rendered ischemic. If recognized, surgeons often insert a gastrostomy tube distally to ensure decompression of the stomach. We have observed several patients in whom the gastrostomy tube migrated superiorly and penetrated through the suture-line or the area of ischemia. Such leaks may be overlooked if the barium is administered through a nasogastric tube or if only a water-soluble material is administered.

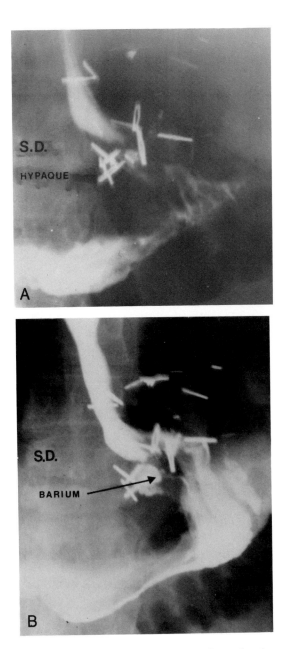

FIGURE 17.3A. Postoperative Gastrografin swallow in a gastroplasty patient suspected of having a leak. No convincing evidence of extravasation. **B.** Study done immediately afterwards using barium. The leak on the lesser curvature is apparent. Patient was taken immediately to the operating-room where the leak was repaired, and her postoperative course was uneventful.

phrenic abscess. Organ displacement by an abscess cavity may also be seen on the upper GI study. Oral contrast medium should be administered to rule out a leak—the most common cause of such collections. Pneumonia and pulmonary embolism are uncommon clinical events, despite the generally held impression that these are "expected" problems in morbidly obese patients, and to assume that the patient has pneumonia or pulmonary embolism rather than a leak is to invite disaster. Mortality from leaks is directly related to the time delayed before re-operation.[10]

NORMAL APPEARANCE

Preliminary spot films are useful for determining the exact position of the staples and therefore the stoma. This allows selection of the best position of the patient during administration of the contrast material. The components of the gastroplasty that should be evaluated are the proximal gastric pouch, stoma and staple-line. After gastric bypass, if distal pouch distention occurs, plain films will demonstrate massive air accumulation in the distal (excluded) pouch.

Following successful gastroplasty, the patient feels full after swallowing one or two ounces of barium. There may be a dilatation of the esophagus and proximal pouch with gastroesophageal reflux and a slow trickle of barium through a 2 to 3 mm edematous channel (Fig. 17.2). The course of the barium should be followed closely under fluoroscopy to allow differentiation between staple disruption and leak. Administration of too much barium, which would obscure the pouch and stoma, is to be avoided for vertical banded gastroplasty according to Agha and co-workers,[11] who found that only 30 to 60 mL of barium gave the best visualization of the pouch. However, this is not a concern if the patient is radiographed in the erect position. The rows of fine staples adjacent to the stoma may be evident only on spot films. After horizontal or vertical gastroplasties, barium will traverse the stoma and partially opacify the distal stomach. The latter cannot be fully distended for complete assessment.[7]

After gastric bypass, the jejunum will fill with barium. Barium seldom flows retrograde into the afferent limb of the Roux-en-Y, although the Roux-en-Y anastomosis can often be visualized. The excluded stomach in gastric bypass cannot be assessed by upper GI study unless a gastrostomy tube had been inserted. Radiographic techniques have been developed to study the duodenum in patients who have undergone Roux-en-Y gastric bypass.[6] However, these techniques are time-consuming, uncomfortable for the patient and rarely delineate the mucosal surfaces of the most distal portions of the excluded stomach. Obstruction of the afferent limb may lead to massve distention and possibly perforation of the excluded distal stomach, heralded by abdominal pain, tachycardia, and a large air collection in the distal pouch. This is avoided if a gastrostomy is routinely inserted to decompress the distal pouch.

Edema around any stoma is common in the early postoperative period. On the initial upper GI study, after gastroplasty there may be some dilatation of the proximal pouch (Fig. 17.5) or after loop gastric bypass there may be dilatation of the proximal pouch and afferent duodenal loop. After a Roux-en-Y gastric bypass, edema of the jejunojejunostomy

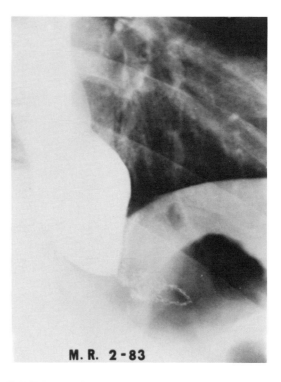

M. R. 2-83

FIGURE 17.5. Severe stomal edema and obstruction in a patient who had vertical banded gastroplasty 5 days previously. The vertical and circular staple rows can be visualized. The patient was fed by a jejunostomy tube, which we inserted per routine during the operation, and his problem resolved over the ensuing months. Re-operation is not necessary for such problems, although frequent dilatations may be required.

may lead to dilatation of the proximal jejunum and gastric pouch and/or the excluded distal gastric pouch.

LEAKS

Intra-operatively, the surgeon should take precautions to detect and deal with leaks. The operative field may be filled with warm saline to observe for air bubbles while the anesthetist injects air down a tube in the channel. Occluding the outlet and esophagus while the anesthetist injects methylene blue through a tube into the gastric pouch is another method.

The incidence of leaks ranges from 1–5%,[12] although rates of <1% have been reported with vertical gastroplasty.[13–16] Leaks were more common with the original loop gastric bypass, particularly before the advent of the special retractors which greatly facilitate exposure. All gastric partitioning procedures are ischemic, in that vessels are ligated (except during vertical gastroplasty) and gastric tissue is crushed by the stapling instruments. The vertical banded gastroplasty removes a doughnut of tissue with the circular stapling instrument. Incomplete rings may lead to leaks adjacent to the lesser curve outlet. Such a leak will produce an inflammatory reaction which may occlude the stoma. As barium flows down the stomach and through the separated staples, the channel so formed may resemble a normal outlet and the leak may go undetected.

Early detection of leaks and re-operation are the key to minimize mortality.[6,10] Clinical recognition of leaks in obese patients can be difficult. Tachycardia, dyspnea and tachypnea are important clinical signs. Symptoms may include abdominal pain, shoulder-tip pain (especially in the recumbent position), back pain, dysuria, diarrhea or vaginal pain due to peritoneal irritation. Abdominal signs are frequently minimal or even absent. The abdominal wall is thick and difficult to examine, especially with a fresh postoperative incision. It is vital that tachycardia, fever, leukocytosis, and all pulmonary symptoms, with or without abdominal pain, be interpreted as leaks until proven otherwise, particularly in the first 2–10 days postoperatively. Such patients must be taken either directly to the operating-room or to radiology for the procedures described above.

Occasionally, a leak may not be demonstrable on upper GI contrast studies even with a proven subphrenic abscess. Presumably such patients had small leaks which sealed spontaneously. Consideration can be given to percutaneous drainage, but due to the patient's size and overlying transverse colon, operative drainage is usually necessary. Direct inspection of the stomach combined with methylene blue injection will ensure that a leak, not detected radiographically, is not overlooked.

Rarely, a clinically unsuspected or asymptomatic leak is demonstrated on a routine postoperative contrast study. Such asymptomatic patients must initially be observed very closely for the occurrence of pain, fever, tachycardia, tachypnea, or elevated white count, while being maintained on intravenous fluids.

STAPLE-LINE DISRUPTION

Staple-line disruption can be distinguished from a leak, in that the contrast medium in the abnormal channel connects with the stomach distally. Staple-line disruption may be partial or complete. It may be seen early or late. The reasons for this are not understood. However, it is believed to be related to technical problems or to the impact of solid food early in the postoperative period.[17–19] With horizontal gastroplasties, animal experiments and clinical observations suggested that disruption began at the stoma and proceeded laterally, as in undoing a zipper.[20,21] Placement of through-and-through non-absorbable sutures on either side of the stoma reduced the incidence of staple-line disruption, but did not prevent the displacement of individual staples within the intact staple-line.[18] The incidence of staple-line disruption may be decreased by: 1) restriction to fluids only, in the early postoperative period; 2) *close* application of *double* staple-lines (each has 2 staggered lines of staples)[10,18] (Fig. 17.6); 3) reinforcement of the stoma to prevent its dilatation; 4) separating the outlet from the partition (as in vertical banded gastroplasty); 5) suture reinforcement of the staple-line; and 6) after gastric bypass, by decompressing the distal gas-

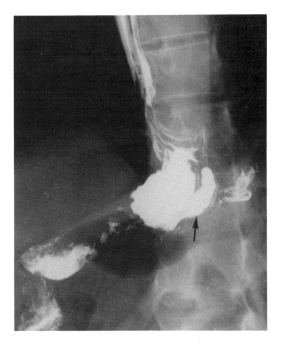

FIGURE 17.6. Vertical banded gastroplasty with disruption of inner row of staples, producing a diverticulum (arrow). It is believed that widely placed staple-lines resulted in a mucous cyst and breakdown. Current single application of TA 90 B or TA 90 BN, which delivers 4 secure equidistant close staple-lines, should obviate this complication.

tric pouch with a gastrostomy and/or dividing between the staple-lines.

Plain films may indicate if staples have migrated. Usually one can see the staple-lines on spot films. The upper GI series may demonstrate complete disruption of the staple-line, in which case no operative deformity of the stomach may be seen[2] (Fig. 17.7). In partial staple-line disruption, one may observe: 1) stomal dilatation (Fig. 17.8); 2) a second stoma, representing staple disruption (Fig. 17.9); or 3) filling of the distal gastric pouch in gastric bypass. With gastroplasties, oblique views[8] will demonstrate filling of the distal pouch through both the disrupted staple-line and the stoma (Fig. 17.10), unless stomal occlusion is present, in which case the staple-line disruption may mimic the normal stoma.[22]

PROXIMAL POUCH

Failure to lose weight after gastric partitioning is related to dilatation of the pouch or outlet, staple-line disruption, type of opera-

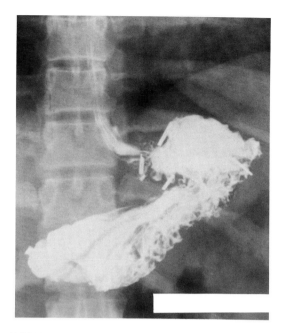

FIGURE 17.8. A patient who lost 61 kg after horizontal gastroplasty and then regained all the weight. The gastroscope passed easily through the stomach. This upper GI series shows massive dilatation of the stoma, which is only recognizable because of the slight indentation (persisting partition) on the lesser curvature.

tion, and patient compliance.[7,22] Radiographic examination of the proximal pouch may be a reliable method of follow-up,[22] although Andersen and Pedersen[23] found that the size of neither the pouch nor the outlet necessarily correlated with the patient's weight loss. A routine postoperative upper GI study performed by ourselves and others[7,8,22,24] serves as a baseline for subsequent comparison (Fig. 17.2). With gastric bypass (or horizontal gastroplasty), the pouch is usually elliptical, but with chronic stomal stenosis, the pouch enlarges and may become globular. All proximal pouches undergo some enlargement due to stretching, which is usually limited.

If there is failure to lose weight and the early radiographic examination was satisfactory, then the follow-up studies will frequently demonstrate dilatation of the proximal pouch (Fig. 17.11) or outlet (Fig. 17.12) or delayed staple-line disruption. Continued overeating may stretch the pouch and not the stoma. Radiologic examination in this situation may be misleading, as a dilated pouch tends to override and obscure the stoma, particularly if too much barium is administered. If this is suspected, endoscopic examination is required for confirmation. Such patients are

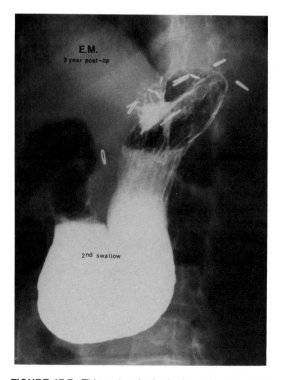

FIGURE 17.7. This patient had a horizontal gastroplasty 2 years previously. Note massive stomal dilatation with stretching of the proximal pouch, resulting in a radiographic picture that nearly resembles a normal stomach. Smaller amounts of barium might have demonstrated the pouch and/or stoma better.

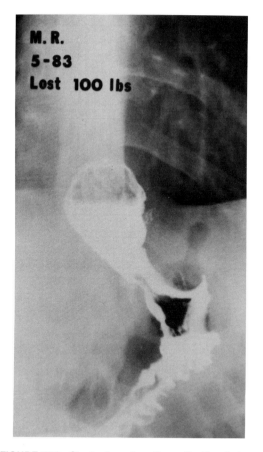

FIGURE 17.9. Staple disruption after vertical banded gastroplasty. This patient lost 45 kg and kept the weight off, despite the appearance of a double-barreled shotgun type of stoma. Staple disruption after horizontal gastroplasty or stapled gastric bypass has a similar radiologic appearance. (Compare to Fig. 17.2A–1.)

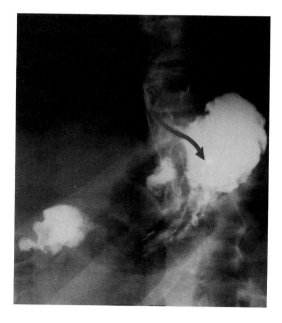

FIGURE 17.10. Patient with vertical banded gastroplasty who regained capacity to eat. Barium promptly passes across breakdown in upper part of partition to fundus and onwards to antrum.

seen because of nausea and vomiting with paradoxical weight gain or at least inadequate weight loss. If the pouch is large and the outlet is of normal caliber, then the patient did not adjust to the small pouch and has been overeating (Fig. 17.13A and B).

Bezoar formation in a proximal pouch may occur and can readily be identified on radiologic or endoscopic examination. It may resolve with enzymatic dissolution (meat tenderizer, cellulase, papain), endoscopic fragmentation, and metoclopramide.[25]

The proximal pouch emptying rate can be studied by ingestion of isotopic-labeled solid or liquid material.[2,26] Such studies are useful in patients who complain of nausea and vomiting but have normal pouches and outlets. Usually such patients are simply eating too much, too rapidly. Alternatively, the vagal nerves may have been damaged or there may

be paraesophageal fibrosis, related to the surgery.

STOMA EVALUATION

Stoma size is critical for weight reduction, in that a stomal diameter >11 mm will probably be inadequate for long-term weight loss. Excessively small stomas probably lead to more complications than to successful weight loss. Many modifications were conceived to obviate stomal dilatation, and these occasionally led to complications secondary to ischemia. Stomal complications recognized radiographically are: 1) early stomal edema; 2) stomal stenosis/obstruction; 3) stomal dilatation; and 4) stomal ulceration (gastric bypass).

1. EARLY STOMAL EDEMA

Stomal edema with obstruction may be secondary to surgical trauma (Fig. 17.5). The most common manifestations are a sensation of substernal fullness and heartburn early postoperatively. These symptoms usually resolve with time and supportive measures, including antacids, metoclopramide and liquid diet. Persistence of such symptoms beyond 6–8 weeks should raise the possibility of true stomal stenosis. The radiographic appearance of early stomal dysfunction and the value of

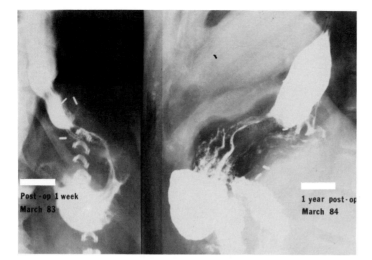

FIGURE 17.11. The postoperative film (left) demonstates a normal vertical banded gastroplasty (the skin clips are still in place). The patient lost >45 kg and then began regaining weight. Repeat upper GI series (right) demonstrates channel (pouch) dilatation, with intact stoma and staple-line. (Compare to Fig. 17.12.)

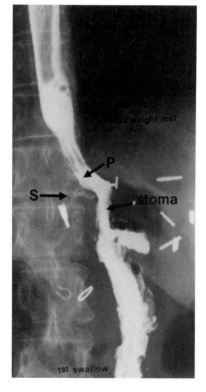

FIGURE 17.12. Stomal dilatation after vertical banded gastroplasty. The pouch (P) is of normal size, but the stoma is nearly 15 mm in diameter. The patient's total weight loss was 23 kg. Note how the careful administration of small amounts of barium with proper positioning shows all components of the operation.

a feeding jejunostomy are discussed in Chapter 18.

2. STOMAL STENOSIS/OBSTRUCTION

Problematic stomal stenosis occurred in about 10% of patients following Gomez horizontal gastroplasty, and is much less frequent after gastric bypass or vertical gastroplasty. Management, including radiologic techniques, is discussed in Chapter 18.

3. STOMAL DILATATION

Stoma size is more critical in gastroplasty than in gastric bypass. Many of the early and late gastroplasty and gastric bypass failures are secondary to stomal dilatation (Fig. 17.12). If the stomal diameter is >12 mm, weight loss will eventually prove inadequate. Not only should a stoma be constructed of 10 mm diameter, but a method of stoma calibration and reinforcement should be used to prevent later dilatation. Patient education regarding tiny meals taken slowly is mandatory. Prevention of stomal dilatation in gastric bypass has been addressed by use of circumferential non-absorbable sutures, Silastic rings, or a 1-cm-wide strip of rectus fascia wrapped around the anastomosis. One reason for the enthusiasm for vertical banded gastroplasty is that it allows a 360° reinforcement of the stoma.

When weight loss is inadequate or the patient starts to regain weight, stomal dilatation should be suspected. An upper GI series with specific measurements of stomal diameter and emptying will demonstrate such dilata-

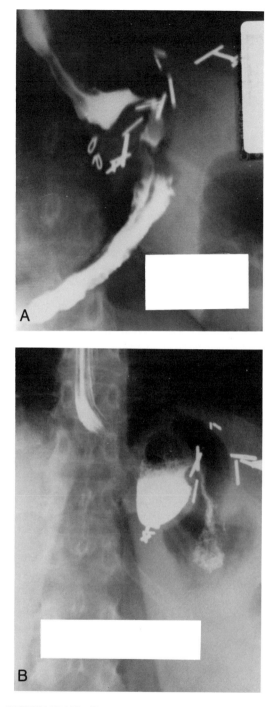

FIGURE 17.13A. The postoperative upper GI series demonstrates a normal Gomez horizontal gastroplasty with a small pouch and a narrow greater curvature channel. The patient lost 21 kg and then began to regain. Despite this, she complained of continual nausea and vomiting. **B.** Repeat upper GI series and endoscopy demonstrated considerable dilatation of the proximal pouch, with an intact stoma and staple-line. This is similar to the findings of Fig. 17.11. These two X-rays demonstrate the syndrome of "nausea and vomiting with weight *gain*".

tion (Fig. 17.12). If there is doubt, the investigation should be complemented by endoscopy.

Messmer et al[24] evaluated 22 patients who had gastric partitioning and subsequent stomal dilatation, using both upper GI series and endoscopy. Both examinations were positive in 8 patients (36%). The remaining 14 patients (64%) had positive endoscopy with negative GI series. Retrospective review of these 14 upper GI examinations showed that, although a normal stoma was reported, the stoma in 9 patients was actually dilated when specific measurements were made. The GI series in 2 of the 14 was technically inadequate to assess stomal diameter. This report stressed the importance of a dedicated radiologist and the need for specific measurement of stomal diameter.

4. STOMAL ULCER

Mason and Ito demonstrated in animals that a two-third distal gastric exclusion was not ulcerogenic.[27] An exclusion of enough stomach to produce weight control will also depress gastrin-mediated secretion in response to a standard meal. Early in the experience with gastric bypass, some gastric pouches were too large and a 3% incidence of stomal ulcer occurred. The problem became rare (0.9%) with construction of a small proximal gastric pouch.[28] In fact, stomal ulceration in gastric bypass with a proximal pouch less than 50 mL indicates a probable underlying ulcer diathesis. The problem is not encountered with gastroplasty, because the antrum is bathed in acid from the proximal stomach, which inhibits gastrin secretion.

Radiographic examination identifies only 50–65% of stomal ulcers. A surgical deformity at the gastrojejunostomy site may mimic stomal ulcer in its absence or conceal it when present. The diagnosis of duodenal ulcer afer gastric bypass cannot be made radiographically, since the distal pouch and duodenum fail to opacify. Thus, endoscopic examination is required to identify stomal or duodenal ulceration.

5. SUTURE-LINE ULCERATION

During endoscopy we have observed staples, polypropylene suture and Marlex in the lumen of the post-gastroplasty stomach. Nunes et al[29] reported two patients with ulcers at the partition-line following horizontal gastroplasty, where the staple-line was reinforced with a non-absorbable suture. The ulcers were identified on upper GI series. At endoscopy, sutures were noted in the center of the ulcers. We have had a referred patient who bled twice from a suture-line ulcer and required a proximal esophagogastrectomy. The radiologist should be aware of the possibility of ulcer occurrence at this site, particularly in a patient being investigated for bleeding or vague abdominal symptoms post-gastroplasty.[30] Such a complication may also herald delayed staple-line disruption.

REFERENCES

1. Freeman JB, Burchett H: Failure rates with gastric partitioning for morbid obesity. Am J Surg 145:113–119, 1983.
2. Agha FP, Harris HH, Houstany MM: Gastroplasty for morbid obesity: roentgen evaluation and spectrum of complications. Gastrointest Radiol 7:217–223, 1982.
3. Menin RA, Malmud LS, Petersen RP: Gastroesophageal scintigraphy to assess the severity of gastroesophageal reflux disease. Ann Surg 191:66–71, 1980.
4. Flickinger EG, Sinar DR, Pories WJ, et al: The bypassed stomach. Am J Surg 149:151–156, 1985.
5. Flickinger EG, Pories WJ, Meelheim HD. et al: The Greenville gastric bypass: progress report at 3 years. Ann Surg 199:555–562, 1984.
6. Mason EE: Surgical Treatment of Obesity. Philadelphia, WB Saunders, 1981.
7. Hammond DI, Freeman JB: The radiology of gastroplasty for morbid obesity. J Can Assoc Radiologists 33:21–24, 1982.
8. Smith C, Gardiner R, Kubicka RA, et al: Gastric restrictive surgery for obesity: early radiologic evaluation. Radiology 153:321–327, 1984.
9. Gallitano AI, Kondi ES, Phillips E, et al: Near fatal hemorrhage following gastrografin studies. Radiology 118:35–36, 1976.
10. Mason EE, Printen KJ, Barron P, et al: Risk reduction in gastric operations for obesity. Ann Surg 190:158–165, 1979.
11. Agha FP, Eckhauser FE, Strodel WE, et al: Mason's vertical banded gastroplasty for obesity: surgical procedure and radiographic evaluation. Radiology 150:825–827, 1984.
12. Cogbill TH, Moore EE: Perforation after gastric partitioning for morbid obesity. Surgery 92:551–552, 1982.
13. Mason EE: Vertical banded gastroplasty for obesity. Arch Surg 117:701–706, 1982.
14. Deitel M, Jones BA, Petrov I, et al: Vertical banded gastroplasty: results in 233 patients. Can J Surg 29:322–324, 1986.
15. Shamblin JR, Shamblin AE: Gastroplasty in morbid obesity: observations in 300 patients. South Med J 78:1036–1040, 1985.
16. Eckhout GV, Willbacks OL: Vertical ring gastroplasty for morbid obesity: five year experience with 1,463 patients. Am J Surg 152:713–716, 1986.
17. Ellison EC, Martin EW Jr, Laschinger J, et al: Prevention of early failure of stapled gastric partitions in treatment of morbid obesity. Arch Surg 115:528–533, 1980.
18. Eskind SJ, Massie JD, Born ML, et al: Experimental study of double staple lines in gastric partitions. Surg Gynecol Obstet 152:751–756, 1981.
19. Strodel WE, Knol JA, Eckhauser FE: Endoscopy of the partitioned stomach. Ann Surg 200:582–586, 1984.
20. Brolin RE, Ravitch MM: Experimental evaluation of techniques of gastric partitioning for morbid obesity. Surg Gynecol Obstet 153:877–882, 1981.
21. Brolin RE: Laboratory evaluation for four techniques of stapled gastroplasty. Surgery 97:66–71, 1985.
22. Grundy A, McFarland RJ, Gazet J-C, et al: Radiological appearance following vertical banded gastroplasty. Clin Radiol 36:395–400, 1985.
23. Andersen T, Pedersen BH: Pouch volume, stoma diameter and clinical outcome after gastroplasty for morbid obesity. Scand J Gastroenterol 19:643–649, 1984.
24. Messmer JM, Wolper JC, Sugarman HJ: Stomal disruption in gastric partition in morbid obesity: comparison of radiographic and endoscopic diagnosis. Am J Gastroenterol 79:603–605, 1984.
25. Winkler WP, Saleh J: Metoclopramide in the treatment of gastric bezoars. Am J Gastroenterol 78:403–405, 1983.
26. Russell COH, Hill LD, Holmes ER, et al: Radionuclide transit: a sensitive screening test for esophageal dysfunction. Gastroenterology 80:887–892, 1981.
27. Mason EE, Ito C: Graded gastric bypass. World J Surg 2:341–349, 1978.
28. Printen KJ, Scott D, Mason EE: Stomal ulcers after gastric bypass. Arch Surg 115:525–527, 1980.
29. Nunes JR, Van Sonnenberg E, Pressman JH, et al: Suture line ulceration: a complication of gastric partitioning. Gastrointest Radiol 9:315–317, 1984.
30. Bass J, Freeman JB: Complications of Surgery of Morbid Obesity. Year Book of Surgery, vol. 18. Chicago, Year Book Medical Publishers, 1984, pp 223–225.

18

Stomal Stenosis After Gastric Restrictive Operations

ZOHAIR Y. AL-HALEES
JOEL B. FREEMAN

Control of pouch size and calibration of the stoma are important steps in achieving a successful gastric operation for weight reduction. If the stomal diameter is >12 mm, the patient will not lose adequate weight. Many failures are secondary to stomal dilatation. Hence, in the evolution of gastroplasty techniques, surgeons concentrated on methods to reinforce the stoma. However, attempts to reduce the stoma to <10 mm may result in obstructions. Stoma size is more important in gastroplasty than in gastic bypass. However, the stoma in gastric bypass is still subject to dilatation or stenosis.

ETIOLOGY

We were unable to find any correlation between the time of surgery and the development of stenosis. Because early stomal dysfunction and staple-line disruption have been related to excessive intake of liquids or solids accompanied by vomiting in the first 6 weeks postoperatively,[1] we performed a feeding jejunostomy routinely with gastric partitioning.[2] Oral intake is not permitted for 4–6 weeks after surgery, and nutrition is maintained via the jejunostomy. All patients are instructed in the use of this tube during their convalescence and are discharged using the tube to provide 600–800 calories and free water daily. The tube is normally removed in 6–8 weeks, after satisfactory oral intake has commenced. Because of this protocol, none of our gastroplasty patients experienced stoma problems of sufficient magnitude to require aggressive intervention in the first 6 weeks after surgery. Intolerance to saliva or substernal fullness is not an uncommon postoperative complaint, but may herald the beginning of stomal dysfunction. Such symptoms are usually secondary to postoperative edema and generally resolve with supportive care. Symptoms of stomal narrowing usually present within the first year and usually within 3 months. However, stomal dysfunction may occur years after gastroplasty.

Some patients develop recurrent stenosis after successful earlier treatment, again without time correlation. Possible explanations for this phenomenon include: a) a stoma which was simply constructed smaller than usual, combined with edema; b) inflammation and/or obstruction caused by certain foods or large pills; c) erosion of suture material, Marlex mesh or a buried Silastic ring through the gastric wall, inciting an inflammatory reaction

and late stenosis;[3] d) patients with a normal postoperative routine upper GI series (see Chapter 17) who develop obstruction 6–12 weeks post-surgery may have had subclinical localized walled-off leaks leading to peristomal inflammation and fibrosis, since this is too soon for suture or Marlex erosion.

PRESENTATION

Symptoms vary with severity of the stenosis, and include substernal discomfort and fullness, nausea, vomiting, and inability to take solids (this usually precipitates vomiting). With severe stenosis, the patient is unable to take fluids orally. With complete obstruction, the patient is unable to swallow saliva.

DIAGNOSIS

Diagnosis is established by symptomatology, complemented by radiographic studies and endoscopy. Radiographic features of stomal stenosis are discussed in Chapter 17. Here, we shall discuss endoscopy of the partitioned stomach.

Fiberoptic endoscopy is an important diagnostic tool for evaluating the patient with upper GI symptoms following gastric bypass or gastroplasty. The patient is prepared with topical oropharyngeal anesthesia, intravenous Demerol and diazepam. A 10 or 11 mm diameter adult gastroscope is used, although occasionally the 9 mm pediatric upper GI endoscope is required.*

Following the now outdated loop gastric bypass, retrograde examination of the duodenum and excluded distal stomach was endoscopically possible. However, after a Roux-en-Y gastric bypass this is usually difficult, requiring patience and skill despite the availability of longer and thinner endoscopes. Flickinger and associates[4] reported a 68% rate of successful completion of retrograde duodenogastrostomy using the pediatric colonofiberscope (Olympus PCF®—external diameter 11 mm and working length >140 cm). They had very few failures in the latter part of their study, as the endoscopist acquired more experience. Patients with gastric bypass who present with active upper GI bleeding should be explored promptly when a proximal source for bleeding has been excluded.

---

*Olympus GIF-Q or -XQ, external diameter 11 or 9.8 mm respectively.

The incidence of gastrojejunal stomal ulcer is <2%.[4] Technetium-labeled red blood cell scans may be of some value. Intra-operative retrograde endoscopy of the Roux limb, duodenum and excluded stomach may help in localizing the bleeding site.

Endoscopy should proceed systematically.[5] With gastroplasties, one examines hypopharynx, esophagus, gastroesophageal junction, proximal gastric pouch (staple-line), stoma, distal stomach and proximal greater curvature (retroflexion of scope), pylorus and duodenum. One should not insufflate too much air, particularly if the examination is done early in the postoperative period. The small proximal gastric pouch collapses easily; this can be overcome by intravenous glucagon and/or Buscopan (hyoscine) if necessary.

Obese patients after gastric partitioning are as susceptible as the non-obese population to develop upper GI lesions such as duodenal and gastric ulceration, gastric carcinoma, gastritis, gastric polyps and gastroesophageal reflux. Specific indications for endoscopic examination of a partitioned stomach include: stomal evaluation in patients who fail to lose adequate weight or who have regained; patients with symptoms of outlet obstruction from channel stenosis or a foreign body; suspected esophagitis in patients with symptoms of gastroesophageal reflux; and suspicion of a marginal ulcer following gastric bypass. Patients who had the old loop gastric bypass are susceptible to bile reflux gastritis and the afferent loop syndrome.

ENDOSCOPIC APPEARANCE

NORMAL

A) VERTICAL BANDED GASTROPLASTY OR SILASTIC RING VERTICAL GASTROPLASTY. The vertical channel permits easy endoscopic visualization. At the lower end of the lesser curvature channel about 7–8 cm distal to the esophagogastric junction, the mucosa tapers to a rosette which represents the stoma. The stoma is usually 0.7–1.5 cm long and 11–12 mm wide, and its endoscopic appearance is similar to the pylorus. The stoma usually accepts the adult upper GI endoscope with slight resistance. Retroflexion of the scope distal to the stoma reveals the partition and greater curvature segment. The appearance of the antrum, pylorus and duodenum is unchanged.

B) HORIZONTAL GASTROPLASTY. The prox-

imal gastric pouch is examined easily. The staple-line is incomplete wherever the channel is located. Air insufflation is required to visualize the channel. Because of the angular orientation of greater curvature outlets, it is frequently difficult to negotiate the gastroscope through such channels. Greater curvature channels are sometimes more easily entered with the patient in the right lateral decubitus position (left side up), so that the greater curvature falls towards midline, thereby bringing esophagus and stoma into alignment.[6] The diameter of the outlet should not be more than 12 mm. Once the endoscope has traversed the outlet, examination of the distal stomach, pylorus and duodenum proceeds easily; retroflexion of the gastroscope allows inspection of the caudal aspect of the staple-line and can demonstrate stomal dilatation if a space >2 mm is seen around the endoscope.

C) ROUX-EN-Y GASTRIC BYPASS. The proximal pouch after gastric bypass is visualized readily. Special attention should be directed to the gastrojejunal anastomosis, especially the jejunal side, to rule out marginal ulcers. Using the pediatric colonofiberoscope for examination of the afferent Roux loop and retrograde duodenogastroscopy, nonerosive gastritis has been observed in 87% with histologic intestinal metaplasia in 10% of patients on mucosal biopsy.[4] The long-term implications of these findings are unknown.

STOMAL STENOSIS

With stomal obstruction, gastroscopic examination may demonstrate:
  A. Proximal gastric pouch dilatation, possibly with hypertrophied rugae.
  B. Undigested food in the proximal gastric pouch, with stasis inflammation.
  C. Phytobezoar formation or foreign material (e.g. chewing gum, a large pill or nut) obstructing the stoma. Upon fragmentation and removal by aspiration or by a Dormia-type wire basket, a narrowed stoma may be seen.
  D. Suture material, Marlex, buried Silastic or a rectus fascial band eroding through the gastric mucosa. Such a finding may explain the stenosis.
  E. A very stenotic stoma which resembles a pinhole. Attempts to pass the endoscope through such a stoma fail because of resistance. Erythema and moderate bleeding may be observed after several attempts.

F. Secondary breakdown of the staple-line partition due to excessive prolonged back-pressure, which, in turn, was caused by the stenosis.

MANAGEMENT

Patients may present with mild symptoms, and as such they can be managed by supportive care using antacids, meat tenderizer, papain, metoclopramide[7] and a liquid high-protein diet or supplement (e.g. Ensure, Sustacal, Meritene, Resource).[8] The jejunostomy or gastrostomy tube, which is routine in our patients,[2] is used to provide fluids and enteral nutrition. Without a jejunostomy tube, a brief hospital admission for rehydration may be required. If symptoms are severe, the patient should be admitted to establish the diagnosis and be managed appropriately. The nutritional status of the patient should be assessed,[9] and one should not hesitate to institute parenteral nutrition, especially in the absence of a feeding jejunostomy tube. Initially however, intravenous fluids should be administered to rehydrate the patient. If nausea and vomiting persist and/or if the patient is unable to swallow saliva, a nasogastric tube should be inserted and connected to low, intermittent suction. After this initial period of stabilization, the patient is studied by a barium upper GI series and endoscopy. The latter can be therapeutic in cases of obstruction by a foreign body, which can be fragmented or removed by grasping forceps at endoscopy. There are two methods for treating severe stomal stenosis: non-operative and operative.

NON-OPERATIVE MANAGEMENT OF STOMAL STENOSIS

In most instances a tight stoma will dilate with repeated dilatation and with time (Figs. 18.1, 18.2 and 18.3). Operation is seldom necessary. Longterm outpatient enteral feeding through a jejunostomy is extremely valuable, since nutrition is maintained and the temptation to operate is much less if the patient is not in hospital.[2,10] Insertion of a feeding jejunostomy, even as a separate procedure, permits treatment at home as well as temporization of reoperation.[11,12] Our suggested protocol for conservative management is as follows.

At time of initial diagnosis, most patients are dehydrated and may be nutritionally depleted. They are admitted to hospital for the initial management. The patient is usually kept on nothing by mouth. Intravenous fluids and total parenteral nutrition and/or enteral feeding via the jejunostomy tube, if it had been inserted at the initial surgery, are started. If the jejunostomy tube had been removed (usually 4–6 weeks postoperatively), the situation is evaluated and consideration given to insertion of a new jejunostomy feeding tube, depending on the severity of the stenosis and the patient's response to conservative therapy.

After rehydration, the patient is taken to the radiology suite for radiologic and endoscopic evaluation. Fluoroscopy will be required. Oropharyngeal anesthesia is performed topically and intravenous Demerol and diazepam are given for sedation. Food particles are lavaged or removed with the biopsy grasping forceps, and the stoma is evaluated. A decision is then made regarding the need for dilatation. If this is required, the stoma is cannulated with a flexible guidewire* inserted through the biopsy channel of the gastroscope and passed gently into the distal stomach. The mobile spring-tip guidewire lessens the danger of perforation. Occasionally, identification of the stoma and cannulation with the guidewire can be laborious and tedious, requiring as long as 45 minutes with repetitive patient repositioning. This is particularly true for patients who have greater curvature channels. The reasons for these difficulties include small size of the proximal pouch, the fact that insufflated air is immediately regurgitated and that the suction of the gastroscope functions poorly when the guidewire is in the biopsy channel. To solve the latter problem, atropine or Buscopan may be used to reduce secretions. Buscopan and glucagon will reduce gastric peristalsis. Under adverse circumstances, dilatation should be attempted again at another time.

If cannulation of the stoma with the guidewire is successful, as demonstrated by fluoroscopy, the endosope is removed and dilatation is commenced with the patient in the supine position using the smallest (12 F) Eder-Puestow dilator.** The procedure is continu-

---

*American Endoscopy Inc., Mentor, OH, U.S.A.; Wilson-Cook Inc., Winston-Salem, NC, U.S.A.: Cook Canada Inc., Markham, Ont., Canada; KeyMed, Southend-on-Sea, Essex, England; Microvasive, Milford, MA, U.S.A.

**American Endoscopy Inc., Mentor, OH, U.S.A.; W. Carson Co., Don Mills, Ont., Canada; KeyMed, Southend-on-Sea, Essex, England.

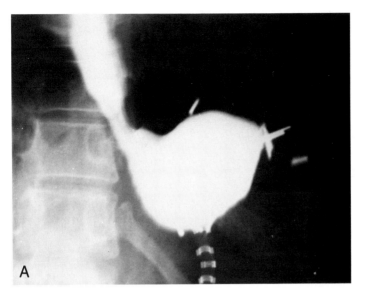

FIGURE 18.1A. Obstruction of a horizontal gastroplasty in the early postoperative period. Patient treated by nasogastric suction and enteral feeding and then discharged on home enteral feedings.

ally monitored under fluoroscopy. Progressively larger metal olives are introduced until the point of resistance. Then the next large dilator is passed and the procedure terminated. Additional sedation is usually required as progressively larger dilators are passed through the stoma. The first dilatation is usually limited to size 27F dilator (27 mm in circumference, *9 mm in diameter*), in order to avoid making the stoma too large, which could result in inadequate weight loss. Usually, more force is required for dilatation if the stoma had been reinforced with Marlex mesh, as in vertical banded gastroplasty.

Following each dilatation, an upper GI series is performed with a water-soluble contrast medium to rule out perforation. If no perforation is shown, this study is followed by a barium swallow, even if the Gastrografin or Hypaque did not pass through the stoma. Barium is heavier and may pass through when Gastrografin or Hypaque did not. Perforation cannot be completely ruled out without a barium study. Placing the patient in the upright position may help in demonstrating the passage of the contrast material distally. If there is still no passage, the contrast material is aspirated via a nasogastric tube and the patient is admitted for observation. Frequently, one is unable to demonstrate passage of the contrast material through the stoma immediately following a successful dil-

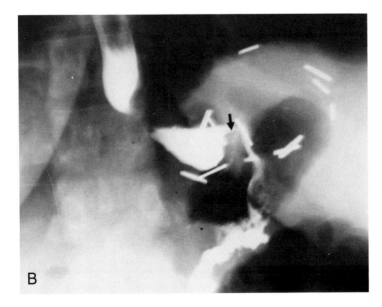

FIGURE 18.1B. Same patient 2 months later, showing normal passage of barium. Dilatations were not required because of increasing ability to tolerate her saliva and sips of fluids with time.

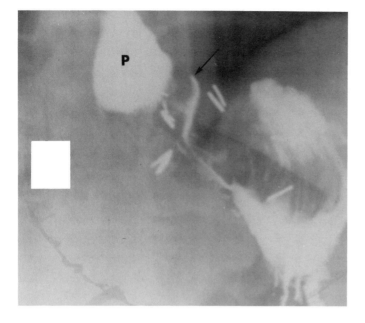

FIGURE 18.2. Typical appearance of early post horizontal gastroplasty obstruction. Note dilated pouch (P) with narrow greater curve channel (arrow). Patient responded well to conservative treatment with enteral nutrition at home and two dilatations.

atation. This is due to edema secondary to dilatation trauma and will resolve in 48–72 hours.

After 2–3 hours of observation, outpatients may be discharged. Longterm nutrition is maintained by enteral feeding through the jejunostomy tube in hospital or at home. Although we have used steroids on occasion in an attempt to reduce the inflammatory reaction, we have not found this particularly helpful. The upper GI study is repeated in 10–14 days. If the stoma is open, no further dilatations are necessary. An oral diet can then be advanced cautiously from liquids to puréed to soft foods. Further dilatations will be required when indicated by symptomatology and/or the radiologic demonstration of persistent stomal obstruction. If a second dilatation is required, it is advisable not to advance more than two sizes larger than the maximum size used in the preceding dilatation. The largest Eder-Puestow dilator is 45 F (15 mm diameter) and is as large as is ever required.[10]

We used the above protocol in managing 33 patients who developed symptoms of stomal obstruction out of 172 gastric bypass and gastroplasty procedures performed over a 6-year period.[11] Initial repletion by combined parenteral and general nutrition was required in 29 patients. Longterm nutrition was maintained enterally through a feeding jejunostomy tube at home. Three patients required insertion of the feeding jejunostomy tube as a separate procedure (Fig. 18.3). Thirteen of

the 33 patients were dilated a total of 36 times. Three patients required 3 to 6 dilatations each. There were no complications. Patients were followed 6–60 months, and 32 did well. Gastrogastrostomy was done in one patient with a stenosis following his second gastroplasty; this was the only reoperation required.

We used Eder-Puestow dilators because of familiarity and experience with the technique and the ability to follow the entire procedure with the fluoroscope. We and others have obtained good results with this dilator.[11,13] The available techniques include:

1. EDER-PUESTOW DILATORS. These stainless steel rigid olives are passed over the guidewire which had been passed through the stoma via the gastroscope, as described above.[14]

2. TRIPLE OLIVE DILATORS. These successively larger 3-olive stainless steel dilators* allow rapid single insertion over the guidewire. Care must be taken not to perforate distally after the third ball has passed into the stricture.

3. SAVARY OR CELESTIN† DILATORS.** These tapered polyvinyl, totally radiopaque, semi-flexible bougies are lubricated and threaded over the guidewire under fluoroscopic surveillance.[15–17] Many workers con-

---

*KeyMed, Southend-on-Sea, Essex, England.
**Wilson-Cook Inc., Winston-Salem, NC, U.S.A.; Cook Canada Inc., Markham, Ont., Canada; American Endoscopy Inc., Mentor, OH, U.S.A.
†American Endoscopy Inc., Mentor, OH, U.S.A.; Porges, Madox, France.

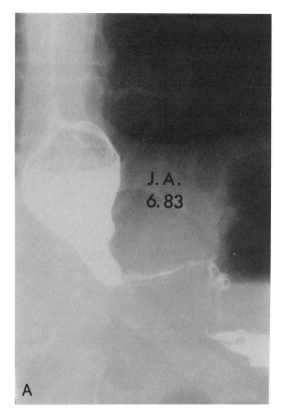

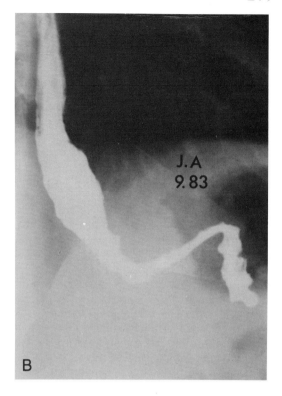

FIGURE 18.3A. Patient with complete obstruction of vertical banded gastroplasty. At the time of this examination, he was 3 months post-op and had been admitted three times for dilatations. Nutritional support was maintained by jejunostomy tube at home. He improved, and the tube was removed. Symptoms recurred one month later. A new tube was inserted and similar treatment continued for an additional 3 months.

FIGURE 18.3B. Same patient 3 months later. He had now been dilated six times. At one-year follow-up, he had attained ideal weight and was eating quite adequately.

sider these safer than the relatively blunt Eder-Puestow dilators, because they are a dilatation cone of increasing bougie caliber, with a maximum taper of 5°. These bougies provide good "tactile feedback" of stenosis resistance, which builds up gradually. Progressive entry into the stenosis provides good judgement from the amount of resistance as to when to stop. These dilators also save time because the taper allows a gradual transition from the small tip to large diameter.

4. BALLOON DILATATION CATHETER. A polyethylene Grüntzig catheter* is passed over the guidewire, which had been introduced endoscopically through the stoma and the

procedure is followed under fluoroscopy.[18] The balloon is inflated with dilute water-soluble contrast medium (50% Gastrografin–50% water).[18] The catheter is withdrawn until a waist is seen in the balloon contour.[19] The prior barium examination is helpful at time of dilatation, indicating the position of the stoma in relation to surrounding surgical clips, creating a road-map for locating the stoma.[20] The balloon is then inflated over the stenotic orifice to 40 lb per sq in (PSI) hydrostatic pressure for 30 seconds to 5 minutes.[19,20] as the waist gradually widens. A dilatation monitor** with a dial indicating PSI can display the dilating (inflation) pressure applied. After dilatation, water-soluble contrast is injected through the catheter tip to evaluate the patency of the stenosis and to document an intact lumen.[20] Redilatation may be necessary later. The balloon method may be the safest technique, as it acts by a radial force against the stenosis, whereas olives and bougies require axial (longitudinal) pushing stresses which can cause tearing.

---

*Inflated balloon diameter 12 or 15 mm, maximum pressure 40 PSI (2.5 atm); balloon catheter 14 F, 95–100 cm long: Wilson-Cook Inc., Winston-Salem, NC, U.S.A.; Cook Canada Inc., Markham, Ont., Canada; Medi-Tech, Watertown, MA, U.S.A.; American Endoscopy Inc., Mentor, OH, U.S.A.

**Rigiflex Dilatation Monitor, MicroVasive, Milford, MA, U.S.A.; Disposable Pressure Gauge, Wilson-Cook, Winston-Salem, NC, U.S.A.

Balloons which inflate up to 15 mm in diameter have been designed to fit directly through the clean 2.8 mm biopsy channel of the gastroscope, avoiding the need for a guidewire, and enabling direct visualization of the stomal dilatation through the scope* (Fig. 18.4). First, silicone liquid or spray is applied to the cleaning or biopsy brush, which is passed throughout the endoscope channel to lubricate and facilitate balloon passage. No gel or oil is used. Then, silicone spray is used to lubricate the fully deflated balloon, which is advanced in short quick pushes down the endoscope channel. The balloon is positioned in the stricture and is inflated with water to the maximum indicated balloon pressure. The inelastic balloon is made of a non-distensible polymer, i.e. excess pressure does not cause greater expansion as with latex balloons. During withdrawal of the catheter, complete deflation is maintained with the 50 mL syringe. If diluted liquid contrast medium had been instilled into the balloon, the reusable catheter must be flushed with water after removal to prevent clogging. The balloon is kept in a sheath when not in use, to maintain compression and avoid deformity. For tortuous strictures, a guidewire and the the dilator are passed through the biopsy channel of the scope.

Radiologists, using angioplasty techniques, have peformed dilatation using fluoroscopy without endoscopy.[20] After pharyngeal anesthesia, an angiographic guidewire is introduced orally and is negotiated through the stoma, the angioplasty catheter is passed over the guidewre, and the 12-mm balloon is inflated in the stoma. The angiographic guidewire may be passed through a nasoesophageal sleeve and be introduced through an open-ended nasogastric tube.

5. ENDOSCOPIC TAPE DILATOR. Paulk[6] and Lehman and O'Connor[21] described a technique using the endoscope itself. The stoma is identified, and if the stoma allows cannulation with the endoscope, the latter is withdrawn. The lower segment of the endoscope is then wrapped with electrical tape, beginning above the flexible steerable tip and extending proximally with a gradually increasing diameter. A fusiform mound 3–4 cm long, 10–15 cm from the tip, with maximal diameter in the center, is thus made just proximal to the directional control section. The dimension of the wrap of the tapered dilator thus created is determined by comparison with Hurst dilators. A water-soluble lubricant is applied to the tape, and the gastroscope is reinserted into the stomach. Using the biopsy forceps as

---

*Rigiflex T.T.S. (Through-the-Scope) Balloon Dilators, MicroVasive, Milford, MA, U.S.A.; HydraCross Coaxial Balloon Catheters (hydrophilic coating—slippery when contacting moisture), American Edwards, 17221 Red Hill Ave., P.O. Box 11150, Santa Ana, CA 92711–1150.

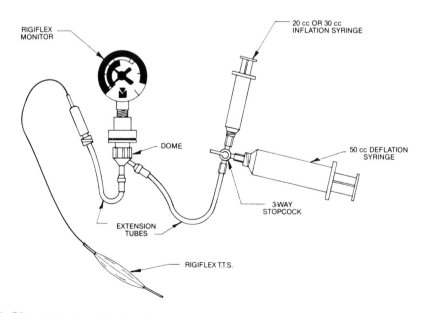

FIGURE 18.4. Dilator is introduced by short, firm pushes down the endoscope channel, while the balloon is maintained deflated by negative pressure with a 50-mL syringe. Once the balloon is in the stricture, it is inflated with water via a hand-held syringe (the smaller of the two), while pressure in the balloon is monitored to the steady state.

a guidewire, the stoma is cannulated and the endoscope is gently advanced over the "biopsy-forceps-guidewire." The tape wrap may be augmented and adjusted as necessary, until a stomal aperture of correct dimension has been obtained. The technique is simple and attractive. However, patients with obstruction have stomas that are very small and may not permit the passage of the pediatric endoscope. Therefore, this technique has limited application.

6. PAPILLOTOME WIDENING OF STOMA. Through the upper GI endoscope, a papillotome* is passed deeply into the stoma to assure proper placement and then is withdrawn until 3–5 mm of wire is visible.[22] Next the endoscope is rotated so that the wire is in the direction desired for the cut. Contact of the papillotome wire with the staples results in destruction of the papillotome. Making the cut just off the staple-line is least likely to result in perforation while preserving the papillotome. A blended current is applied in short bursts, while watching the progression of the cut.

This technique was successful in 6 of 8 patients with no complications.[22] There is the possibility of overheating a staple, thereby causing a deeper burn and hence a perforation. It requires more experience and still has the limitation of occasionally not being able to pass the papillotome through the stoma. The safety of applying the technique more than once, if the first time fails, has not been determined, compared to the feasibility of multiple dilatations when needed.

General Principles

The patient is generally kept NPO for 6–8 hr before a dilatation. Certain danger signals indicate that a dilatation should be stopped: a) if pain occurs; b) if blood is present on the bougie; c) if there is excessive resistance. After the dilatation, a contrast study with Gastrografin (meglumine diatrizoate) should be done.

The choice of a contrast agent after endoscopic dilatation is somewhat problematic. Most surgeons and radiologists prefer to use a water-soluble agent first and then to follow such a study with barium. However, there is a small but definite danger of aspiration after these procedures, especially if a large amount of local anesthetic had been used. If one feels that the pharynx is still anesthetized, then

one should either wait for the gag reflex to return or else use barium.

Although no leaks occurred in our series, we have seen postoperative patients with surgical leaks that were not visualized with water-soluble agents. Therefore, each study done with such a water-soluble agent must be followed by a barium study in order to completely rule out a leak.

Longterm enteral nutrition at home will allow multiple dilatations over a long period of time.[11] The stoma is frequently a rigid fibrosed tube, which may remain stenosed even when suitably sized dilators have been passed. Repetitive dilatations are required to gently fracture these fibrotic bands, being careful not to erode through to a Marlex or Silastic band. Some patients will require 6–8 months of conservative management before they become completely asymptomatic. This can be frustrating to the patient, and psychiatric support is occasionally of value.

OPERATIVE MANAGEMENT

Patients who develop stomal obstruction after a second gastroplasty are a more difficult group to treat conservatively, probably because the stoma has been devascularized. However, a short trial of conservative management is worthwhile, before subjecting them to an often difficult and hazardous reoperation. Certain features are associated with a difficult and prolonged management course (Table 18.1).

When conservative management fails, the simplest operation with horizontal staple-lines is an anterior gastrogastrostomy between proximal and distal stomach. If the proximal pouch is dilated, it can be amputated with stapling instruments to a size of two ounces, leaving enough anterior wall to easily construct the anastomosis. Gastrogastrostomy will not result in adequate longterm weight loss. Moreover, a gastrogastrostomy of 3 cm is often constructed to obviate all obstructive and nutritional symptoms. An obstructed gastroplasty is best converted to a Roux-en-Y gastric bypass. This procedure, while more complex, offers a chance of permanent weight loss while still rectifying the problem.

Reoperation on an obstructed vertical gastroplasty should be undertaken only after careful consideration, since these channels are often easily dilated and surgery was seldom required in our series.[11] Anterior gastro-

---

*Wilson-Cook, Winston-Salem, NC, U.S.A.

TABLE 18.1. PROGNOSTIC FEATURES IN POST-GASTROPLASTY OBSTRUCTION

Favorable	Unfavorable
First gastroplasty	Revision gastroplasty
Gradual increase in tolerance to saliva, leading to ability to sip water	Unable to tolerate saliva or liquids
Small amount of barium passing through stoma or appearing in small bowel on delayed films	No passage of barium after 8–12 weeks of conservative therapy

gastrostomy over the vertical staple-lines will relieve obstruction but is followed by regain of weight. Deitel et al[3] recommend anterior freeing and division of the Marlex collar, passage of a 34 F bougie and suture of a short Marlex strip to both edges of the severed mesh. As an alternative, they have cut the polypropylene sutures, freed the anterior overlapped portions of the mesh, and sutured the *edges* together over a 34 F bougie.[3] After a Silastic ring vertical gastroplasty, the tubing is usually replaced by a larger 43–46 mm ring, which is not buried.[23]

Cowan and associates[24] found oral bacteria, likely introduced via the bougie, contaminating the stomach contents of 61% of patients undergoing vertical banded gastroplasty; 43% of all patients grew multiple bacteria. This suggests that bacteria can contaminate the mesh, lie dormant, and cause inflammatory narrowing later. The narrowing may be remedied by surgical enlargement of the collar.

An obstructed gastric bypass can be treated either by gastrogastrostomy or by revising the gastrojejunal anastomosis. The former procedure is simpler, but unlikely to maintain weight loss.

The most important principle of reoperative surgery is to wait as long as possible. Reoperations within the first 3–6 weeks are often very long and difficult. The mortality rate is about 4%, and the longterm success of revisionary surgery with respect to weight loss is poorly documented. Gastrostomies to assure decompression and feeding jejunostomies are important adjuvant procedures with reoperation.[3] Leaks and restenoses are not uncommon due to the additional devascularization which occurs at the second operation. For procedures in proximal greater curvature, care is required to avoid splenectomy, since this will further devascularize stomach in addition to exposing the patient to the complications of splenectomy.

REFERENCES

1. Ellison EC, Martin EW Jr, Laschinger J, et al: Prevention of early failure of stapled gastric partitions in the treatment of morbid obesity. Arch Surg 115:528–533, 1980.
2. Makarewicz PA, Freeman JB, Burchett H, et al: Vertical banded gastroplasty: assessment of efficacy. Surgery 98:700–707, 1985.
3. Deitel M, Jones BA, Petrov I, et al: Vertical banded gastroplasty: results in 233 patients. Can J Surg 29, 322–324, 1986.
4. Flickinger EG, Sinar DR, Pories WJ, et al: The bypassed stomach. Am J Surg 149:151–156, 1985.
5. Freeman JB: The use of endoscopy after gastric partitioning for morbid obesity. Gastroenterol Clin N Am 16:339–347, 1987.
6. Paulk SC: Formal dilatation after gastric partitioning. Surg Gynecol Obstet 156:503–504, 1984.
7. Winkler WP, Saleh J: Metoclopramide in treatment of gastric bezoars. Am J Gastroenterol 78:403–405, 1983.
8. Deitel M, McArdle AH, Brown R, et al: Elemental and liquid diets in surgery. In Deitel M (ed): Nutrition in Clinical Surgery, second edition. Baltimore, Williams & Wilkins, 1985, pp 44–49.
9. Dudrick SJ, O'Donnell JJ, Weinmann-Winkler S, et al: Nutritional assessment: indications for nutritional support. In Deitel M (ed): Nutrition in Clinical Surgery, second edition. Baltimore, Williams & Wilkins, 1985, pp 24–43.
10. Al-Halees ZY, Freeman JB: 21. Nonoperative management of stomal stenosis after gastric partitioning. Can J Surg 27:232–233, 1984.
11. Al-Halees ZY Freeman JB, Burchett H, et al: Nonoperative management of stomal stenosis after gastroplasty for morbid obesity. Surg Gynecol Obstet 162:349–354, 1986.
12. Freeman JB, Fairfull-Smith RJ: Feeding jejunostomy under local anesthesia. Can J Surg 24:511, 1981.
13. Keshishian JM, Smyth NPD, Maxwell DD, et al: Dilatation of difficult strictures of the esophagus. Surg Gynecol Obstet 158:81–85, 1984.
14. Royston CMS, Dowling BL, Gear MWL: Esophageal dilatation using the Eder-Puestow dilators. Am J Surg 131:697–700, 1976.
15. Monnier P, Hsieh V, Savary M: Endoscopic treatment of esophageal stenosis using Savary-Gilliard bougies: technical innovation. Acta Endoscopica 15:1–5, 1985.
16. Celestin LR, Campbell WB: A new and safe system for oesophageal dilatation. Lancet 1:74–75, 1981.
17. Fellows IW, Raina S, Holmes GKT: Celestin dilatation of benign esophageal strictures: a review of 100 patients. Am J Gastroenterol 81:1052–1054, 1986.
18. Lee CS, Perry AJ, Arate JE: Endoscopic treatment of

gastric stenosis secondary to gastric partition for morbid obesity (abstract). Gastrointest Endoscopy 28:136–137, 1982.

19. Taub S, Rodan BA, Bean WJ, et al: Balloon dilatation of esophageal strictures. Am J Gastroenterol 81:14–18, 1986.

20. Rankin RN, Ford J, Grace DM: Intestinal stomal dilatation. J Can Assoc Radiologists 35:332–334, 1984.

21. Lehman GA, O'Connor KW: Endoscopic tape dilator—a simple and inexpensive method to dilate upper gastrointestinal strictures. J Clin Gastroenterol 7:208–210, 1985.

22. Goff JS: The non-operative widening of obstructed gastroplasties with a papillotome. Gastrointest Endoscopy 30:32–34, 1984.

23. Shamblin JR, Shamblin AE: Gastroplasty in morbid obesity: observations in 300 patients. South Med J 78:1036–1040, 1985.

24. Cowan GSM Jr, Duralde RA, Ring WL: Presence of intragastric organisms in the bariatric surgical field. Proceedings of the Third Annual Meeting, American Society for Bariatric Surgery, Iowa City, June 18–20, 1986, pp 211–212.

19

Silastic Ring Vertical Gastroplasty

GIFFORD V. ECKHOUT
OTTO L. WILLBANKS

MATERIAL AND METHODS
  Technique
  Patient Data
RESULTS
COMMENTS
SUMMARY

Morbid obesity presents a serious health hazard.[1] Because of the almost total failure of medical treatment for morbid obesity, surgical procedures have been developed in an effort to relieve this devastating condition. Intestinal bypass produced satisfactory weight loss, but has been abandoned by most surgeons due to serious complications.[2]

In 1967, Mason[3] introduced gastric bypass and produced satisfactory long-term weight loss with a low complication rate and a low mortality rate, but the operation did not become popular until 1977, when Alden[4] adapted stapling instruments to Mason's gastric bypass. The addition of this stapling technique greatly simplified the operation, reduced the operating time by two-thirds, decreased the mortality to <0.5% and also yielded satisfactory long-term weight loss of 35 to 38% of the patient's initial weight. Because of some long-term problems of gastric bypass, such as marginal ulcer in 3%, vitamin B_{12}, folic acid, iron, and calcium deficiencies,[5] and the inability to examine the distal bypassed stomach, the authors, as well as other surgeons, began studies in 1979 of various gastroplasty procedures in an attempt to develop an operation which would be safer than gastric bypass and still produce satisfactory weight loss.

For a gastroplasty operation to be successful, several criteria must be met: a less than one ounce size gastric reservoir is established, with a 10–12 mm outlet which is stabilized by a non-absorbing material, and with a permanent gastric partition that will not break down.[6] Most of the first various gastroplasty operations employed a transverse staple-line across the upper portion of the stomach to form a small gastric pouch. Unfortunately, transverse staple-line gastroplasties have been associated with failure to produce permanent adequate weight loss in up to 70–80%.[7–11] With these objectives in mind, in 1979 we began a study of vertical gastroplasty (VG).

MATERIAL AND METHODS

Our experience involves 1463 VG patients with 3 methods of support to the outlet of the pouch: 192 patients with a chromic ring (CRVG), 157 patients with a *covered* silastic ring, and 1114 patients with a *non-covered* silastic ring to support the outlet.[12]

TECHNIQUE

The first step in VG is to make a window in the gastrohepatic ligament close to the stomach (Fig. 19.1) midway between the pylorus and cardia and another window above the greater curvature close to the esophagus. The two windows are connected with an 18 F urethral catheter for safe passage of a 90 mm stapler (Fig. 19.2). A directly superimposed or immediately adjacent double (4-row) staple-line is placed vertically, parallel to the lesser curvature of the stomach, forming a less than one ounce size proximal gastric pouch with an outlet located also on the lesser curvature. The staple-lines are made with two firings of a special notched TA-90™ (Autosuture) or PI-90™ (3M Surgical Division) stapler using 4.8 mm staples. More recently, the TA-90-BN™ has been used to place 4 equidistant staple-lines with one firing (Fig. 19.3).

In order to leave a portion of the gastric lumen along the lesser curvature open to form the outlet of the pouch, it is necessary to employ a modified 90 stapler with a "notch" built into the heel to leave the channel unstapled. In 1979, a TA-90™ stapler was modified for this purpose. In 1984, notched instruments became commercially available specifically to perform VG.

The CRVG patients were done using a no. 1 chromic suture tied down over either a 30 or 32 F dilator in the lesser curvature channel to form a 10–11 mm stoma. A pseudopylorus was made with running 2-0 polypropylene covering the chromic suture and a layer of silk lemberts to accentuate the pseudopylorus. Early weight loss was satisfactory with the chromic ring, but with absorption of the chromic ring, dilation of the stoma occurred, allowing weight gain. This experience led to the use of the silastic ring, which is a non-expandable permanent support for the stoma. The technique for the use of the silastic ring was described by Laws.[13]

Our first group of 157 silastic ring vertical gastroplasty (SRVG) patients with covered rings had a 40 to 43 mm length of silastic tubing (Heyer-Schulte, Silicone Elastomer) size 7–10 F tied over a 30 or 32 F dilator. The silastic ring is held in place with a double strand of 2-0 polypropylene, using a Keith needle to pass through the stomach to the left of the staple-lines (Fig. 19.4). The silastic ring was then covered (i.e., buried) with a running 2-0 polypropylene suture, following Laws' technique.[13]

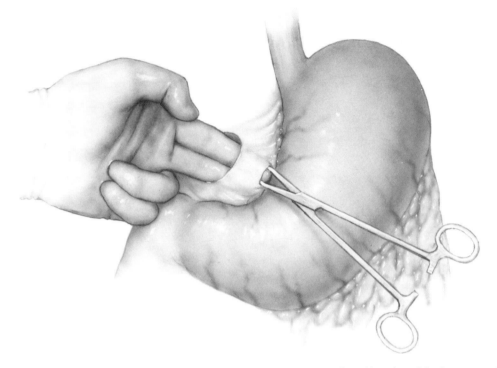

FIGURE 19.1. With the finger through the opening in the lesser omentum, at the mid-portion of the lesser curvature a window is made close to the gastric wall through which the notched 90 stapler is introduced.

To increase the strength of the staple-lines, a running 2-0 polypropylene suture was placed through-and-through the gastric wall to encircle and reinforce the staple-lines (Fig. 19.5).

It soon became evident that some patients with a covered silastic ring developed erosion of the silastic ring into the lumen of the stomach. This erosion was a benign event, not accompanied by a leak, but resulted in loss of effectiveness of the support, allowing dilation of the stoma with resultant weight gain. In 1984, a collected series* of 2515 SRVG patients was reported in which there were 1014 patients with covered rings and 1501 with non-covered rings.[14] In this collected study there were 29 known erosions of the silastic ring in the covered SRVG group and only one known erosion in the 1501 patients with the non-covered silastic ring. Therefore, our next 1114 SRVG patients were done with the same technique but without covering the silastic ring (Fig. 19.5).

PATIENT DATA

Preoperative evaluation included study of the gallbladder, upper gastrointestinal tract,

thyroid, and bleeding and clotting parameters. The age range was 15 to 68 years (mean 40.4 years). The average weight for women was 241 lb (109.5 kg) and for men 329 lb (149.5 kg). All patients were at least twice ideal weight or 100 lb (45 kg) above ideal weight, using the Metropolitan Life Insurance Company tables.[15–17] All patients were unable to lose weight by medical means, had no medical disease that would contraindicate major surgery, and had been morbidly obese for several years. Several patients were <100 lb above ideal weight but were accepted for surgery because of medical problems which would be improved by weight loss, such as debilitating osteoarthritis of weight-bearing joints. Absolute contraindications to surgery included alcoholism, active peptic ulcer disease and recent myocardial infarction.

Early frequent ambulation was encouraged and continued throughout the first postoperative night. The nasogastric tube was removed either in the recovery room or 24 hours after surgery, and oral fluids were started at 48 hours. On discharge, the diet was restricted to full liquids for the first 90 days. Two chewable multiple vitamin pills were taken daily.

*Eckhout GV, Fox SR, Willbanks OL, Fabito DC, Kane JM, Laws HL, Shamblin JR, Shamblin W, Alston JL.

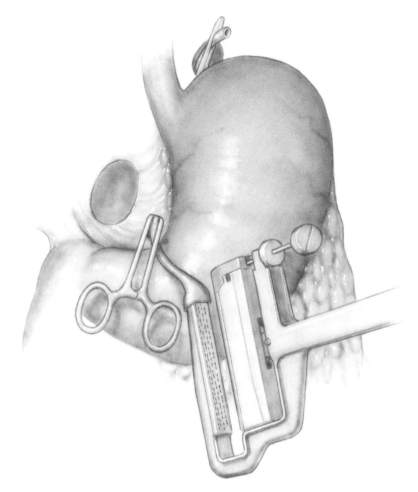

FIGURE 19.2. An 18 F urethral catheter is passed to guide placement of the notched 90 stapler. (Copyright United States Surgical Corporation, 1986. Used by permission.)

Peri-operative antibiotics were used as well as low dose heparin. The average patient was discharged on the fifth postoperative day. Frequent explicit diet counselling was given both before and after surgery and continued for the first 12 months. All patients were encouraged to attend our gastric stapling support group meetings both before and after surgery. Walking up to 2 miles per day by the end of 6 weeks was encouraged.

RESULTS

The mortality rate for the 1463 patients was 0.13%. There was one death from pulmonary embolism and one from cardiac arrhythmia (Table 19.1). There was one leak which occurred in a patient with a CRVG. A lesser sac abscess was noted in three patients. A leak could not be demonstrated in any one of the three patients. One patient in the series developed an obstruction of the stoma and required reversal of the gastroplasty. This patient was on high doses of anti-inflammatory drugs, which contributed to the stricture.

Revisions were necessary in 14.1% of the CRVG patients for dilation of the stoma with weight gain. Dilation of the stoma did not occur with SRVG unless the silastic ring eroded into the lumen of the stomach, which occurred only in the covered silastic ring group. Of the 1114 patients with a non-covered silastic ring, no erosions of the ring have been observed. Of the non-covered SRVG patients, revision was required in 14 patients: 13 for staple-line disruption resulting in failure to lose an adequate amount of weight, and one for stomal narrowing causing inability to tolerate meat. Rehospitalization for excessive vomiting has been much less frequent with the non-covered silastic ring. This is thought to be due to less edema of the stoma

NASOGASTRIC
TUBE

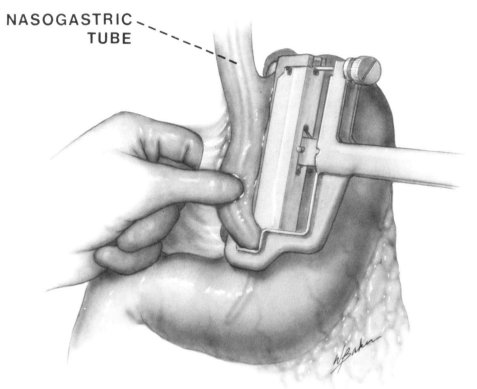

FIGURE 19.3. The notched 90 stapler is applied vertically parallel to the lesser curvature, forming a <30 mL pouch. Note the nasogastric tube out of harm's way, held firmly in the notch. 4.8 mm staples are used.

with the non-covered ring. CRVG produced the least weight loss while non-covered SRVG gave the best, which was equivalent to that reported for gastric bypass (Table 19.2).

COMMENTS

A gastroplasty operation must have an outlet which will not dilate, if weight loss is to be permanent. The high failure-rates of gastroplasty with a transverse staple-line are largely due to dilation of the outlet and lack of any satisfactory technique to stabilize the stoma. Many investigators have tried various sutures, meshes, Teflon pledgets, and other devices without success, due to erosion, migration, obstruction or other problems when attempting to stabilize the outlet with a transverse staple-line.[18,19]

When SRVG was first introduced, there was apprehension that the same fate would befall the silastic ring. Indeed, when the first erosions of the silastic ring were encountered with the covered silastic ring technique, there was concern that all silastic rings would eventually erode and migrate. However, with the report of the collected series of 2515 SRVG

patients in 1984, showing only one erosion when a non-covered silastic ring was used,[14] enthusiasm for non-covered SRVG gained momentum. The absence of erosion of the silastic ring when the ring is not buried is borne out by our series of 1114 non-covered SRVG with no erosions encountered. It is postulated that erosion of the silastic ring occurs when the ring is covered by inverting the gastric wall with sutures which are too tight, causing pressure on the ring. The initial technique of using the silastic ring introduced by Laws unfortunately suggested that the ring be covered to prevent leaks. With experience in the use of the silastic ring, it has been found that leaks when the ring is left uncovered are extremely rare.[20]

Patients with uncovered SRVG have comparatively less vomiting, and the majority of patients state that eventually they are able to eat a regular diet including meat and fresh vegetables. All gastroplasty patients report epigastric pain and vomiting if food is not well masticated or is consumed rapidly.

It is important that all patients take multiple vitamins daily to avoid symptomatic avita-

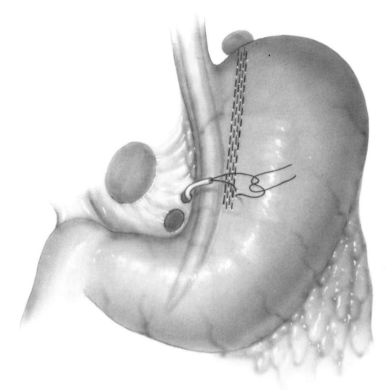

FIGURE 19.4. A 4.3 cm length of silastic tubing size 7–10 French is threaded twice over a strand of 2-0 polypropylene which passes through-and-through the gastric wall on the greater curvature side of the staple-line, inserted about 1 cm cephalad to the lower end of the staple-line. Keith needle is used on 2-0 polypropylene.

minosis. Close follow-up with frequent dietetic counselling is important, as well as daily exercise to achieve adequate weight loss. In general, medical problems are improved after surgery as weight loss continues. Diabetics required less or no insulin. Anti-inflammatory and antihypertensive medications were reduced or discontinued in most patients. Symptomatic relief of lower extremity vari-

cosities and osteoarthritic back, hip and knee pain was noted.

SUMMARY

Vertical gastroplasty is a safer and simpler operation than gastric bypass for morbid obesity, but to produce permanent weight loss, a permanent support is needed for the outlet

TABLE 19.1. SURGICAL COMPLICATIONS

No. of Patients	CRVG 192	Silastic Ring VG Covered 157	Uncovered 1114
Deaths	0%	0%	0.17%
Staple-line failure	2.6%	3.8%	1.16%
Stomal dilation	14.1%	17.2%	0%
Erosion of silastic ring		17.2%	0%
Revised	14.1%	15.3%	1.25%
Splenectomy	1.6%	0.6%	0.40%
Wound infection	7.3%	3.8%	0.90%
Rehospitalized—vomiting	8.3%	7.0%	1.00%
Gastric hemorrhage	1.0%	0%	0.10%
Pulmonary embolus	0.5%	0.6%	0.10%
Leaks (proven)	0.5%	0%	0%
Abdominal abscess (leak?)	0%	0%	0.30%
Stomal obstruction	0%	0%	0.10%
Reversal—psychological?	0.5%	1.3%	0.30%

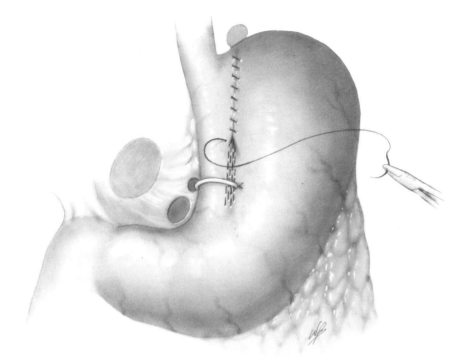

FIGURE 19.5. 2-0 polypropylene suture is tied down over 30 or 32 F bougie in lesser curvature channel, with ends of the silastic ring gently touching the gastric wall anteriorly and posteriorly. Running 2-0 polypropylene suture encircles all staple-lines and includes anterior and posterior gastric wall bites. The bougie is removed and replaced by a nasogastric tube.

TABLE 19.2. COMPARISON OF 24-MONTH AVERAGE WEIGHT LOSS

		Pounds	% Excess Wt. Loss	% Pre-op Wt. Loss
Chromic ring VG	(192 patients)			
24 mo	72 patients	67.4	50.6	25.5
Covered SRVG	(157 patients)			
24 mo	77 patients	75.4	59.3	29.9
Uncovered SRVG	(1114 patients)			
24 mo	325 patients	100.9	63.4	36.7

of the gastric pouch. The important development in this study of 1463 VG patents is the safe and practical use of a silastic ring to permanently support the outlet. Weight loss at 2 years was only 25.5% for CRVG and 29.9% for buried SRVG. However, using a non-covered silastic ring in 1114 patients, erosion of the ring has not been observed and the long-term weight loss of 36.7% of original weight or 63.4% of excess weight is equivalent to that for gastric bypass or other gastric reduction procedures, with a lower mortality and morbidity rate. SRVG with an uncovered ring is the safest and most effective of the gastric reduction operations for morbid obesity.

REFERENCES

1. Drenick EJ: Risk of obesity and surgical indications. Int J Obesity 5:387–398, 1980.
2. Griffen WO, Young VL, Stevenson CC: A prospective comparison of gastric and jejunoileal bypass procedures for morbid obesity. Ann Surg 186:500–509, 1977.
3. Mason EE, Ito C: Gastric bypass in obesity. Surg Clin North Am 47:1345–1351, 1967.
4. Alden JF: Gastric and jejunoileal bypass. Arch Surg 112:799–803, 1977.
5. Halverson JD, Zuckerman GR, Koehler RE, et al: Gastric bypass for morbid obesity. A medical-surgical assessment. Ann Surg 194:152–160, 1981.
6. Willbanks OL: Gastric restrictive procedures: gastroplasty. Gastroenterol Clin North Am 16:273–281, 1987.

7. Linner JH: Comparative effectiveness of gastric bypass and gastroplasty. Arch Surg 117:695–700, 1982.

8. Pories WJ, Flickinger EG, Meelheim D, et al: The effectiveness of gastric bypass over gastric partition in morbid obesity. Consequences of distal gastric and duodenal exclusion. Ann Surg 196:389–399, 1982.

9. Lechner GW, Callender AK: Subtotal gastric exclusion and gastric partitioning: a randomized prospective comparison of 100 patients. Surgery 90:637–644, 1981.

10. Laws HL, Piantadosi S: Superior gastric reduction procedure for morbid obesity. A prospective, randomized trial. Ann Surg 193:334–336, 1981.

11. MacLean LD, Rhode BM, Shizgal HM: Gastroplasty for obesity. Surg Gynecol Obstet 153:200–208, 1981.

12. Eckhout GV, Willbanks OL, Moore JT: Vertical ring gastroplasty for obesity: five year experience with 1463 patients. Am J Surg 152:713–716, 1986.

13. Laws HL: Standardized gastroplasty orifice. Am J Surg 141:393–394, 1981.

14. Eckhout GV: Vertical gastroplasty with chromic or silastic ring vs gastric bypass. Proceedings, 1st Annual Meeting, American Society for Bariatric Surgery, Iowa City, June 4–5, 1984, pp 191–196.

15. Metropolitan Life Insurance Company: New weight standards for men and women. Statistical Bulletin, 40:1, 1959.

16. Buchwald J: True informed consent in surgical treatment of morbid obesity. Am J Clin Nutr 33:482–499, 1980.

17. Statistical Bulletin, vol 64, no 1, Metropolitan Life Foundation, New York pp 2–9, 1983.

18. Linner JH: Surgery for Morbid Obesity. New York, Springer-Verlag, 1984, p 61.

19. Smith LB, Fricke FJ, Graney AS: Results and complications of gastric partitioning: four-year follow-up of 300 morbidly obese patients. Am J Surg 146:815–819, 1983.

20. Willbanks OL: Long-term results of silicone elastomer ring vertical gastroplasty for the treatment of morbid obesity. Surgery 101:606–610, 1987.

20

Gastric Banding

LUBOMYR I. KUZMAK

Gastric banding is a less invasive procedure than any other gastric restriction operation. When the band is placed around the stomach, a small pouch and a small reinforced stoma are created in one step. The stomach is not cut or crushed by staples, no anastomoses are made and there are no changes made in the food passage.

INTRODUCTION

The concept of using gastric banding for treatment of obesity originated in 1976, when Wilkinson performed the first such operation (see Chapter 21). He used a strip of Marlex mesh as the banding material. Because the patient experienced poor weight loss, Wilkinson did not pursue this concept.

In 1980–1981, the gastric banding operation was independently introduced by Marcel Molina (Houston, USA) and Knut Kolle (Oslo, Norway). The first written reports about the technique were presented by Kolle.[1-3] Initially, Kolle used a self-lockable nylon band (personal communication) (Fig. 20.1). Later, the band was enclosed in a Dacron arterial prosthetic graft[2,4] (Fig. 20.2), and eventually a Dacron arterial graft 14-mm-wide without the self-lockable band was used at the Ulleval University Hospital in Oslo, Norway and by other surgeons[5] (Fig. 20.3).

Molina has used the Dacron arterial graft as his banding material from the beginning. Molina's surgical technique differs significantly from all the other surgical techniques used in gastric banding. His technique involves a very small skin incision and blind blunt dissection of the tunnel under the stomach toward the avascular ligament of the fundus with the fingers, as a preparation for gastric banding.[6] He does the procedure largely by palpation.

Gastric banding has become the prevailing procedure for controlling severe obesity in the Scandinavian countries and Australia. Also, it is an accepted operation in the United States, Poland, Czechoslovakia and other countries.

Since 1981, Lars Backman and Lars Granström have been using a strip of Marlex mesh 2.5 cm-wide for gastric banding.[7,8] They were the first to measure the tension applied to the band by using a dynamometer.

Since 1983, Ingmar Näslund of Sweden has performed 55 gastric bandings using the polytetrafluoroethylene (PTFE, Gore-Tex or Impra) band (personal communication). James

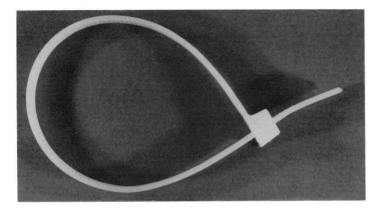

FIGURE 20.1. Self-lockable nylon band.

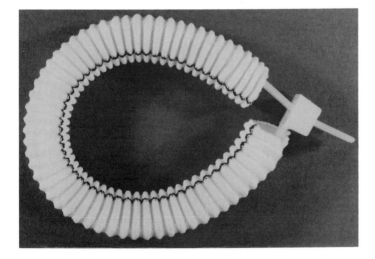

FIGURE 20.2. Self-lockable nylon band covered with Dacron vascular graft.

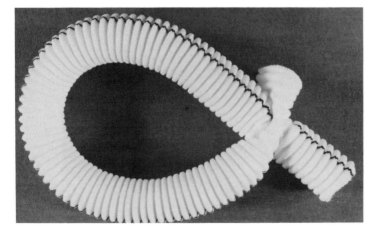

FIGURE 20.3. Dacron vascular graft band.

Ritchie of Australia also has been performing gastric banding since 1983 and utilizes the technique recommended by Molina with a Dacron vascular graft (personal communication).

David M. Steinberg and Harry B. Frydenberg, both from Australia, also started performing gastric banding in 1983. Steinberg has been using the Dacron arterial graft (personal communication). Frydenberg uses a 1.5 cm-wide silicone band reinforced with a single layer of mesh (personal communication), over a 36 or 38 Fr bougie. The silicone band has serrated edges, with the narrowest part 8 mm. The serrated edges make the band self-lockable.[9] Excess band is cut off, the band sutured together, and the stomach imbricated anteriorly over the band.

Gastric wall erosions by the band following gastric banding (Fig. 20.4) have been reported by other surgeons in personal communications with the author. However, there is no published statistical information on the subject. Näslund, through personal contacts with the other Swedish bariatric surgeons, reviewed over 250 patients with gastric banding procedures (personal communication). These patients had been followed for up to 3 years and represented approximately 60% of all such operations performed in Sweden during that time period. He found that the incidence of stomach wall erosion in gastric banding was 4%. Marlex mesh, Dacron vascular graft and PTFE had been used as the banding material. The highest incidence of gastric wall erosions occurred with the PTFE band. The

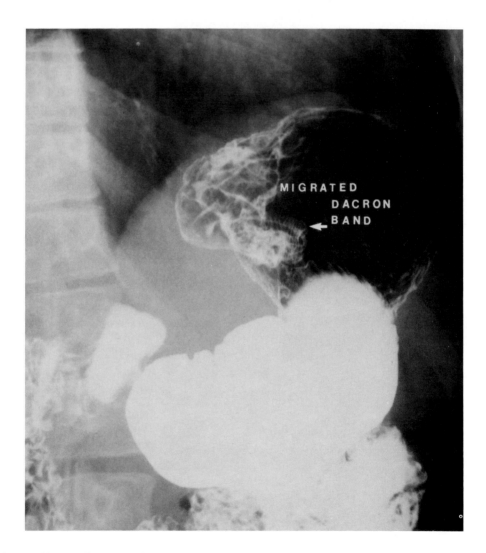

FIGURE 20.4. Migrated Dacron band.

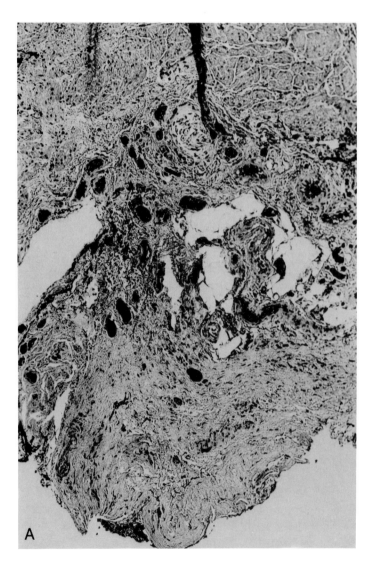

FIGURE 20.5-A. Serosal fibrosis in full-thickness biopsy, 39 months after SGB.

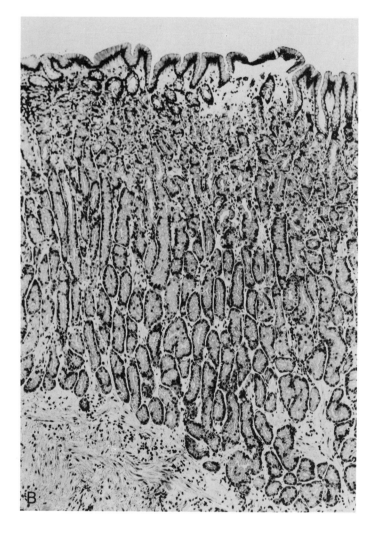

FIGURE 20.5-B. Normal gastric mucosa in full-thickness biopsy, 39 months after SGB.

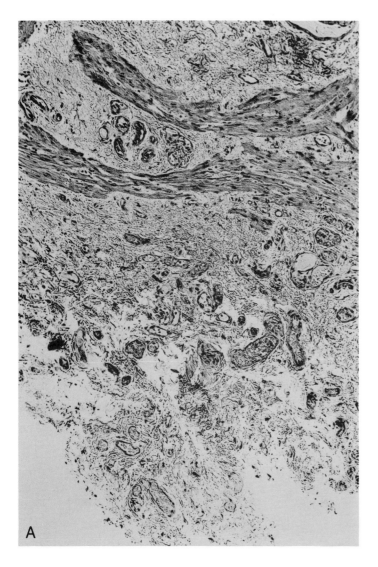

FIGURE 20.6-A. Serosal fibrosis in full-thickness biopsy, 36 months after SGB.

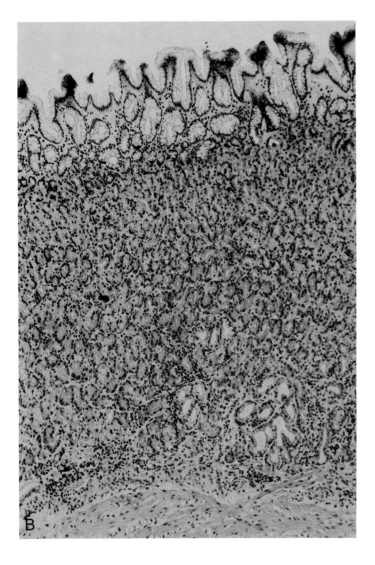

FIGURE 20.6-B. Normal gastric mucosa in full-thickness biopsy, 36 months after SGB.

mechanism that causes stomach wall erosion is not clear. Although banding creates an hour-glass configuration of the stomach, it does not constrict the stomach to the point that ischemia may develop at the banding site. While the chemical composition of the band may be a very important factor, most likely a combination of factors leads to the gastric wall erosion.

The author uses a silicone band, since silicone is one of the most inert materials used in the medical field.[10,11] In more than 4½ years of experience with more than 240 **silicone gastric bandings (SGB)**, there has not been a single incidence of the band eroding into the stomach wall. Full-thickness biopsy of the area where the band had been placed, performed 39 months after banding during a patient-requested take-down of SGB, revealed only serosal fibrosis (Fig. 20.5-A) and normal mucosal surface (Fig. 20.5-B). In another patient undergoing revision of SGB at 36 months after banding, similar results were found when a full-thickness biopsy was done (Fig. 20.6-A, 20.6-B). To date, a total of 7 patients with varying lengths of follow-up have had full-thickness biopsies. None of the biopsies have shown any pathological findings indicating impending gastric wall erosion. No giant or inflammatory cells were found in any of the biopsies. This is contrary to the experimental findings in studies with Dacron graft and Marlex mesh,[8,12] where giant and inflammatory cells were found in all specimens. It appears that the silicone band is safe for use in gastric banding.

MATERIALS AND METHODS

The first SGB operation was performed by the author in January 1983 and since then 244 SGB have been done. The operation was done to revise failed other gastric restriction operations in 60 patients. The new inflatable band was used in 32 patients. The remaining 152 were primary patients. The silicone band, which is 1-cm-wide and soft, but reinforced with two layers of Dacron mesh (Fig. 20.7), was made to the author's specifications (originally by Mentor Corporation). The band is covered by a silicone drain-like cover which smooths the edges and reduces the possibility of gastric wall erosion. At one end there is a buckle to facilitate the tightening of the band. The band is radiopaque for easy radiological evaluation.

It is generally accepted in gastric bariatric surgery that the pouch and stoma must be properly measured and calibrated in order to ensure a good result. In gastric banding, the diameter of the stoma depends both on the diameter of the calibrating tube and, even more importantly, on how tightly the band is placed around the stomach. Granström in his study of three different band tensions measured during the operation with a dynamometer, confirmed that the tension applied to the band when it is placed around the stomach has a direct effect on postoperative weight loss.[8]

From the beginning of his series, the author has been developing and testing different calibrating devices to determine how tight the band should be placed around the stomach and how that tightness corresponds with the diameter of the stoma. As a result of this research, a calibrating tube and an electronic sensor were developed by the author (Fig. 20.8). The calibrating tube has two independent compartments. One is an inflatable balloon to measure the capacity of the pouch and the other is an air-chamber that connects to the electronic sensor. The outside diameter of the air-chamber is 13 mm. Compression of the air-chamber by tightening the band will turn on sequential lights on the sensor. These lights correspond to the diameter of the stoma. In the recently redesigned electronic sensor, the first light indicates that the sensor is set at point zero. The second light corresponds to a stoma-diameter of 13 mm, and the third light indicates that the stoma is between 12 and 13 mm. The fourth light corresponds to a 12-mm diameter stoma. By reading these lights, the surgeon can easily select the desired diameter of the stoma.

In order to tighten the band around the stomach and hold the desired tightness until the band is sutured, a banding instrument (Pilling Company) was designed by the author (Fig. 20.9). Once the desired stoma-diameter has been achieved, by fastening the screw on the handle, the desired tension of the band can be held, while the band is sutured together.

While the calibrating devices and other instruments were developed gradually and changed as needed, the basic design and composition of the silicone band has not changed since 1983. However, in 1985, the band was modified by adding a small inflatable part. Since June 1986, 32 patients received this modified band. The surgical technique, com-

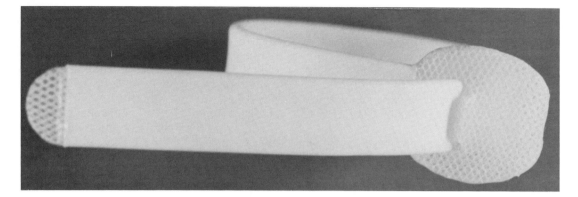

FIGURE 20.7. Dacron reinforced silicone band designed by author.

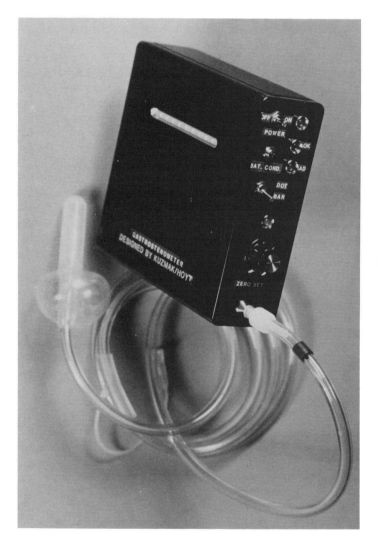

FIGURE 20.8. Pouch and stoma calibrating tube and electronic sensor.

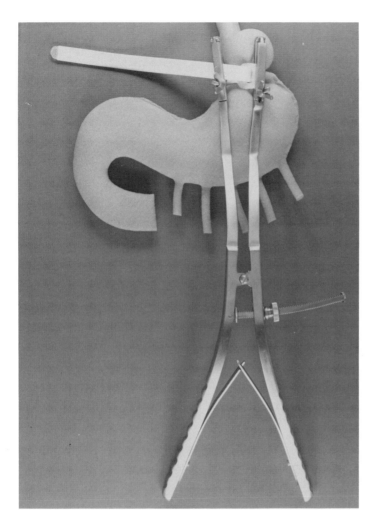

FIGURE 20.9. Banding instrument designed by author.

plications and results of both the non-inflatable and inflatable SGB will be discussed.

PRE-, PERI- AND POSTOPERATIVE MANAGEMENT

Preoperative Evaluation of a Candidate for SGB

Prospective patients contact the office and request information about SGB. Those candidates who according to the guidelines established by the American Society for Bariatric Surgery qualify for SGB (see Chapter 7), receive a preliminary booklet through the mail. This booklet contains both an extensive questionnaire pertaining to the patient's medical history and obesity-related problems and general information on the SGB operation. After receiving this booklet, people who are still interested in this operation are requested to return the questionnaire and call the office for an appointment.

Prospective patients are required to visit the office twice. The first visit is with the patient care coordinator who obtains detailed information on the patient's background and medical, psychiatric, and obesity history, to accompany information from the questionnaire. The patient than receives a second booklet with various articles regarding obesity surgery, the health risks related to obesity, information on postoperative lifestyle changes and a copy of the post-gastric-banding diet.

During the second visit, the candidate views a videotape presentation. In the videotape are sections on the operative risks and the changes in lifestyle and eating habits that will result from the surgery. Following the video, a discussion is conducted with the surgeon and the dietitian. During this session, the surgeon discusses the SGB operation, long-term results, possible complications and operative risk. The dietitian stresses the changes in eating habits that will accompany the surgery.

Medical and psychosocial information about each candidate is carefully reviewed and analyzed before the operation is scheduled. An ultrasound scan and GI series are performed before admission to hospital, while other laboratory tests and consultations are obtained on admission. If a cholecystectomy is needed, it is performed simultaneously with the SGB operation. Due to the potential risk of silicone implant infection, we believe that neither intraoperative cholangiogram nor common bile duct exploration should be done. Results of all preadmission consultations and tests are reviewed before the patient's admission to the hospital.

Hospital Stay

ADMISSION DAY. Routine preoperative tests are done. A pulmonary consultation and an anesthesia consultation are obtained for all patients. A full liquid diet is given. Heparin 5000 units subcutaneously is given every 12 hours to patients weighing <300 lb (136 kg) and every 8 hours to patients weighing >300 lb. Routine preparation for major surgery is carried out.

DAY OF SURGERY. A. BEFORE THE OPERATION. Prophylactic doses of antibiotics, heparin and preanesthesia medications are given as ordered. Athrombic calves connected to a pump are used in all patients during the operation and for the following 24 hours. Antiembolic stockings were found to be too small for most of the morbidly obese patients and are not used.

B. AFTER THE OPERATION. Sips of water are permitted. A small cocktail straw is used to diminish the amount of swallowed air. A nasogastric tube is not inserted. Pulmonary care orders are given by the pulmonary consultant. Heparin, prophylactic antibiotics and in-

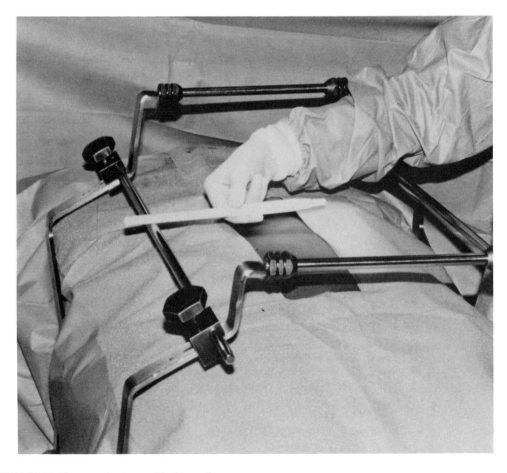

FIGURE 20.10. Gomez retractor modified by author.

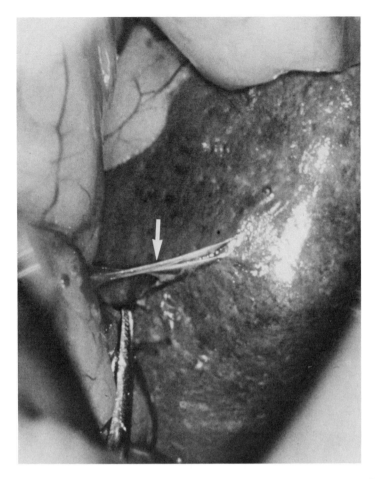

FIGURE 20.11. Adhesions to the spleen.

travenous infusion are continued. An over-head trapeze is mounted for all patients.

FIRST POSTOPERATIVE DAY. The patient is ambulated. Athrombic calves connected to the pump are removed.

SECOND POSTOPERATIVE DAY. Intravenous infusion, prophylactic antibiotics and the Foley catheter are discontinued. The patient is ambulated outside the room. "Second Day" post-gastric-banding diet is started and progressed daily. Dulcolax suppository is given. Heparin is continued until the day of discharge from the hospital.

DAY OF DISCHARGE. Before discharge, a GI series is done. Also pulmonary and surgical evaluations of the patient are done. Instructions about activities and follow-up visits are given by the surgeon. The post-gastric-banding diet,* changes in eating habits and the importance of vitamin supplements are discussed by the dietitian.

---

*Post-gastric-banding diet plan, available from L.I. Kuzmak, M.D., 340 E. Northfield Road, Livingston, NJ 07039.

Postoperative Follow-up

The first office visit is scheduled for 3 weeks after discharge. Monthly visits are strongly suggested for local patients. Out-of-state patients receive a supply of questionnaires that are to be mailed by the patient at 3-month intervals. Patients who do not return for scheduled visits are contacted by telephone or mail. All office visits are free of charge indefinitely.

During the first 1–3 months after surgery, over-eating, too frequent eating or eating solid foods should be avoided; all solid food should be ground or pureed. Intake is restricted to 600–800 (maximum 1000) calories per day. Vitamins with minerals are prescribed. High caloric liquids should be avoided, and the patient should eat only three meals per day. After 1–3 months, solid food may be taken slowly if thoroughly chewed. The patient should stop eating at the first feeling of fullness to avoid vomiting.

A follow-up GI series is requested yearly after SGB to evaluate the position of the band, the pouch size and the incidence of esopha-

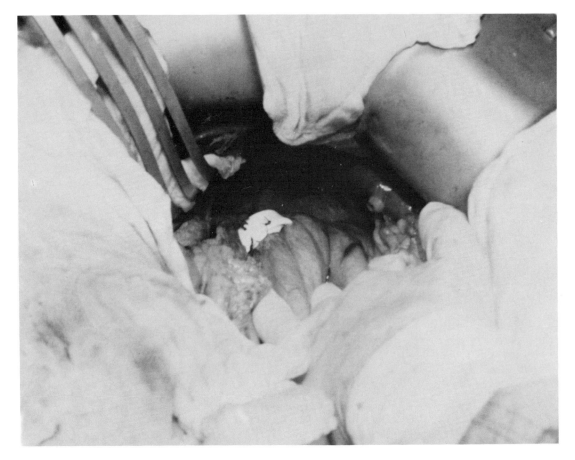

FIGURE 20.12. Exposure of the gastroesophageal junction. Liver retractor modified by author. Note completed SGB.

geal reflux. Laboratory work-up is done at the same time. While the pre-, peri- and postoperative care is the same regardless of whether the band is non-inflatable or inflatable, the operative techniques for non-inflatable and inflatable are considerably different. For this reason, the technique and results of each type will be discussed separately.

NON-INFLATABLE SGB

SURGICAL TECHNIQUE

Following the usual preparation and draping for an abdominal procedure, a Gomez retractor modified by the author (Pilling Company) (Fig. 20.10) is fastened to the operating-table. An upper midline incision is made and the abdomen is explored. Adhesions to the spleen are secured and transected to prevent injury to the spleen (Fig. 20.11). The Gomez retractor is then assembled using three blades. The first blade lifts the sternum, while the second retracts the left rib cage, and the

third retracts the liver. To provide better exposure to the gastroesophageal junction and subdiaphragmatic space, the author modified the fingers of the liver retractor by making them longer and slightly curved (Pilling Company) (Fig. 20.12). When the retractor assembly is completed, the gastrohepatic ligament is opened in the avascular area (Fig. 20.13). Then using blunt dissection with fingers, a tunnel is formed under the stomach and through the avascular gastrophrenic suspensory ligament of the fundus (Fig. 20.14). The tunnel is started at midportion of the lesser curvature of the stomach. For traction, a Penrose drain is placed around the stomach, the gastric vessels and branches of the vagus nerve (Fig. 20.15). The fundus is further mobilized to obtain the correct pouch volume. Once the fundus has been adequately mobilized, a small opening is made next to the lesser curvature, 3 cm below the gastroesophageal junction and medial to the gastric vessels and branches of the vagus nerve. The silicone band is then threaded through that opening and around the stomach (Fig. 20.16).

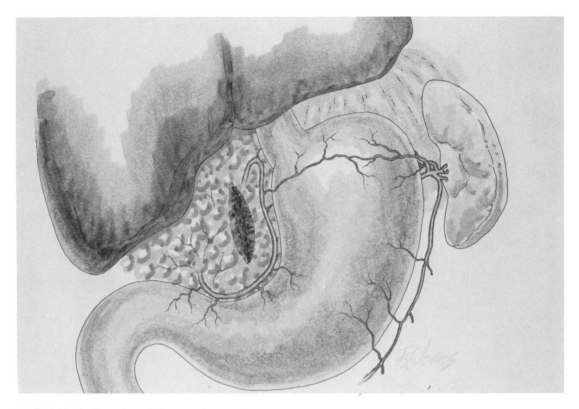

FIGURE 20.13. Gastrohepatic ligament is opened in the avascular area. Reproduced with permission from Kuzmak, LI: Silicone gastric banding: a simple and effective operation for morbid obesity. Contemp Surg 28:13–18, 1986.

Care must be exercised when placing the band. It should not be placed over the gastric vessels, since the circulation of the stomach wall could be impaired. More importantly, the fat within the gastrohepatic ligament under the band will undergo atrophy which will lead to stomal enlargement. Compression of the vagus nerve may cause pylorospasm.

After the silicone band has been guided into place around the stomach, the anesthesiologist inserts the calibrating tube. The volume of the pouch is then calibrated by inflating the balloon with 20 mL of saline. The silicone band is tightened to the desired stoma-diameter, using the previously described banding instrument. In patients weighing <300 lb (136 kg), a 13-mm stoma is created. In patients weighing ≥300 lb, a 12-mm stoma is suggested. As mentioned previously, the diameter of the stoma can be selected by reading the lights on the sensor. At the correct tightness, the band is sutured together with four nonabsorbable 2–0 sutures. The buckle and the redundant portion of the band are excised. The previously mobilized greater curvature is sutured over the band to

the pouch with three to four 3–0 silk sutures (Fig. 20.17). The position of the band and hemostasis are checked. The abdomen is irrigated with antibiotic solution. The incision is closed in the usual fashion for abdominal procedures.

RESULTS

Non-inflatable SGB has been performed in 212 patients since January 1983. Of these patients, 152 were undergoing their first, or primary, bariatric operation. The other 60 patients had SGB as a revision for failed other gastric restriction operations. Only the results of the primary non-inflatable SGB will be discussed in this section. The early results from the use of the inflatable SGB and the results of SGB as a revision operation for other failed gastric restriction procedures will be discussed in later sections.

Of the 152 patients, 140 (92.1%) are still being followed. Only 11 (7.2%) of the patients have been lost to follow-up. There was one operative death. Analyses of the remaining 140 patients that have been followed include average excess weight loss, early and late

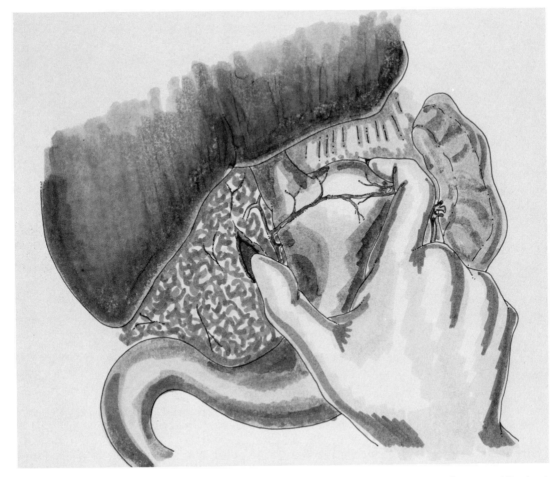

FIGURE 20.14. A tunnel is made behind the stomach and through the avascular suspensory ligament of the fundus using blunt dissection with fingers.

complications and/or reoperations, and long-term follow-up evaluation with GI series.

The average preoperative weight was 293 lb (133 kg), with the heaviest patient weighing 510 lb (231 kg). The average percent of excess weight lost at 1 year postoperatively was 42.1 ± 25.5%. The average excess weight loss at 2 years was 60.1 ± 27.3%, at 3 years 72.0 ± 26.5% and at 4 years 76.0 ± 22.8%. At 55 months, the longest follow-up, the average is 72.7 ± 36.6%. Slightly more than 28% of the patients have reached a weight that is less than 30% above their estimated ideal weight.

Early Complications and Reoperations (Table 20.1)

The one operative mortality (0.7%) was due to massive pulmonary embolism. This was the only mortality in the author's series of SGB operations.

TABLE 20.1.   EARLY COMPLICATIONS AND REOPERATIONS IN 152 PRIMARY NON-INFLATABLE SILICONE GASTRIC BANDINGS

Complication	Type of Reoperation	No. of Patients	%
Pulmonary embolism, fatal	—	1	0.7
Mortality	—	1	0.7
Femoral artery embolism	Femoral Embolectomy	1	0.7
Obstruction of stoma from:			
edema	—	3	2.0
migration of band over cardia	Banding Revised	1	0.7
Minor pulmonary complications	—	6	3.9

TABLE 20.2. LATE COMPLICATIONS AND REOPERATIONS IN 152 PRIMARY NON-INFLATABLE SILICONE GASTRIC BANDINGS

Complication	Type of Reoperation	No. of Patients	%
Persistent excessive vomiting	Stoma size enlarged	3	2.0
No feeling of satiety leading to excessive eating	Stoma size decreased	3	2.0
Late stomal obstruction	Banding revised	4	2.6
Excessive enlargement of pouch	Banding revised*	3	2.0
Incisional hernia	Hernia repair*	3	2.0

*Only 2 of 3 reoperated.

One patient developed an embolism of the femoral artery, requiring femoral embolectomy. Three patients developed obstruction of the stoma due to edema (2.0%), and all 3 patients were successfully treated with intravenous infusions and nasogastric tube.

Another patient drank a large amount of water on the third postoperative day and developed violent vomiting (0.7%). The severity of the vomiting caused the band to migrate over the cardia. Revision of the SGB was done on the sixth postoperative day.

Six patients had minor pulmonary complications (3.9%); none required extension of their hospital stay. There were no wound infections or dehiscences, intraabdomial infections or splenic injuries.

Late Complications and Reoperations (Table 20.2)

Persistent and excessive vomiting in three patients (2.0%) was caused by a too small stoma. All three patients were among the first patients who had SGB, when the stoma-diameter was calibrated to 11 mm. Surgical enlargement of stoma diameter was required. Three other patients (2.0%) from this very early group had stomas that were too large and required surgical revision of the stoma.

Four patients (2.6%) developed late obstruction of the stoma due to edema caused by excessive vomiting. Of the four patients, one patient that was operated on in 1983 requested that the band be removed 6 weeks after the operation. The other three patients were operated on in 1986. In one of these patients, the stoma was obstructed one month after gastric banding. Edema was caused by forced eating. In the other two patients, 4 and 6 months after banding respectively, the obstruction of the stoma was caused by excessive vomiting that was induced by a viral infection. Conservative treatment with nasogastric tube and intravenous infusions failed and all three patients required revision of their SGB with an inflatable silicone band.

Excessively enlarged pouches were found in three patients (2.0%). Two of these patients required a revision. These patients were given an inflatable silicone band.

Three patients (2.0%) developed an incisional hernia. The incisional hernia was repaired in two of the patients.

An upper GI series was done to evaluate the size of the pouch and change in the size of the stoma in 89 patients that were at least 12 months after banding. In addition, the incidence of esophageal reflux was evaluated. The results of this study are presented in Table 20.3.

Postoperative clinical observations in 140 patients revealed that SGB patients did not suffer from metabolic complications. To date, there has been no evidence of anemia, malnutrition, vitamin B_{12} or iron deficiency, electrolyte imbalance and dehydration. Also, there has been no evidence of peptic ulcer or gastritis. Six patients (3.9%) have experienced regurgitation, mainly at night.

As of August 1987, there has not been a single incidence of erosion of the stomach wall by the band, disruption of the band, intraabdominal infection or adverse reaction to the silicone band.

INFLATABLE SGB

A well calibrated and reinforced stoma in gastric restriction operations for obesity is a must. Yet, even with a properly calibrated and reinforced stoma, some individuals will be able to eat more than others. This suggests that for some patients the stoma must be individually "tailored." Näslund, by endoscopically measuring the diameter of the stoma in patients with gastric restriction operations, found that the stoma enlarges over time.[13,14]

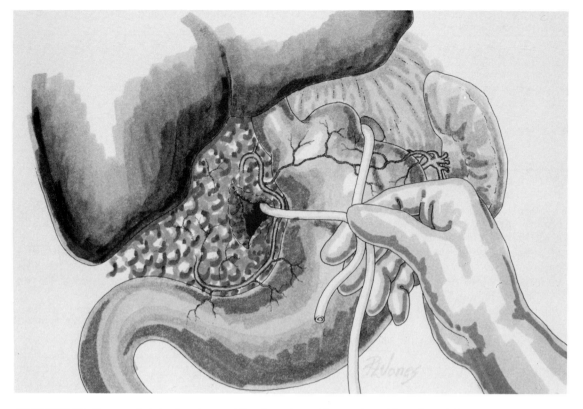

FIGURE 20.15. Penrose drain is placed around the stomach, gastric vessels and branches of the vagus nerve.

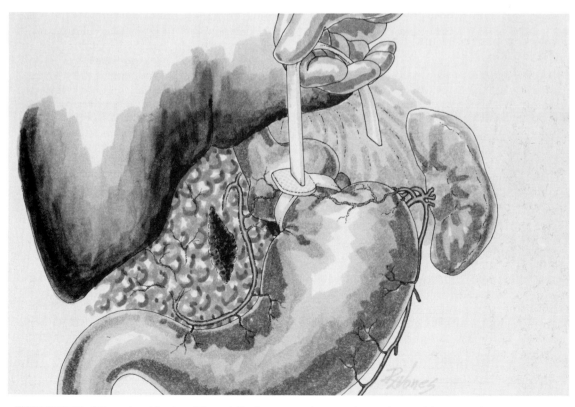

FIGURE 20.16. Silicone band is placed through the lesser curvature opening and around the stomach.

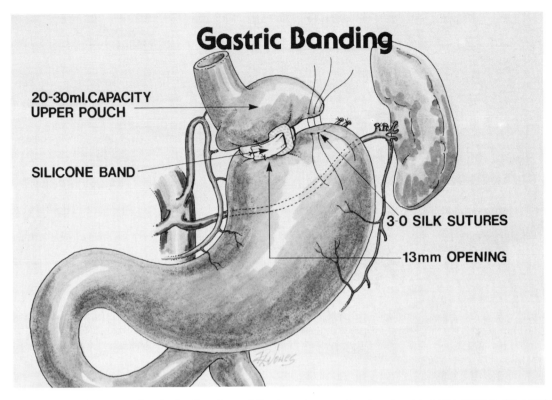

Gastric Banding

20-30ml.CAPACITY UPPER POUCH

SILICONE BAND

3-0 SILK SUTURES

13mm OPENING

FIGURE 20.17. To prevent band migration, the mobilized greater curvature is sutured over the band to the pouch. Reproduced with permission from Kuzmak, LI: Silicone gastric banding: a simple and effective operation for morbid obesity. Contemp Surg 28:13–18, 1986.

It was felt that if the size of the stoma could be changed without having to reoperate, such a change would provide better control over individual patients and improve postoperative weight loss in general without any increased risk to the patient. It was for these reasons that modifications were made to the silicone band in 1985. The modifications consist of adding to a small part of the band an inflatable balloon (Fig. 20.18) which is connected to a self-sealing reservoir by thin tubing (Fig. 20.19). The reservoir is implanted within the right rectus sheath (Fig. 20.20).

QUALITY CONTROL

The basic design and composition of the Dacron reinforced silicone band used by the author since 1983 was not changed except for the addition of an inflatable part to the band. The inflatable segment is 4 cm long and can be inflated safely with 3.5 mL of saline. Infla-

TABLE 20.3.   154 PATIENTS WITH PRIMARY NON-INFLATABLE SILICONE GASTRIC BANDING HAVE BEEN FOLLOWED FOR ≥12 MONTHS. 89 (58.5%) HAVE HAD A FOLLOW-UP UPPER GI SERIES AT THEIR 12-MONTH CHECK-UP—RESULTS LISTED BELOW

	No. of Patients	%
Percent of Pouch Enlargement		
0	28	31.5
30–50	21	23.6
51–100	22	24.7
101–200	15	16.9
>200	3	3.4
Changes in Stoma Size		
Enlargement	3	3.4
Decreased	3	3.4
Esophageal Reflux	6	6.7

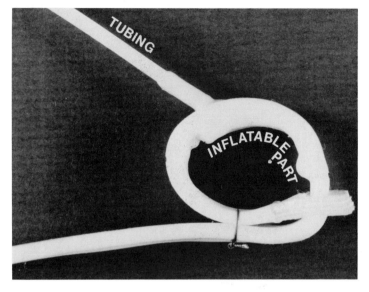

FIGURE 20.18. Inflatable balloon part of the modified silicone band.

tion with this amount of saline will decrease the diameter of the stoma approximately 4 mm (Fig. 20.21).

The balloon is made from the same type of of silicone that has been used for some time in skin expanders. The non-kinking tubing connecting the band with the reservoir and the reservoir are also made of silicone. All parts of the band, the tubing and the reservoir are radiopaque (Fig 20.22). By adding a "funnel-like" stainless steel based covered with silicone, the reservoir has been redesigned to

prevent penetration of the side of the reservoir by the needle and possible leakage of the saline injected into the band under pressure.

SURGICAL TECHNIQUE

When the inflatable band is used, the patient is prepped as previously described for the non-inflatable band. An upper midline incision is made through the skin and subcutaneous tissue. At about 10 cm below the rib cage, subcutaneous fat is dissected from the

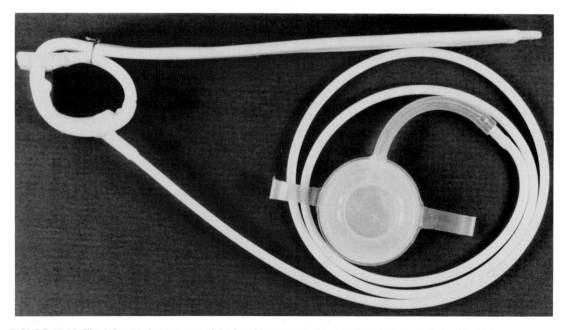

FIGURE 20.19 The inflatable balloon part of the band is connected to a self-sealing reservoir by thin tubing.

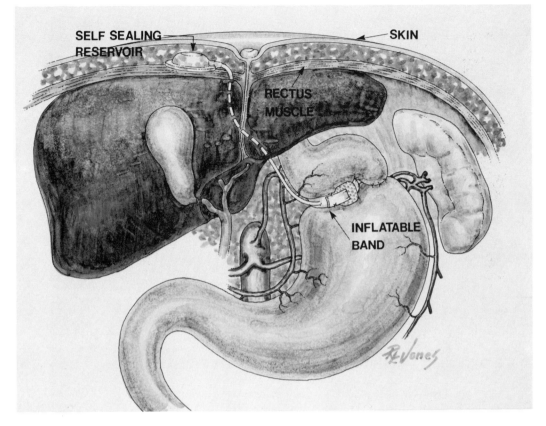

FIGURE 20.20. Diagram showing implantation of inflatable SGB.

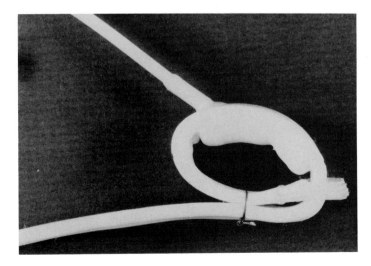

FIGURE 20.21. Inflatable silicone band inflated.

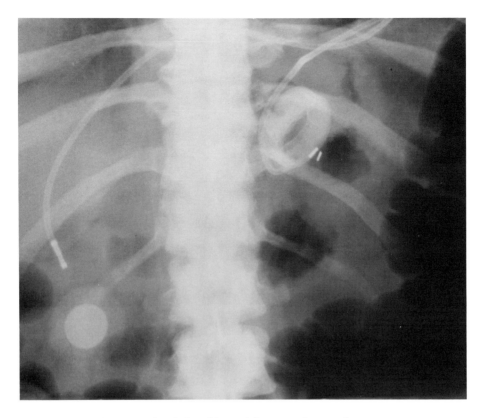

FIGURE 20.22. All parts of the silicone band, the tubing and the reservoir are radiopaque.

right rectus sheath. The right anterior rectus sheath is cut transversely and part of the rectus muscle is transected to prepare the space for the reservoir.

The midline incision is then made in the linea alba and the abdomen is entered. The general technique of banding with an inflatable band is performed as previously described for the non-inflatable band[15,16] with a few exceptions. The inflatable band is irrigated with saline to drain out the air from the balloon and the tubing. The placement of the band is done in the same fashion as when the non-inflatable silicone band is used. The calibrating tube and the electronic sensor are used to calibrate the pouch and the stoma.[15,16] The band should be partially preinflated, so that the surgeon has the choice of increasing or decreasing the stoma by inflating or deflating the band. When the calibration is completed, the band is sutured together. Markings on the band locate the balloon portion of the band and prevent the balloon from being punctured by the sutures.

The non-kinking tubing is placed loosely over the pouch, under the diaphragm and into the prepared space within the right rectus sheath where the reservoir is to be implanted. The position of the tubing is secured with loosely applied 3–0 chromic catgut sutures. Any excess length of the tubing is excised and the tubing is connected to the reservoir filled with saline. The reservoir is implanted (Fig. 20.23) and the anterior rectus sheath is sutured. All incisions are closed in the usual fashion.

RESULTS

Since the introduction of the inflatable silicone band in 1986, 32 such procedures have been performed. Of the 32 patients, 21 had the inflatable SGB as their primary procedure and 11 patients had inflatable SGB as a revision operation for a failed other gastric restriction operation. There was no operative morbidity or mortality. Analyses of the patients included average excess weight loss, early and late complications and/or reoperations.

The average preoperative weight in the 21 primary patients was 313 lb (142 kg), with the

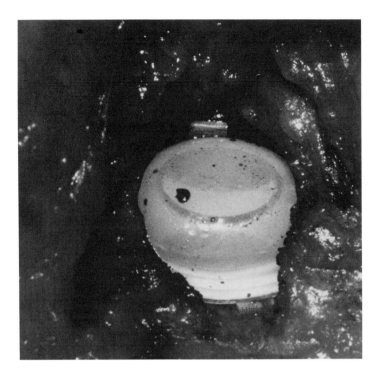

FIGURE 20.23. Implanted reservoir within right rectus sheath.

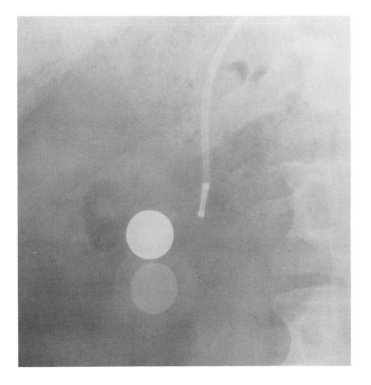

FIGURE 20.24. A penny is used to locate the center of the reservoir.

heaviest patient weighing 566 lb (257 kg). The average per cent of excess weight loss in the six primary patients who are ≥10 months postoperative is 80.0 ± 22.8%.

Early Complications and Reoperations

Six patients, all who were revision operations, have required adjustment of their stomas. In two patients, the preinflated band was percutaneously deflated because of excessive vomiting. In the other four patients, the band was percutaneously inflated to reduce the diameter of the stoma. The desired stoma size was achieved in all the patients.

Inflation or deflation of the band was done percutaneously with x-ray localization of the reservoir. The technique is simple. Placing a penny on the abdomen (Fig. 20.24) and eventually positioning it exactly over the center of the reservoir (Fig. 20.25) allows the surgeon to insert a 22-gauge spinal needle into the reservoir. Before inflating or deflating, the po-

sition of the needle should be confirmed with an x-ray (Fig. 20.26).

Late Complications and Reoperations

One patient, who had a prior horizontal gastroplasty revised with the inflatable SGB, was reoperated 4 months after the banding because of obstruction of the gastric banding stoma by the staples (Fig. 20.27-A). The GI series which had been done on discharge from hospital had shown proper passage of barium through the stomach (Fig. 20.27-B). However, the patient lost her dentures and was unable to chew food properly, which led to excessive vomiting. The vomiting, we believe, caused the stoma to become obstructed by the staples from the gastroplasty.

SGB AS A REVISION OPERATION FOR FAILED GASTRIC RESTRICTION PROCEDURES

The various gastric restrictive operations will fail to produce or maintain the desired

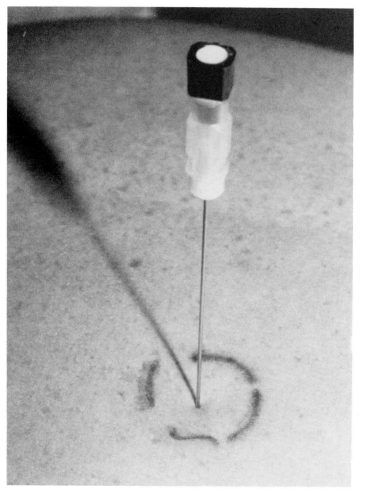

FIGURE 20.25. 22-gauge spinal needle used for inflation or deflation of band.

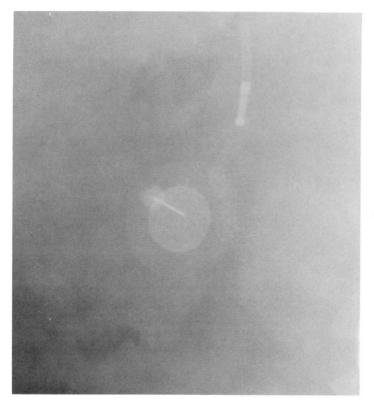

FIGURE 20.26. Position of the needle is confirmed by an x-ray.

weight loss in some patients. We have performed 60 SGB to revise other failed gastric restriction operations.

REVISION OF HORIZONTAL GASTROPLASTIES

Operation for a failed horizontal gastroplasty was performed in 50 patients (Fig. 28.28). With a large proximal pouch, the revision is relatively simple. Before the banding is done, the fundus and proximal stomach are dissected and mobilized. The silicone band is placed proximal to the staple-line (Fig. 20.29). However, when the proximal pouch is small, the staple-line may be so close to the gastric banding stoma that obstruction may occur. In this instance, the staples and the stapling septum should be transected before or after SGB is performed (Fig. 20.30).[17]

REVISION OF VERTICAL NON-BANDED GASTROPLASTY

Three patients presented with failed vertical gastroplasty which had a polypropylene suture reinforced stoma. In two, the silicone band was placed over the staple-line (Fig. 20.31). The other had partial transection of the staples and the stapling septum to prevent obstruction of the SGB stoma.

REVISION OF THE ORIGINAL LOOP GASTRIC BYPASS

A loop gastric bypass with a transected stomach was revised in one patient. The pouch and gastrojejunostomy were mobilized, and the silicone band was placed around the pouch, and the stoma was calibrated. The band was sutured together and also to the stomach wall to secure its position (Figs. 20.32-A and B).

REVISION OF LOOP GASTRIC BYPASS WITH CROSS-STAPLED STOMACH

This operation had failed due to enlargement of the stoma and partial disruption of the staple-line. The gastrojejunostomy was double stapled with a TA-30 stapler and transected between the staple-lines. The staples and septum dividing the pouch from the rest of the stomach were also transected. SGB was then done in the usual fashion (Fig. 20.33).

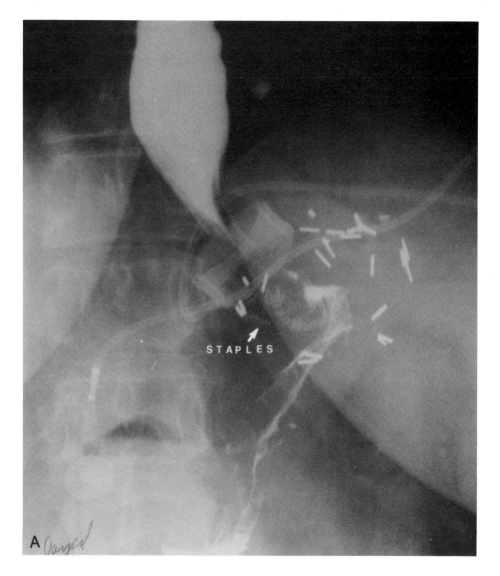

FIGURE 20.27-A. Obstruction of stoma is confirmed by GI series (delayed film).

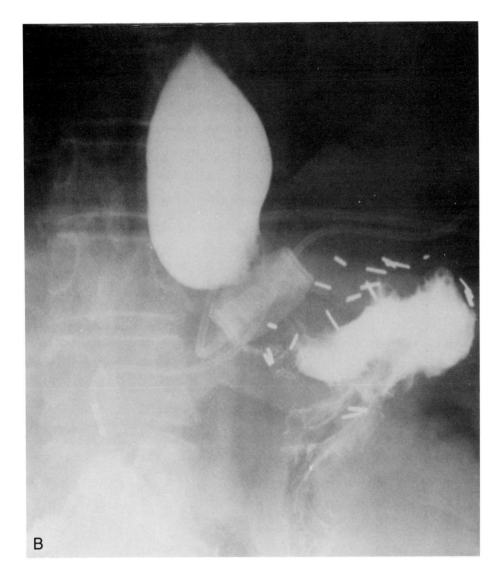

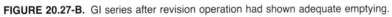

FIGURE 20.27-B. GI series after revision operation had shown adequate emptying.

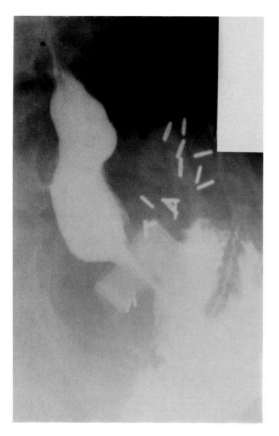

FIGURE 20.28. Horizontal gastric partitioning revised with SGB.

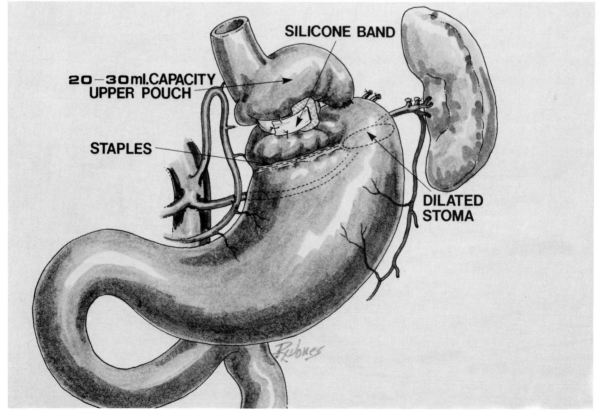

FIGURE 20.29. Horizontal gastroplasty with large pouch revised with SGB.

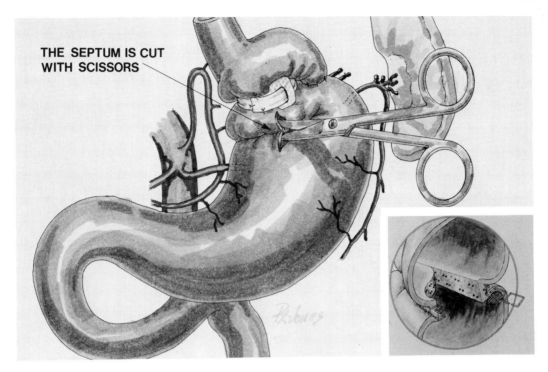

THE SEPTUM IS CUT
WITH SCISSORS

FIGURE 20.30. Staples and stapling septum are transected.

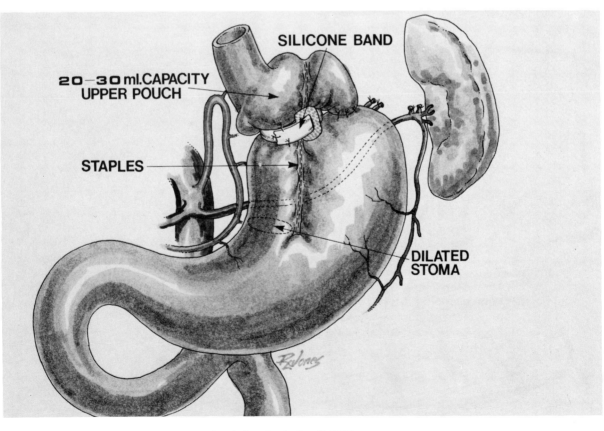

SILICONE BAND

20–30 ml.CAPACITY
UPPER POUCH

STAPLES

DILATED
STOMA

FIGURE 20.31. Revision of vertical non-banded gastroplasty with SGB.

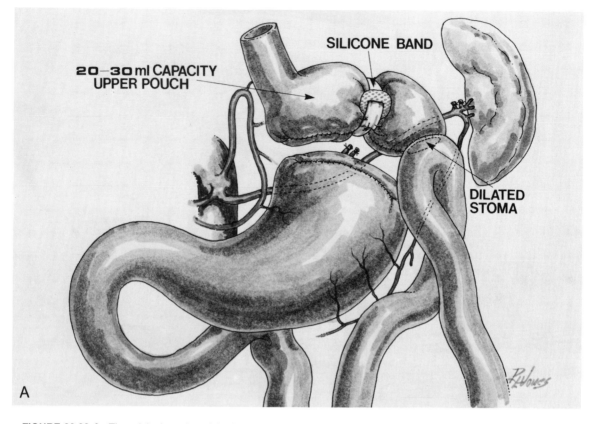

FIGURE 20.32-A. The original version of the loop gastric bypass, revised with SGB.

REVISION OF GASTRIC BYPASS WITH ROUX-EN-Y GASTROJEJUNOSTOMY AND CROSS-STAPLED STOMACH

Roux-en-Y gastric bypass had failed in two patients. In both, the stoma and pouch had enlarged. Essentially the same technique as that for revision of loop gastric bypass was used; however, the Roux-en-Y loop of jejunum was left in situ (Fig. 20.34).

REVISION OF GASTRIC WRAPPING

One patient presented with a gastric wrapping in which the Teflon mesh had disrupted at the suture-line. Nissen fundoplication had been done before the stomach had been wrapped with Teflon mesh. This fundoplication and tight wrapping did not allow the pouch or stoma to be calibrated with the calibrating tube and electronic sensor used in SGB. Accordingly, the silicone band was placed around the stomach distal to the fundoplication, and the pouch capacity was estimated with the inflatable balloon on the calibrating tube. The stoma diameter was then calibrated with a Hegar dilator inserted through a small gastrotomy.

REVISION OF DACRON ARTERIAL GRAFT GASTRIC BANDING

Two patients who had undergone gastric banding with a Dacron vascular graft have been revised. In both patients, the Dacron graft was found to be severely adherent to the stomach. In one, the stoma was obstructed and the band was dissected and removed. In the other, the Dacron graft had eroded partially into the stomach (see Fig. 20.4). This band was also dissected, transected and removed, and openings in the gastric wall caused by the erosion were sutured. SGB was then performed proximal to the area where the Dacron arterial graft banding had been done. Both patients received the inflatable SGB.

RESULTS

Of the 60 revision patients, 56 (93.3%) have been followed. Mean preoperative weight was 243 lb (110 kg), with the heaviest patient weighing 374 lb (170 kg). Mean loss of excess weight was 45.4% at 12 months, 54.4% at 24 months, 56.4% at 36 months and 58% at 48

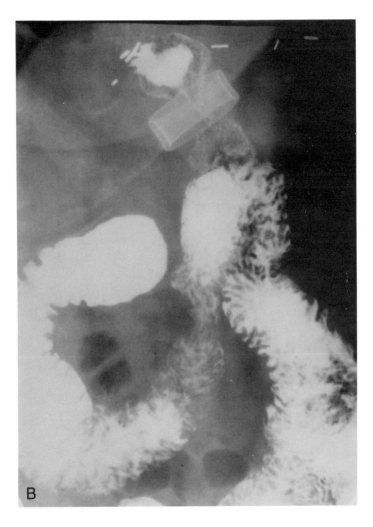

FIGURE 20.32-B. GI series after SGB revision of original loop gastric bypass.

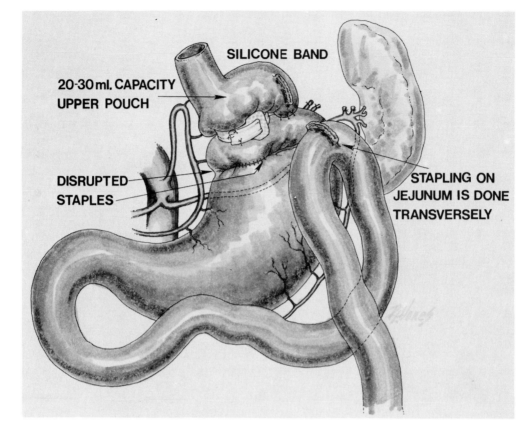

FIGURE 20.33. Gastric bypass with loop gastrojejunostomy revised with SGB.

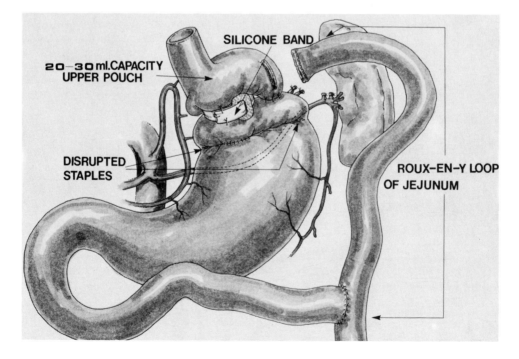

FIGURE 20.34. Gastric bypass with Roux-en-Y gastrojejunostomy after revision with SGB.

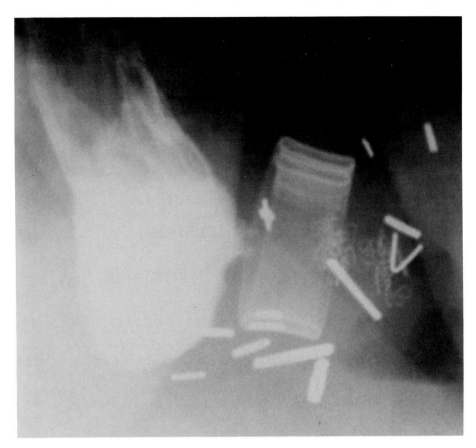

FIGURE 20.35. Stoma obstructed by staples after revision of failed horizontal gastroplasty by SGB.

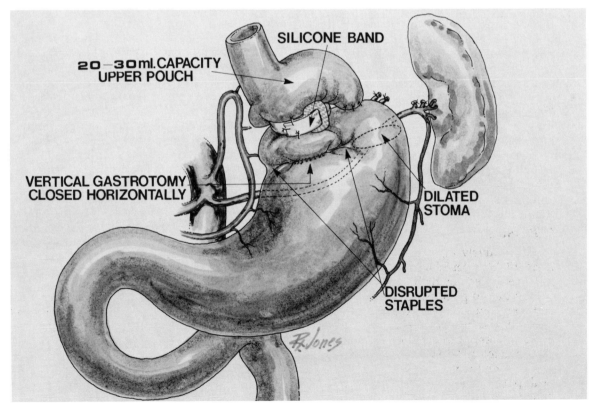

FIGURE 20.36. Revision of SGB after the stoma was obstructed by staples. This is a sequel to Fig. 20.30.

257

months. Presently, 29% of the patients are <30% above their ideal weight.

COMPLICATIONS AND REOPERATIONS

Early Complications

Four patients developed postoperative stomal obstruction. All were successfully treated with nasogastric suction and intravenous fluids with an average of 3 days treatment.

Late Complications

All of the late complications occurred in prior horizontal gastroplasty patients. Three patients developed partial stomal obstruction caused by the staples (Fig. 20.35). All required further operation, consisting of transection of the staples and the stapling septum (Fig. 20.36).

The silicone band migrated over the cardia in two patients. In one, the migration was caused by abdominal trauma that occurred 3 weeks after SGB, and the second band migration occurred 6 weeks after SGB. Both patients required a revision of their SGB.

One patient developed excessive vomiting because the stoma was too small. The stoma diameter was enlarged surgically.

Six patients who initially had a well functioning SGB gradually lost the feeling of satiety and started to gain weight. All 6 had their stoma diameter surgically decreased. The late stomal enlargement was caused by pressure atrophy of the thick scarring of the stomach wall from previous gastric procedures and revision. Full thickness gastric wall biopsy has shown it is the scarring, and not the stomach wall, that undergoes atrophy leading to the enlargement of the stoma.

There have been no adverse reactions to the band, no disruptions of the band, no erosions of the band through the stomach wall, no intraabdominal infections and no mortalities.

DISCUSSION

The relatively high incidence of re-operations, 18.3%, after SGB as a revision operation for other failed gastric bariatric operations is mainly due to pioneering work. Most re-operations were done in the earlier patients whose horizontal gastroplasty had been revised. Presently, to avoid stomal obstruction by the staples, transection of the staples is routinely done in patients with a small proximal pouch. Such transections have been done in 26 patients.

Migration of the band over the cardia was due to disruption of the sutures used to suture the greater curvature over the band to the pouch. Three or four sutures are now used instead of the one or two used initially.

It is safe if necessary to open the stomach when the silicone band is used. Transection of staples requiring opening of the stomach were done in 26 patients, without intraabdominal infection.

Some may consider the 4-year average excess weight loss of 58% to be only a good result. However, in 48.3% of the patients the weight at revision was less than 100 lb (45 kg) above ideal weight. The criteria to qualify for a primary operation for obesity does not apply to patients undergoing revision procedures.

In 4 years of follow-up, SGB has proven to be an effective revision operation for any type of gastric restriction operation that has failed. To eliminate re-operations for late stomal enlargement, use of the percutaneously inflatable band is now recommended in all SGB procedures performed as a revision.

SUMMARY AND CONCLUSION

With over 4½ years of follow-up, SGB has proven to be a simple and effective operation for controlling severe obesity. The use of silicone has eliminated adhesions of the band to the gastric wall, erosions of the band and the unpredictable stretching of the band. Revision and even removal of the silicone gastric band is relatively simple, since the band is encapsulated and does not adhere to the stomach wall. The inertness and softness of the silicone band probably contribute to the fact that there has not been a single incidence in our patients of erosion by the band into the gastric wall. This is contrary to the 4% incidence of erosion in gastric bandings when Dacron graft, Marlex mesh or PTFE graft was used as the banding material (Näslund, personal communication).

The pouch and stoma calibrating devices and other instruments developed by the author make the SGB procedure reproducible and simple. Use of the inflatable silicone band will permit percutaneous adjustment of the stoma diameter and is expected to further improve postoperative weight loss and reduce the incidence of reoperation. Whether with the non-inflatable or inflatable band, silicone gastric banding is a truly totally reversible operation.

REFERENCES

1. Kolle K: Gastric banding. OMGI 7th Congress, Stockholm, 1982, Abstract No. 145, p. 37.
2. Kolle K, Bö O, Stadaas J: "Gastric banding": An operative method to treat morbid obesity. CICD 7th World Congress, Tokyo, 1982, Abstracts Vol 1, p 184.
3. Check WA: Yet another variation on surgery for obesity. JAMA 248:1939–1943, 1982.
4. Bö O, Modalsli O: Gastric banding, a surgical method of treating morbid obesity: preliminary report. Int J Obes 7:493–499, 1983.
5. Solhaug JH: Gastric banding: a new method in the treatment of morbid obesity. Curr Surg 40:424–428, 1983.
6. Molina M, Oria HE: Gastric banding. Program, 6th Bariatric Surgery Colloquium, Iowa City, 1983, p 15 (abstract).
7. Backman L, Granström L: Initial (1-year) weight loss after gastric banding, gastroplasty or gastric bypass. Acta Chir Scand 150:63–67, 1984.
8. Granström L: Gastric banding: study of one method for surgical treatment of massive obesity. Acta Chir Scand, Supplementum, 1987, pp 1–48.
9. Frydenberg H, Gordon R: Easy to Stomach: Gastric Stapling & Banding. René Gordon Publishing Pty Ltd, North Balwyn, Australia, 1986, pp 26–27.
10. Habal MB: The biologic basis for the clinical application of the silicones. Arch Surg 119:843–848, 1984.
11. Nelbandiam RM, Swanson AB, Manpin BK: Long-term silicone implant arthroplasty: implications of animal and human autopsy findings. JAMA 250:1195–1198, 1983.
12. Greisler HP, Kim DU, Prince JB et al: Arterial regeneration activity after prosthetic implantation. Arch Surg 120:315–323, 1985.
13. Näslund I: The size of the gastric outlet and the outcome of surgery for obesity. Acta Chir Scand 152:205–210, 1985.
14. Näslund I: Gastric bypass versus gastroplasty: a prospective study of differences in two surgical procedures for morbid obesity. Acta Chir Scand, Supplementum 536, 1987, pp 1–60.
15. Kuzmak LI: A preliminary report on silicone gastric banding for obesity. Clin Nutr (suppl) 5:73–77, 1986.
16. Kuzmak LI: Silicone gastric banding: a simple and effective operation for morbid obesity. Contemp Surg 28:13–18, 1986.
17. Kuzmak LI: A simple technique to reverse stapling gastric restriction operation. Curr Surg 44:462–466, 1987.

21

Gastric Wrapping (Gastric Reservoir Reduction)

LAWRENCE H. WILKINSON
OLE A. PELOSO
ROBERT L. MILNE

Many morbidly obese patients convinced us that they had tried every regime which seemed reasonable and yet were unable to maintain significant weight loss. In some massively obese individuals, the fat appears fairly evenly deposited while in others it is distributed mostly in the upper half of the body or mostly in the lower half of the body. Furthermore, many humans are unable to become significantly obese no matter what or how much they ingest. These observations suggest that at least many morbidly obese individuals have a genetic or acquired endocrine or metabolic abnormality. People afflicted with morbid obesity eat too much for their metabolic requirement. It was our belief that the safest operation for morbid obesity would be one which achieves early satiety and limits intake without altering the continuity of the GI tract, and this led to our studies.

ANIMAL STUDIES

Our studies commenced in 1974 with 4 mongrel dogs. Our objective was to reduce the size of the dog's stomach so that less could be eaten. We found that the greater curvature was easy to mobilize, and inverted the greater curvature with polypropylene sutures to reduce stomach size. Observations of the dogs early after gastric inversion indicated that the ability to eat large amounts had been significantly reduced. After a few weeks, however, the dogs began to eat more, and barium contrast studies revealed that the dogs' stomachs had returned towards normal size.

It was reasoned that the initial results could be maintained by wrapping the inverted stomach with a nonabsorbable material. Marlex (knitted polypropylene) mesh was the most frequently used material at the time. Thus, the same 4 dogs were reoperated, the greater curvature was again inverted, and the stomach was wrapped with Marlex mesh. X-ray studies after part of the stomach had been wrapped revealed that the wrapped portion remained as reduced, but the remaining part of the stomach became greatly dilated. Various degrees of gastric wrapping were then studied in additional dogs.

In order to achieve permanent reduction of the amount that the dog was able to eat, we completely wrapped a dog's stomach with a Marlex sheet. The dog was was unable to eat very much and lost weight rapidly (Fig. 21.1). However, barium GI series revealed that the

wrap about the dog's stomach was causing a significant amount of pyloric obstruction. The dog was returned to surgery and the distal 1 cm of the mesh was removed from around the pylorus, which corrected the problem. The dog was still unable to eat very much but enough that 6 months later, he had regained his strength sufficiently to jump a 4-foot-high fence and became lost to follow-up. By April 1976, it had been observed in dogs that there was no ulceration or other deleterious effect of greater curvature inversion and complete wrapping with Marlex mesh (excluding the pylorus) (Fig. 21.2), with weight loss maintained.

APPLICATION IN THE HUMAN— EARLY TECHNIQUE

SELECTION OF PATIENTS FOR GASTRIC RESERVOIR REDUCTION

A. Age 18–50 yr, with exceptions for medical indications.
B. 45 kg (100 lb) above ideal weight for >5 yr.
C. Sincere efforts to lose weight by attending weight loss clinics and similar programs and doctors' supervised regimes.
D. Prolonged and often repeated interviews by the surgeon preoperatively, and agreement to lifelong follow-up postoperatively.

In 1976, a registered nurse was referred for reversal of a jejunoileal bypass which had been performed in 1972. Although she had lost only 15 kg, her blood chemistries were very abnormal; she had developed gallstones and renal stones and was quite anemic. She requested that we do something at the time of the reversal operation which would help her lose weight, and we discussed Marlex wrap of the stomach which had been performed in animals only. The patient requested that we apply the Marlex to her inverted stomach at the time of reversal of the intestinal bypass, although we explained that, although Marlex had been used for other purposes for more than 15 years, Marlex had never been used to wrap the stomach in humans, it would become incorporated into the gastric wall and it could become infected.

In June 1976 she underwent gastric reservoir reduction. We initially divided the adhesions about the small bowel anastomoses to be certain that they could be taken down

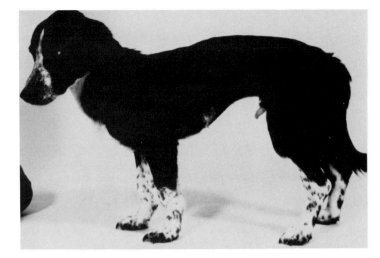

FIGURE 21.1. Dog with complete stomach wrap 2 months postoperatively.

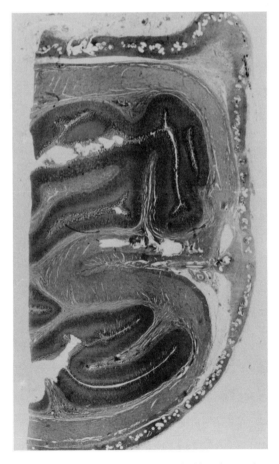

FIGURE 21.2. Dog stomach wrapped with polypropylene mesh, sacrificed at 6 months for study.

and the continuity of the small bowel reconstructed without difficulty. We then mobilized the stomach and inverted the greater curvature (Fig. 21.3-A), which reduced the stomach to a tubular organ. We wrapped the stomach with a sheet of polypropylene mesh (Fig. 21.3-B), with a 36-French lavacuator (hollow bougie) passing from the esophagus along the lesser curvature to the pylorus to prevent making the wrap too tight. The gastrocolic omentum was sutured to the right crus of the diaphragm to completely cover the foreign body around the stomach. The gallbladder was then removed and the jejunoileal bypass reversed. It is important to stress that the small bowel anastomoses were done after the nonabsorbable material had been covered with omentum.

This procedure was then performed with careful follow-up on a series of patients. The GI series showed the anticipated change in the shape of the stomach, but the only blood chemistry changes were those of improvement with decrease in weight. The first 7 patients had greater curvature inversion. The 8th patient to be accepted for this operation had a hiatus hernia with significant reflux. We feared increased reflux, and therefore when we mobilized the stomach, we performed a floppy Nissen fundoplication (lesser curve inversion) instead of greater curvature inversion, and the wrapped the stomach with the rectangular polypropylene mesh sheet. The Nissen fundoplication with lesser curvature inversion extending down to the left gastric artery was used in future patients, and seemed satisfactory except when the patient had esophagogastric dysmotility or the wrap was tight at the esophagogastric junction. In

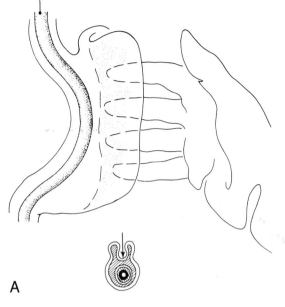

FIGURE 21.3-A. Inversion of greater curvature. 36-Fr bougie traversing stomach. **B.** Greater curvature inverted and stomach wrapped with polypropylene mesh.

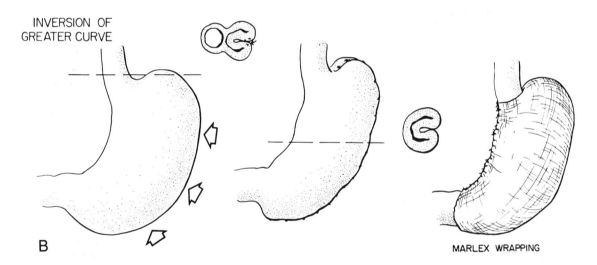

a few patients the wrap had to be loosened at the esophagogastric area a few years after placement.

OTHER PROCEDURES DEVELOPED IN THE HUMAN

In 1978, the horizontal gastroplasty was being widely performed, although it was not infrequently failing because of dilatation of the upper gastric pouch, possibly due to the thin muscle layers in the wall of the fundus, and dilatation of the outlet. Although we were doing gastric reduction, it was difficult without a pre-formed pouch, and we also de-

sired to keep an open mind about the best operation. Because of the more complete three muscle layers of the gastric wall along the lesser curvature, starting May 1978, 3 patients underwent complete stapling along the lesser curvature which contained a 36-French hollow bougie. A posterior gastroenterostomy was created to empty the greater curvature portion of the stomach (Fig. 21.4), and the fundus was wrapped about lesser curvature to prevent a leak. However, the third patient developed a staple-line leak near the upper end of the stomach resulting in a subphrenic abscess. Although the patient maintains weight 30 kg below her preoperative

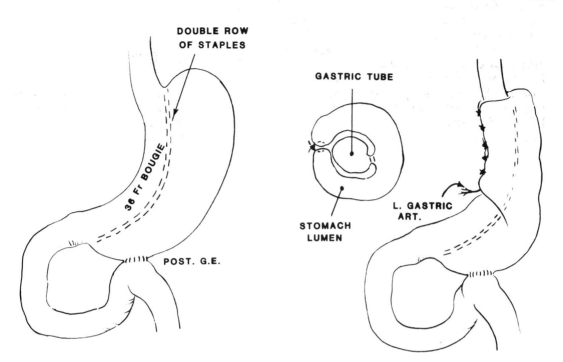

FIGURE 21.4. Vertical stapling with 36-Fr bougie traversing the human stomach. Gastroduodenostomy to drain greater curvature portion of stomach.

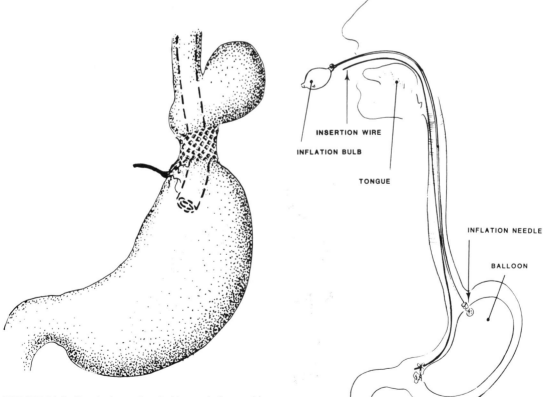

FIGURE 21.5. Band of nonabsorbable mesh 2 cm wide wrapped about stomach above left gastric artery, with 36-Fr bougie traversing stomach.

FIGURE 21.6. Intragastric balloon design, 1979.

weight (loss of 54% of her excess weight), we concluded that, for us, staples were not as safe as wrapping the stomach.

Also in 1978, we attempted gastric reservoir reduction by applying a 2-cm-wide band of Marlex mesh around the upper part of the stomach, between the upper short gastric vessels on the greater curvature and above the left gastric vessels on the lesser curvature. The band was snugly sutured to itself over a 36-French bougie (Fig. 21.5). However, the upper pouch dilated or the stoma was too large to reduce intake sufficiently for the desired weight loss. We thus abandoned this approach, although others subsequently have had good results with gastric banding.

In 1979, we devised an intragastric balloon (Fig. 21.6). However, at that same time, we removed a very large trichobezoar, which extended from diaphragm to pelvis (Fig. 21.7 A and B) from a 25-year-old veterinarian who had a habit of swallowing his hair and who had been asymptomatic until just before surgery. The bezoar had caused multiple gastric ulcers. Because of the great ability of the stomach to dilate, we abandoned the idea of a balloon as a method of achieving long-term weight loss.

FURTHER EXPERIENCE WITH GASTRIC WRAPPING

After these experiences, we decided to continue with gastric wrapping. The polypropylene sheet was difficult to place about the stomach, especially at the cardia, because the stomach is a pyriform organ. To remedy this, we then inserted a yoke, which is a circular piece of material with a hole in the center the diameter of the esophagus, sutured to the esophageal collar and the body of the wrap (Fig. 21.8-A). This enabled us to prepare preoperatively a hand-sewn **pouch** made of polypropylene mesh, which conformed to the shape of the stomach after completion of a Nissen fundoplication (Fig. 21.8-B).[2,3]

In March 1981 we discontinued the use of polypropylene mesh. Up to that time, 7 polypropylene sheets wth greater curvature inversion, 53 polypropylene sheets with Nissen fundoplication and 73 pre-formed polypropylene pouches with Nissen fundoplication

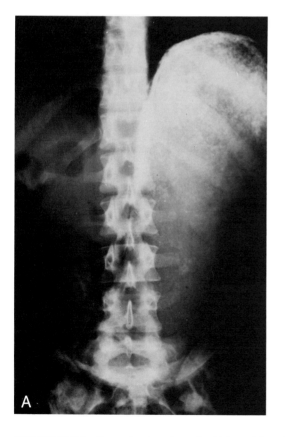

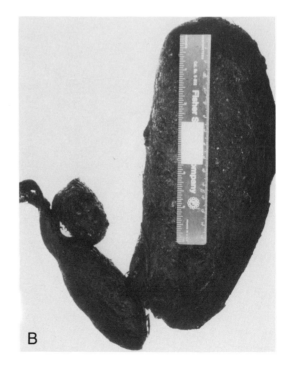

FIGURE 21.7-A. X-ray showing stomach which contains giant trichobezoar. **B.** Trichobezoar removed from stomach.

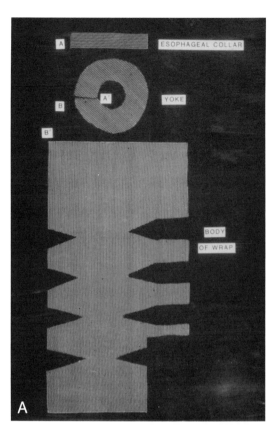

FIGURE 21.8-A. Design of polypropylene mesh to make hand-sewn pouch. Esophageal collar A is sutured to yoke A[1], and outer margin of yoke B is sutured to body of wrap B[1] with continuous 3–0 polypropylene sutures. Edges of darts are overlapped 5 mm and sutured together with continuous 3–0 polypropylene sutures. Frequent chain-stitch knots avoid wrinkling (1).

had been applied. Of the total 126 patients who underwent Nissen fundoplication and wrapping with Marlex, 15 wraps have been removed to date, because of perforation in the area of the Nissen fundoplication, possibly due to inadequate blood supply resulting from division of the short gastric arteries.

It has been reported that 3% of patients undergoing Nissen fundoplication (without wrapping) develop significant morbidity as a result of ulceration developing.[4] It is possible that this ulceration represents at least a part of the cause of our perforations which were in the Nissen portion of the stomach under the polypropylene mesh. No gastric perforations have been observed in the first 7 patients who underwent polypropylene mesh wrapping where only the greater curvature was inverted.

USE OF TEFLON

We used Teflon mesh on 6 patients, but 2 of these developed a perforation while the other 4 have remained well (see Table 21.1).

The first commercially prepared gastric pouch was made of Teflon mesh by the C.R. Bard Company, and was designed to fit the stomach which had undergone a Nissen fundoplication. From 1980 to 1983, 150 gastric reductions were performed using the Teflon pouch applied over the stomach which had undergone Nissen fundoplication. There were four complications in these 158 patients. One was readmitted 8 days postoperatively with rectal bleeding and succumbed to disseminated intravascular coagulation and acute respiratory distress syndrome 13 days postoperatively before a duodenal ulcer was diagnosed. Another was readmitted to the hospital 13 days postoperatively and succumbed to alcoholic pancreatitis following exploratory laparotomy 19 days postoperatively. One patient developed a perforation in the Nissen portion of the stomach 6 months postoperatively.

The fourth patient had the pouch removed 49 days after placement, because of esophagogastric dysmotility.[5] Upper GI barium x-rays revealed no narrowing at the esophagogastric junction and no excessive narrowing of the stomach, but the barium remained in the distal stomach without advancing. Esophagogastroscopy revealed no narrowing.

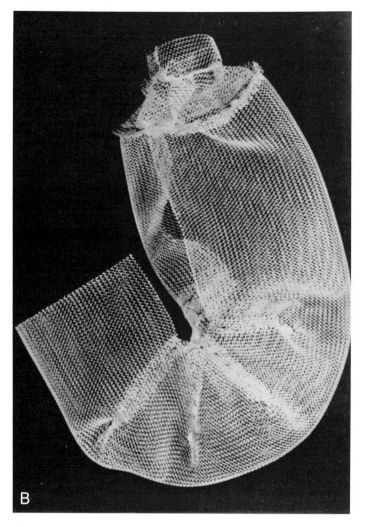

FIGURE 21.8-B. Hand-sewn pre-formed pouch made from polypropylene mesh, utilizing yoke.

The wrap about the distal half of the stomach was enlarged surgically 33 days postoperatively, but did not result in any improvement. The patient requested that we remove the pouch, which was performed on the 49th postoperative day, with uneventful recovery except for some symptoms which we felt were due to esophagogastric dysmotility which she had apparently had for a number of years. The remaining patients who have Teflon pouches have maintained an average loss of excess weight of 68.1%.

FURTHER ANIMAL STUDIES

In 1982, the Bard Company financed a study at the Animal Resources Center of the University of New Mexico, to determine the effect of Teflon mesh when applied to the external surface of the stomach. The greater curvature of the stomach was inverted and wrapped in 18 dogs: a) 6 wrapped with Teflon mesh; b) 6 wrapped with Teflon mesh with 3-mm openings in the mesh; c) 6 wrapped with Teflon mesh which had been impregnated with silicone and which had 3-mm openings. Three of the dogs in each group were sacrificed at 42 days and 3 in each group at 180 days postoperatively, and the gastric wall was studied grossly and histologically. No complications were noted following the use of any of the three different pouches, but it was believed that the Teflon mesh with 3-mm fenestrations, impregnated with silicone, would lessen the reaction, although no difference was revealed at 180 days study.

FURTHER PATIENT EXPERIENCE

In June 1983, Teflon pouches which had 3-mm openings became commercially available,

TABLE 21.1. EXPERIENCE WITH THE GASTRIC RESERVOIR REDUCTION OPERATION

No. of Patients	Material	Method of Gastric Reduction	Type of Wrap	Follow-up No.	Follow-up %	Follow-up Years	Complications	% Loss Excess Weight
7	Polypropylene	Greater curvature inversion	Sheet	4	57	9–11	0	72
53	Polypropylene	Nissen fundoplication	Sheet (last used 5-14-80)	26	49	9–9	16 (30%)	76
73	Polypropylene	Nissen fundoplication	Pouch hand-sewn (last used 3-3-81)	57	78	6–7	6 (8%)	67
6	Teflon	Nissen fundoplication	Sheet	4	67	7–8	2 (33%)	66
158	Teflon	Nissen fundoplication	Commercial pouch	142	90	4–7	4 (3%)	68
1	Silicone	Greater curvature inversion	Commercial pouch (collar) 1980	1	100	7	1	65
12	Silicone	Nissen fundoplication	Commercial pouch	10	83	6	9 (75%)	75
27	Silicone	Greater curvature inversion	Commercial pouch (fenestrated) 1982–1983	27	100	4–5	3 (11%)	72

and 6 were applied over stomachs which had undergone Nissen fundoplication (Fig. 21.9). All of these have done well to the present time. Subsequently, Bard has made available a Teflon pouch with 3-mm openings designed to fit the stomach which has undergone greater curvature inversion only (Fig. 21.10).

SILICONE-IMPREGNATED DACRON MESH POUCHES

In November 1980 we used the first gastric pouch made of Dacron mesh impregnated with silicone, designed by Heyer-Schulte Corporation (now Mentor Corporation), on the 112th patient to undergo gastric reservoir re-

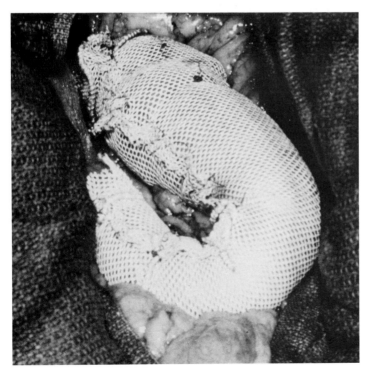

FIGURE 21.9. Bard Teflon pouch (1983) on stomach which has undergone Nissen fundoplication at surgery. 3-mm openings in mesh.

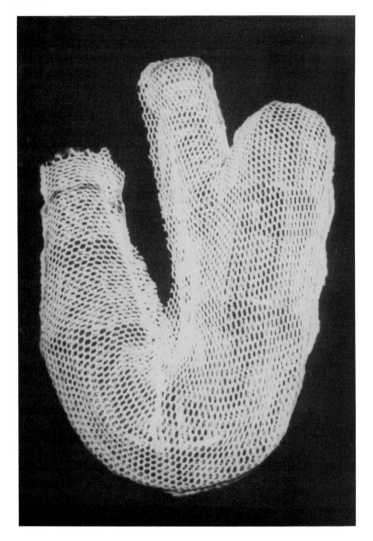

FIGURE 21.10. Teflon mesh pouch with 3-mm openings, designed to cover stomach with greater curvature inversion. Not used in humans yet.

duction. It was designed to fit the stomach which had undergone greater curvature inversion only, and had a silicone collar affixed to the edge of the esophageal opening which likely prevented reflux (Fig. 21.11 A and B). This patient lost 10 lb per month for 6 months. However, loss of fat about the external gastric surface permitted the stomach to move about inside the pouch so extensively that the fundus dropped down and herniated up through the esophageal opening, causing esophageal obstruction which required further surgery. Had we made a 3–4 mm opening in the fundus of the pouch and pulled the gastric fundus to this opening and affixed it there with seromuscular sutures, we likely could have saved the pouch. We were pleased that the silicone did not adhere to the tissue.

We then designed a second generation, silicone-impregnated Dacron pouch to fit the stomach which had undergone a Nissen fun-

doplication, reasoning that this would prevent the slippage which occurred with the first silicone pouch (Fig. 21.12). This second generation silicone pouch was applied to 12 patients, with losses of 58–93% of excess weight. However, all but 3 of these patients eventually had the pouch removed because of excessive movement of the stomach inside the non-fenestrated pouch.

The Heyer-Schulte (Mentor) Corporation produced a third generation silicone pouch which had 3-mm openings in the walls and was designed for greater curvature inversion only (Fig. 21.13 A and B). The fenestrations are for adhesions to hold the stomach in place. The silicone collar was not available on this model, but the walls of the pouch extended up 1.5 cm to enclose the esophagus and impede reflux. Such pouches were applied in 27 patients from 1982 to 1983, and the results are shown in Table 21.2.[6] The

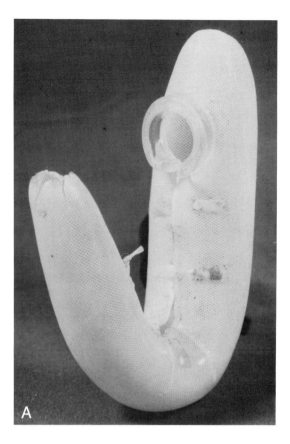

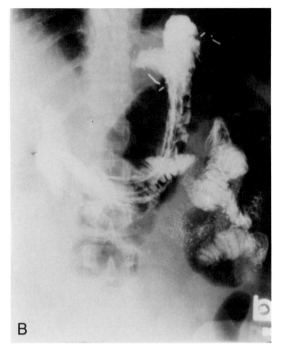

FIGURE 21.11-A. First generation silicone pouch. **B.** Barium study of stomach wrapped with the silicone pouch.

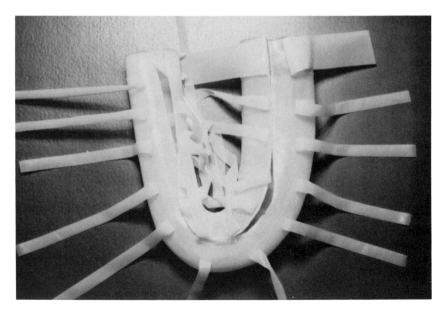

FIGURE 21.12. Second generation silicone pouch designed to fit stomach which has undergone Nissen fundoplication.

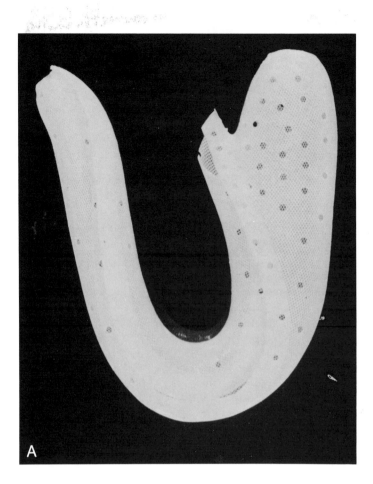

FIGURE 21.13-A. Third generation silicone pouch with 3-mm fenestrations. **B.** Upper GI X-ray of stomach enclosed in third generation silicone pouch. Enlarged view on right demonstrates mucosal folds as barium is leaving stomach.

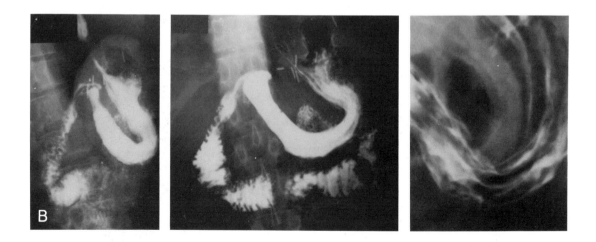

TABLE 21.2. COMPLICATIONS IN THE 27 PATIENTS WHO RECEIVED THIRD GENERATION SILICONE POUCH, NOW FOLLOWED >4 YEARS

Death	0
Wound infection	0
Intra-abdominal infection	0
Perforation	0
Incisional hernia	3
*Demand for removal of pouch	3
†Capsule formation	1
Weight loss failure	0

*Patients understood removal of silicone pouch is not difficult and refused to eat slowly.

†Removal of pouch required.

pouch was removed in one patient 8 months postoperatively due to capsule formation about the entire silicone pouch, preventing the patient from eating adequately. After the pouch was removed, there was sufficient perigastric fibrosis to enable the patient to maintain near normal weight to the present time. The average loss of excess weight in the 27 patients wrapped with the third generation silicone pouch followed for >4 yr is 71.8%.

Fig. 21.13-B is from a patient who underwent gastric reduction with the third generation fenestrated silicone pouch. Her upper GI series reveals no esophageal dilatation, narrowing or reflux and no gastric narrowing or dilatation. The Dow Corning Corporation is presently developing a fourth generation silicone pouch, which like the third generation is fenestrated and is applied to the stomach which had undergone greater curvature inversion only (Fig. 21.14 A and B). However, this pouch again has the silicone collar.

RESULTS

Our results are summarized in Table 21.1. More than 500 patients have undergone gastric wrapping, including patients of Drs. Charles E. Lucas and Ann Ledgerwood in Detroit and Dr. Edward Dainko in San Bernardino, California. Over 1,000,000 silicone devices have been implanted in the human body without any reported incidence of rejection. Teflon appears to be equally inert, but is more difficult to remove if required. We believe that greater curvature inversion, rather than Nissen fundoplication, is the best method of reducing the gastric reservoir. No herniations have occurred when the pouch is fenestrated near the collar. No gastric perforation has occurred in any of the total of 40 patients whose stomach has been wrapped with a silicone pouch. The application of a silicone-impreg-

nated Dacron pouch fenestrated with 3-mm openings appears to be the best method of maintaining reduced gastric volume indefinitely, because of its ease of removal if required. Patients who have a hiatus hernia undergo approximation of the diaphragmatic crura anterior to the esophagus.

CURRENT TECHNIQUE FOR THE GASTRIC RESERVOIR REDUCTION OPERATION

The patient is supine on the operating table. Bilateral shoulder braces are securely placed. The patient is then placed in 20° Trendelenberg position so that the foot-board can be fixed to the table as far superiorly as possible, which prevents the body from moving as the table is changed from 20° Trendelenberg to 20° reverse-Trendelenberg position during the operation.

A midline incision is made from xiphoid to umbilicus. The subcutaneous tissue is pulled apart, a maneuver which is usually bloodless and leads accurately to the linea alba (Fig. 21.15). We use the Pilling Polytract (Gomez) retractor (Fig. 21.16), although other excellent retractors may be employed. The gastrocolic omentum is opened into the lesser sac at the junction of the right and left gastroepiploic vessels at the midpoint on the greater curvature, and the dissection is continued inferiorly at the outer border of the right gastroepiploic vessels, removing as much fat as possible while leaving the right gastroepiploic vessels intact attached to the stomach. The posterior peritoneal attachments to the posterior wall of the antrum are pushed away. The right hand, palm up, is inserted behind the stomach and the fingers tear through the lesser omentum to the right of the nerves of Laterjet, and the lesser curvature is mobilized down to the region of the right gastric artery.

Every 30 minutes the operating-table is placed in 20° Trendelenberg position for 30 seconds to permit drainage of the lower extremity and lower abdominal veins,[7] which we believe has contributed to the fact that we have not recognized thrombophlebitis or pulmonary embolism in the last 324 patients. Routine prophylactic subcutaneous heparin has not been given.

As dissection under the ribs is commenced, the operating-table is placed in 20° reverse-Trendelenberg position so that the intestines will fall away from the diaphragm. The peritoneum over the left gastric vessels and

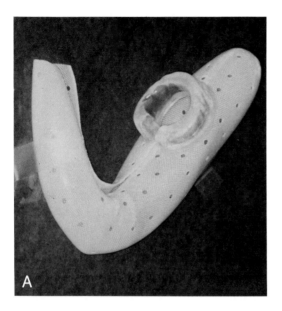

FIGURE 21.14-A. Fourth generation silicone pouch designed with soft collar. **B.** Procedure entails mobilization of stomach, inversion of greater curvature and application of pouch. The 3 gastric vessels shown are preserved.

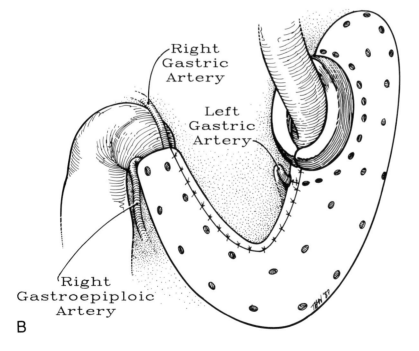

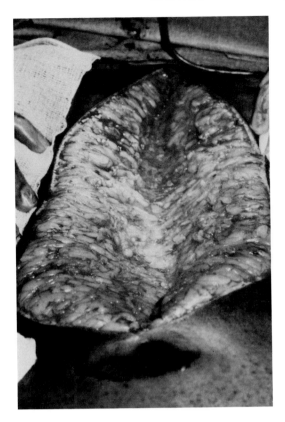

FIGURE 21.15. Subcutaneous tissue of upper midline incision pulled apart to linea alba.

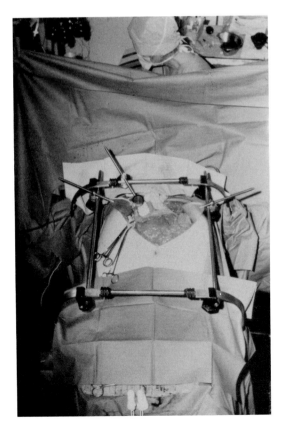

FIGURE 21.16. Gomez modification of Polytract retractor used in gastric reservoir reduction operation.

esophagogastric area is incised, and the left gastric vessels identified and a medium Penrose drain passed around them for identification. Downward traction on the stomach is effected with the left hand while the short gastric vessels are divided between clips until the esophagus is reached. When the fundus is mobilized, the metal clips on the gastric side are later replaced with 2–0 plain catgut ties quite easily, since enclosing these inside the wrap may lead to gastric perforation.

Dissection in the esophageal hiatus above the left gastric vessels is just enough to permit the collar about the esophageal opening of the gastric pouch to pass behind the esophagus. A 36-French hollow bougie is passed transorally down to the pylorus.

The greater curvature is then inverted and held with 8–12 interrupted seromuscular sutures of 3–0 chromic catgut.

The gastric pouch is inspected to make certain there are adequate 3-mm fenestrations (1 every 2–3 cm) especially near the collar and in the fundus. The pouch is applied, and a horizontal cut is made 1.5–2.0 cm with the scissors in the posterior wall and a 1-cm circle cut out, to permit passage of the left gastric artery and coronary vein through the wall of the pouch (see Fig. 21.14-B). The opening around the vessels is made sufficiently large to prevent occlusion or erosion of the vessels, and the cut in the posterior wall is closed with 2–0 polypropylene sutures up to the opening for the vessels.

The anterior and posterior edges of the pouch are approximated or overlapped with 2–0 polypropylene sutures. If the curve of the pouch does not fit the curve of the stomach satisfactorily, simply cut the walls of the pouch transversely at the edge of the opening along the middle of the lesser curve. The overlapping which then occurs achieves a satisfactory covering of the stomach, and is secured with 2–0 polypropylene sutures. The closure of the pouch along the lesser curve should be sufficiently tight that the index finger inserted under the pouch is just comfortable, with the 36-French bougie in place. The pouch is cut off distally so that the lower end is 1–2 cm proximal to the pylorus.

If the esophageal hiatus is enlarged or a hiatus hernia is present, the diaphragmatic crura are approximated anterior to the esophagus. The gastrocolic omentum is brought anterior to the pouch and anchored to the right crus with 2–0 chromic catgut sutures. A nasogastric tube is not inserted.

If there is a further abdominal procedure to be performed, e.g. cholecystectomy or reversal of jejunoileal bypass, these are performed after the pouch has been covered with omentum, to avoid contamination. However, before doing the gastric procedure, the adhesions about an intestinal bypass are taken down, in order to be sure that the reversal will be able to be performed. In closing, through-and-through button retention sutures are used generously to assure no wound disruption.

POSTOPERATIVE CARE

The patient receives a first generation cephalosporin intravenously at the beginning of the operation and 6–8 hours postoperatively. When the patient reaches the recovery-room, an 18-inch-high wedge which extends from the elevated feet up to the hips is placed under the mattress.[8] This wedge is not removed until the patient is able to lift each leg for 30 seconds; this is repeated hourly while awake. A trapeze hangs over the bed so that the patient will pull the chest one inch off the bed and take a deep breath through the mouth and cough each hour while awake; in this position, only diaphragmatic respiratory motion is possible, so atelectasis of the lower lobes is prevented. The incentive spirometer is used. As the patients are escorted to the bathroom on call to the operating-room, catheterization is rarely required. Continuous intravenous narcotics are administered under careful supervision, and the dose decreased if the respiratory rate falls below 18 per minute. Early ambulation is encouraged. Clear liquids are begun after flatus is expelled.

POSTOPERATIVE COURSE

The gastric reduction operation usually produces a 60–90 cc pouch which cannot enlarge except for the perigastric fat which is lost. Early satiety is achieved, and discomfort and emesis will occur if the patient overeats. Patients must eat slowly with small bites and chew well. If the patient begins a meal with a salad or other high fiber food, adequate weight loss is generally achieved. Continuous ingestion of high calorie liquids can defeat the operation. A multiple vitamin and nutritional guidance are mandatory. Patients must avoid ulcerogenic drugs.

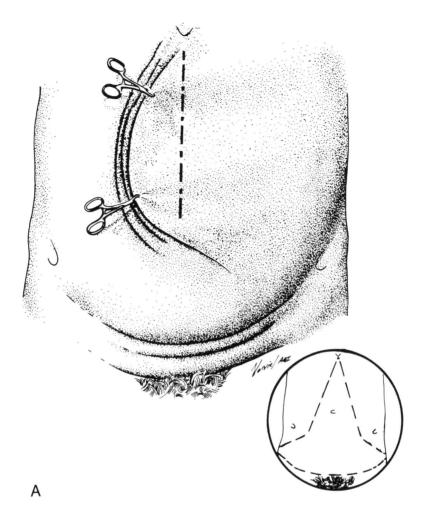

A

FIGURE 21.17-A. Towel clips pulling skin to right. Vertical line indicates amount of skin to be excised on each side. The inset shows area of skin and subcutaneous tissue to be excised.

TECHNIQUE OF REMOVAL OF THE REDUNDANT ABDOMINAL SKIN AFTER WEIGHT LOSS

We do not encourage the patient to have excision of the excess skin-folds until the patient has lost 65% of excess body weight. We apply towel clips to the skin to the left of the midline and pull the skin taut towards the right, and draw a straight line from xyphoid to the umbilical area (Fig. 21.17-A). We then remove the towel clips and allow the skin to relax, and measure on the right side the same distance away from the midline. This assures symmetrical removal of skin on each side.

We then draw a transverse line 1 cm above the pubic hairline, which is curved slightly superiorly as it ends outwards below and lateral to the anterior superior iliac spines. From the end of this incision on each side, a line is drawn superiorly and medially to join the previously drawn ellipse. By pulling down towards the pubis on this skin on one side of the umbilicus and pulling the pubic skin superiorly, we can mark out where these two lines should intersect (Fig. 21.17-A, inset).

Thus, we have an outline of the skin to be removed, which consists of a transverse suprapubic ellipse which joins a vertical subxiphoid half ellipse. A 2.5-cm-diameter periumbilical incision is deepened to the linea, which protects the blood supply to the umbilicus. We then make the skin incisions, undermining usually to the costal margins and beyond the lateral border of the rectus muscles, leaving a 2-cm thickness of fat attached to the skin of the flaps. The large area of skin and subcutaneous fat outlined inside the incisions is excised, along with the subcutane-

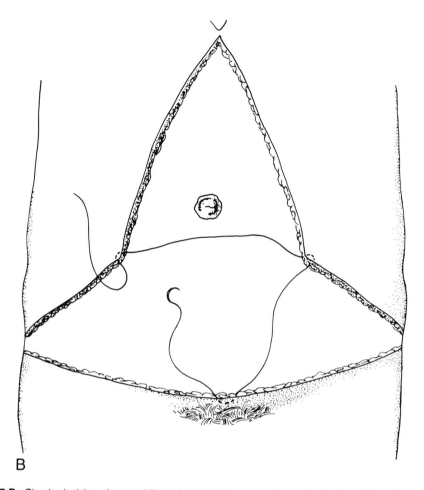

B

FIGURE 21.17-B. Circular incision about umbilicus. Horizontal suture in dermis beginning at the obtuse flap-angle on patient's right, crossing to left and then down to pubis in midline.

ous fat left on the fascia when the flaps were undermined.

A suture of 2–0 polyglactin 910 is placed in the dermis at the angle on the right side, and is brought across to the angle on the left side and then down to the dermis of the midline of the pubic area, and tied (Fig. 21.17 B and C).

The subcutaneous tissue is closed. The umbilicus is brought out in proper location, and where it comes through the vertical portion of the wound, a circular incision is made, with half of the circle in each flap (Fig. 21.17-C). The dermis is approximated with continuous 4–0 polyglactin 910. Drains or suction catheters are inserted.

SUMMARY

We have performed gastric reservoir reduction on 336 patients since 1976. Of the

patients, 31 had previous operations which failed to correct morbid obesity. There have been 33 complications[9] related to the gastric wrap; only 5 complications have occurred in the last 165 patients. In the series, one death occurred in the initial hospitalization (pulmonary embolus), 3 deaths occurred during the first postoperative month, and 6 deaths occurred from 3 months to 9 years of other causes. Deep wound infection or disruption did not occur. Splenectomy was not required. A total of 285 patients, including 21 failures (6.3%—failures lost <40% excess weight), are still wrapped and being followed 4–11 years, with average loss of excess weight 69.4%.

We believe that the best long-term weight loss is achieved by enclosing the stomach, which has undergone greater curvature inversion with absorbable seromuscular sutures, with a pouch made of Dacron mesh impregnated with silicone and fenestrated

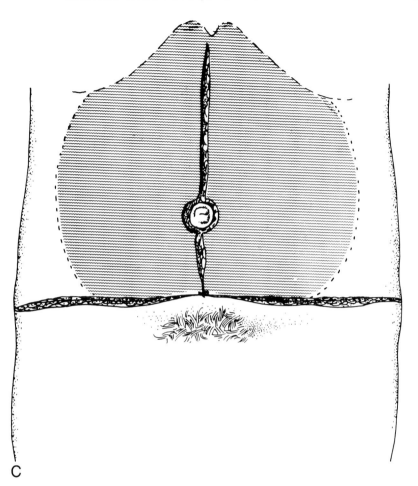

FIGURE 21.17-C. Suture in dermis tied. Circular removal of skin to provide exit of umbilicus. Shaded area indicates extent of undermining.

with 3-mm openings to form adhesions to hold the stomach in place. A gastric pouch achieves: a. reservoir reduction without entering, distorting or rearranging the GI tract; b. a sense of satiety which lasts a number of hours; c. prevention of late dilatation of the stomach; d. an average loss of 70% of excess weight; e. easy removal of the pouch if required, leaving a stomach which is not deformed or partially removed.

REFERENCES

1. Peloso OA, Wilkinson LH: The chain stitch knot. Surg Gynecol Obstet 139:599–600, 1974.
2. Wilkinson LH: Reduction of gastric reservoir capacity. J Clin Nutr 33:515–517, 1980.
3. Wilkinson LH, Peloso OA: Gastric (reservoir) reduction for morbid obesity. Arch Surg 116:602–605, 1981.
4. Maher JW, Cerda JJ: The role of gastric stasis in the genesis of gastric ulceration following fundoplication. World J Surg 6:794–799, 1982.
5. Pelligrini C, Ryan T: Management of gastric motility disorders. Contemp Surg 11:15–26, 1983.
6. Wilkinson LH, Peloso OA, Milne RO: Gastric reservoir reduction. Paper presented at the First International Symposium on Obesity Surgery. Genoa, Italy, October 3, 1984.
7. Lewis CE, Mueller CF, Jr, Edward WS: Venous stasis of the operating table. Am J Surg 124:780–784, 1972.
8. Solomon J, Hamadey C: Preventing gastric wrap complications. Dimensions of Critical Care Nursing 4:18–23, 1985.
9. Curley SA, Weaver W, Wilkinson LH, et al: Late complications after gastric reservoir reduction with external wrap. Arch Surg 112:781–783, 1987.

22

Gastro-Clip Gastroplasty

SAMUEL B. BASHOUR

Gastro-clip* gastroplasty is an alternative surgical gastric reduction procedure for patients with chronic intractable morbid obesity. This gastroplasty has been found to be effective, safe and requires less time to perform. Its follow-up is equally dependable and rewarding in the routine postoperative management of the loss of weight. Operating surgeons may be refocusing their expertise on this method as a surgical management.

MATERIAL

The Gastro-clip is made of medical grade polypropylene, and is impregnated with steel implants for radiologic postoperative follow-up. It is 10.5 cm in length, weighs 8.3 g and the inside diameter of the clamp stoma is 1.25 cm. It causes a uniform pouch of 50 mL and an unchangeable and permanent stoma (Fig. 22.1). It has been used in 77 patients since January 1983. The average age of the patients was 38 years, the youngest being 18 and the oldest 62 years.

PATIENT WORK-UP

General work-up is mostly done on an outpatient basis in the pre-admission period in order to limit hospital expense.

The routine tests are as follows:
1. CBC and urinalysis
2. Blood gases (when patient weighs >300 lb)
3. SMA-12, serum electrolytes, free T4, PTT, PT, PCHE

*Patented and made by Irving Surgical Instruments Inc., 2105 W. Airport Freeway, Irving, Texas 75062, U.S.A.

4. Spirometry
5. Incentive spirometry (q.i.d. for hospitalized patients >300 lb)
6. Chest X-ray
7. EKG
8. 2 hr postprandial plasma glucose
9. Sonography of gallbladder and upper GI series
10. Lipoprotein profile, HDL and LDL (blood drawn at 0700 hr day of surgery)
11. Amino acid assay

Two variables in pre-operative hospital orders are noted: (1) miniheparinization is administered only to patients who weigh >300 lb; (2) prophylactic antibiotic is used in the same weight category or in patients with a past history of upper respiratory infections, pulmonary infections, thrombophlebitis, urinary infections, diabetes or any other pertinent problem.

TECHNIQUE OF APPLICATION OF THE GASTRO-CLIP

Under general endotracheal anesthesia, the abdomen which has been surgically prepped and draped is opened through a midline incision commencing at the xyphoid and extending inferiorly to the umbilicus. The incision is deepened in the subcutaneous tissue, at which point the subcutaneous fat is stretched manually apart and the rectus sheath is reached. The sheath is opened by electrocautery and the peritoneum by blade and scissors. The peritoneal cavity is first explored, noting the pelvis, sigmoid colon and large bowel, putting emphasis on possible pa-

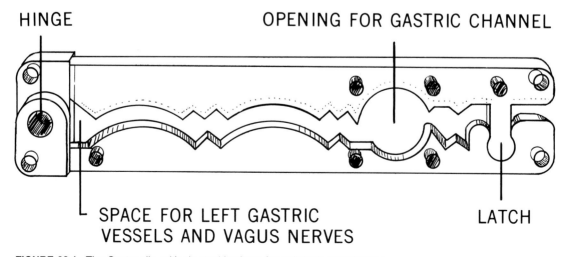

HINGE   OPENING FOR GASTRIC CHANNEL

SPACE FOR LEFT GASTRIC VESSELS AND VAGUS NERVES   LATCH

FIGURE 22.1. The Gastro-clip, with six steel implants for radiologic identification.

thology of the gallbladder where stones or adhesions are noted.

Traction of the wound for exposure is done by the "Iron Intern" retractor (Automated Medical Products, 2315 Broadway, New York 10024) or the Gomez retractor (Pilling, 420 Delaware Dr., Fort Washington, PA 19034). The stomach is approached and examined. The gastrohepatic ligament is opened through its bare area, and the index and middle fingers are passed behind the posterior wall of the stomach to ensure freedom from adhesions and to align the future passage of the posterior blade of the Gastro-clip to the greater curvature of the stomach, essentially proximal to the first and highest vasa brevia.

At this point, an opening is made in the peritoneal coverage of the greater curvature for implantation of the clip. At this time the modified Pingree-Jack nasogastric gastroplasty tube* (which has two lumina, a larger lumen for suction and a smaller lumen leading to a 50 mL balloon at the end of the tube) is passed by the anesthesiologist. The modification was made to extend the nasogastric lumen 5 cm beyond the balloon. This extended part of the tube serves as a palpable guide to the future stoma in the clip and also permits the clip to be immediately subjacent to the inflated balloon which is below the gastroesophageal

---

*Wilson-Cook Inc., Winston-Salem, NC 27105.

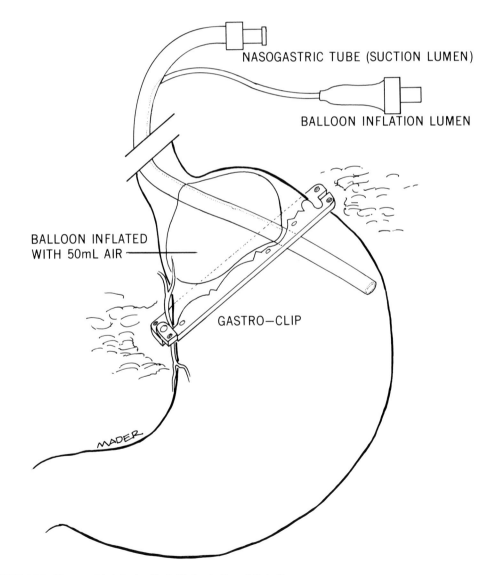

NASOGASTRIC TUBE (SUCTION LUMEN)

BALLOON INFLATION LUMEN

BALLOON INFLATED WITH 50mL AIR

GASTRO—CLIP

MADER

FIGURE 22.2. Nasogastric tube in situ (with the balloon inflated).

junction. The balloon is inflated with 50 mL of air, and the clip is introduced around the stomach walls at this site and closed (Fig. 22.2).

The eye in the posterior blade of the clip is threaded with a 30-inch polypropylene or Gore-Tex suture which is tied at the midpoint of the suture. A Satinsky or a right-angled clamp is used to clamp the ends and pass the two 15-inch strands of suture through the tunnel behind the stomach to the greater curvature (Fig. 22.3). The suture is used to lead the posterior blade of the clip behind the posterior wall of the stomach and onto the greater curvature. When the blade has traversed the posterior gastric wall and is latched at the greater curvature, one end of the suture is threaded into a curved needle and passed through the eye in the anterior blade; four throws of tying are made to the other end of the suture, which ensures that the clip re-

mains securely closed. One end of the same suture is brought with the curved needle seromuscularly through the greater curvature of the stomach below the clip, to anchor the clip and prevent displacement. Sometimes an extra suture is taken through the posterior eye and seromuscularly through the gastric wall above the clip for further anchorage. At the completion of this procedure with anchorage completed, the balloon of the nasogastric tube is deflated and the nasogastric tube is removed.

A similar suture is used at the lesser curvature. This suture is passed through the eye in the anterior blade of the clip, brought through a piece of gastrohepatic omentum at the lesser curvature, and tied, so that omentum covers the hinge of the clip, thus creating a buttress between the clip and liver or any other adjacent structure. Occasionally this suture is brought through the omentum as a

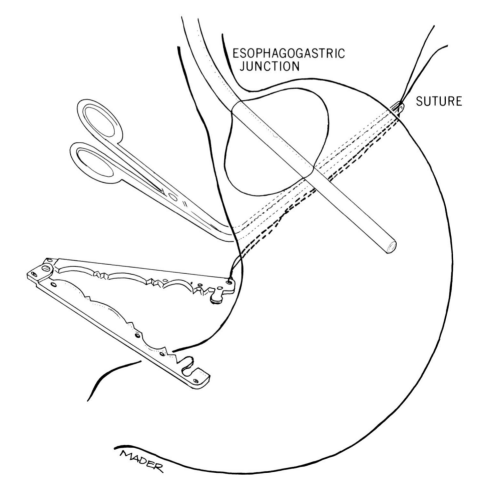

ESOPHAGOGASTRIC
JUNCTION

SUTURE

FIGURE 22.3. A suture is passed through the posterior eye and tied at its midpoint. The two ends of the suture are grasped with a right-angled clamp, for retrogastric passage.

figure-of-eight, to entirely cover the hinge. If the posterior eye is accessible, the suture can be brought through it and omentum, for further coverage. The lesser curvature suture is not brought through the stomach wall, as slippage will not occur here and a gastric hematoma could result.

Implanting the clip in this fashion avoids injury to the left gastric vessels, the nerve of Latarjet, or the vasa brevia at the greater curvature (Fig. 22.4). Because of the varied stomach angulation in different patients at the angle of His, one vasa brevia might have to be sacrificed and secured.

The abdominal incision is closed by using a No. 2 polypropylene continuous suture on the rectus sheath, reinforced by 4 to 6 interrupted traction sutures of the same. The subcutaneous fat is irrigated with saline and the skin approximated with staples. A dry dressing of Telfa and sterile gauze is used to cover the wound.

An added step is the injection of 20 mL of 0.25% Marcaine (bupivacaine) subcutaneously on both sides of the wound. This procedure diminishes incisional pain and was found to be a definite factor in decreased demand for narcotics postoperatively.

RESULTS

Clip gastroplasty follow-up is as follows:

1 month:	Upper GI (Fig. 22.5)
	Vit. B_{12} 2 mL I.M.
2 months:	SMA-12
	Electrolytes
	CBC
4 months:	Vit. B_{12} 2 mL I.M.
6 months:	Upper GI
12 months:	Upper GI
	Electrolytes
	SMA-12
	CBC
24 months:	Same as 12 months

Mortality in 77 cases is 0.

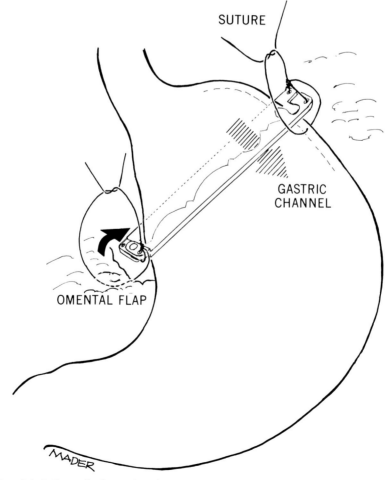

SUTURE

GASTRIC CHANNEL

OMENTAL FLAP

MADER

FIGURE 22.4. Completed clip application and anchorage.

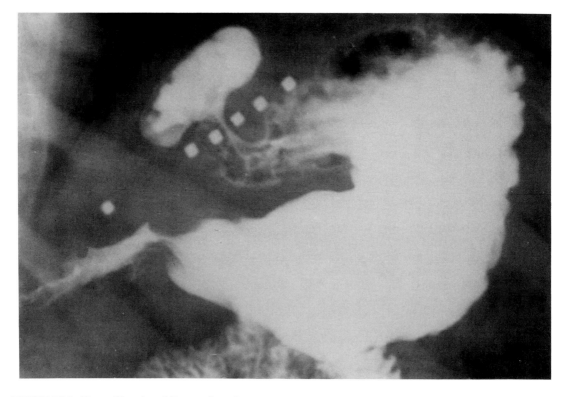

FIGURE 22.5. Upper GI series of Gastro-clip patient one month postoperatively.

Figure 22.6 compares mean pre- and postoperative weights of three groups of female patients during three time periods. These groups were chosen after passing the "t" test and found to be homogeneous. The "t" test showed no statistical difference between average pre- and postoperative weights in each group.

The average yearly loss of weight is about 68 lb, as noted in group 1 on the graph. A second group of 11 such patients showed the same mean loss at one year. A third group of 11 patients showed an average loss of 57 lb when followed for only 8.5 months. It is predicted that this group will continue to lose the same average weight in the remaining 3.5 months of their studied year, to compare with the groups 1 and 2. Furthermore, the patients in group 1 (19 patients) were followed for 21.6 months postoperatively, and did not regain any of their lost weight, as shown in Figure 22.6.

This study indicates that the clip maintains the constructed pouch and the size of the stomal opening. By radiologic upper gastrointestinal study, the stomal size established by the clip continues its net diameter of 9 mm.

CONTRAINDICATIONS TO THE USE OF THE GASTRO-CLIP

The following conditions contraindicate the use of the Gastro-clip:

1. Failure in psychologic clearance, where patients are not likely to follow the small-size meals or to change their lifestyle. A psychologist is consulted preoperatively. A megaesophagus or a perforation of the pouch could result from overeating.

2. Jejunoileal bypass patients should not have clip surgery at the same time as take-down of their jejunoileal bypass. Clip gastroplasty can be done at a later date, when the patients have shown restoration of their proteins and essential amino acids (by serum chromatography), 6 to 12 months after their anatomic restoration. One such patient had perforation in the hospital 5 days post gastroplasty.

3. Previous gastroplasty failure after vertical banded gastroplasty, gastrojejunostomy procedures or any other stomach resectional procedures. One such patient had perforation 2 weeks post clip

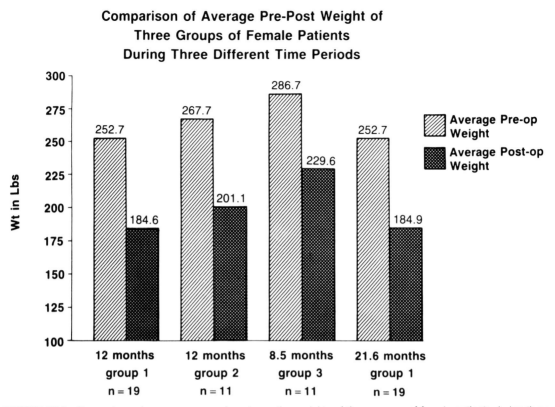

Comparison of Average Pre-Post Weight of Three Groups of Female Patients During Three Different Time Periods

FIGURE 22.6. Comparison of average pre- and postoperative weights of three groups of female patients during three different time periods.

gastroplasty, after staple gastroplasty had failed and the patient had regained most of her weight. The clip was removed and the patient had an uneventful recovery.

CONCLUSIONS

A Gastro-clip gastroplasty has been devised and found effective and safe in morbidly obese patients who have not had previous gastric restrictive operations. It is done in place of the more complicated invasive resectional procedures, and reduces hospital and operating-room expenses as compared with the other procedures. The intensive care unit has not been required postoperatively. Nutritional food is recommended directly after discharge from the hospital, thus eliminating

any protein or electrolyte deficiencies that are commonly seen following other procedures. Only beef is not tolerated and thus not allowed, on account of indigestion due to low acidity in the pouch. Follow-up shows marked acceptance of the procedure.

Editor's Note: Further follow-up and caution on this procedure[1] is warranted, as four patients with late erosion of the clip have been reported.[2]

REFERENCES

1. Bashour SB, Hill RW: The gastro-clip gastroplasty: an alternative surgical procedure for the treatment of morbid obesity. Tex Med 81:36–38, 1985.
2. Aquirre JM, Reid RM Jr: Complications of gastro-clip gastroplasty for morbid obesity. Tex Med 82:4–5, 1986.

23

Intragastric Balloon

CLAUDE P. LIEBER
URSULA L. SEINIGE
DAHLIA M. SATALOFF
HU A. BLAKE II
PETER F. ROVITO

Most morbidly obese individuals have failed to have sustained weight loss with multiple conservative measures for weight control. The implication is that special therapeutic modalities are needed to manage their weight problem. One potential therapeutic method is the intragastric balloon, which is inserted as an outpatient procedure. Balloon therapy is combined with a calorie-restricted diet and behavior modification plus an exercise program, in an attempt to alter lifestyle permanently. The balloon functions as an artificial bezoar which decreases available stomach volume. This is intended to produce early satiety and suppress appetite. We will review the subject of intragastric balloons and present our experience.

ANIMAL STUDIES

In 1979, Miller inserted a 250-mL polyethylene bottle into the stomach of dogs via a gastrotomy at laparotomy.[1] The device occupied 75 to 90% of the dogs' stomachs. Postoperatively, dogs were given access to food and water ad libitum. While the dogs showed a temporary decline in weight in the first 2–3 weeks, beyond this period there was no difference in weight compared to the control dogs. At sacrifice at 5–16 weeks, some of the dogs showed superficial gastritis.

Geliebter et al[2] studied a gastric balloon in rats. The balloon (modified from a Foley catheter) was inserted orally into the stomach of obese rats, inflated with 7 mL of water and then detached. The inflatable balloon occupied 33% of estimated stomach capacity. Rats with inflated balloons consumed 30% less and after 2 months weighed 19% less than controls. No histologic change was found in gastric mucosa.

Yang and co-workers[3] passed spherical silicone balloons with a one-way valve into pigs noninvasively under intravenous pentothal anesthesia. A blunt needle connected to a catheter containing an intraluminal stiff guide was placed in the one-way valve, and the balloon was wrapped around the tip of the catheter. The semipermeable balloon was filled with fluid of a proper osmolarity to maintain balloon volume, and the catheter was withdrawn, leaving the balloon free in the stomach. The balloons had 600 mL volume each, and either two (1200 mL) or three (1800 mL) were inserted in each pig. The pigs were then fed ad libitum. The food intake of the experimental pigs was inhibited for less than one

week, and the pigs with three balloons ate less than controls but showed no significant difference in weight loss. Stomachs in the experimental pigs dilated and frequently showed ulcerations at sacrifice at 6 weeks.

DEVELOPMENT OF GASTRIC BALLOONS

In 1979, Wilkinson devised an intragastric balloon with the intent of achieving long-term weight loss (see Chapter 21, Fig. 21.6). At the same time, however, a patient presented with a huge trichobezoar in a dilated stomach showing secondary gastric erosions. Because that patient had been asymptomatic until just before surgery, Wilkinson abandoned the concept of a bolus. However, some surgeons have noted anorexia, small intake and weight loss to be a feature in 38% of patients with gastric bezoars.[4]

Since 1980, Percival has used balloons which had been glued and tied around the distal part of fine nasogastric tubes, in massively obese patients.[5] Some metallic mercury was instilled in the balloon for weight in order to make it easier to swallow. The balloon was passed nasally, swallowed into stomach, and inflated with 200 mL of air and 150–200 mL of water through the narrow catheter. The catheter was then plugged and taped to the cheek or side of the nostril with skin-colored tape or looped over an ear. Initially toy-store balloons were used, which generally broke after a few weeks, but were replaced as desired. After the first 43 patients, a spherical silicone mammary implant (Dow Corning) has been used, lasting an average of 10 weeks. Because the silicone is semipermeable, it has to be refilled on a regular basis.

Percival's patients experienced initial satiety and learned to eat small meals. The balloon was part of a behavior modification and exercise program, aimed at changing the patient's lifestyle. The external portion of the connecting catheter was generally not uncomfortable, but was inconvenient and visible, and had occasional traction on the nostril. Percival subsequently reported the use in 200 patients, but unfortunately he has not given data regarding patient weight loss.[6] In 10% of patients the tubes were completely swallowed into the stomach, and were retrieved gastroscopically. One patient required removal for hemorrhage from a gastric erosion. Another patient developed small-bowel obstruction due to balloon dislodgement, with swallowing of the thin connecting catheter.[7]

Deitel and co-workers[8] also reported the introduction of intragastric balloons transnasally in five morbidly obese patients. A toy balloon (which broke readily), condom or latex balloon from a Blakemore tube was glued and sutured, so that the attachment was airtight around the lower end of a fine nasogastric tube, with the feeding-hole in the balloon. The patient swallowed water which facilitated passage of the balloon, the lubricated guidewire was removed from the narrow tube[9] and the balloon was inflated with 200 mL of air. The external end of the tube was tied shut and taped over the ear (Fig. 23.1A and B).[10] The tube enabled control over the volume of air in the balloon, and 50 mL increments of air weekly were instilled as necessary to maintain satiety. It appeared that the pliable stomach enlarged progressively and required a progressively larger bolus to produce satiety. All balloons broke after a variable length of time, and then travelled into duodenum from which they were removed promptly by gastroscopic retrieval, and were frequently replaced. Weight losses were variable, but after discontinuance of this treatment, ultimately all patients regained any weight lost.

A commercial balloon has been made available in Europe by the William Cook company (Denmark). The balloon is the shape of the stomach, and 300 mL of air are introduced through a tube which exits through the nostril, is plugged with a stopcock and is brought over the ear. Because the stomach dilates, air has to be added to the balloon to maintain satiety. Dr. Lizbet Mathus-Bligcen of Amsterdam has reported on preliminary weight losses of up to 45 kg in 62 patients.[11]

FREE-FLOATING GASTRIC BALLOONS

In 1982, Nieben and Harboe in Denmark reported on the use of an oval latex-rubber intragastric balloon in 5 obese women.[12] The balloon was attached to two catheters, one within the other, and was passed orally into the stomach and inflated with 250 mL of air via a valve in the mid-portion of the side of the oval. The tube system was then pulled back to the cardia, detaching it from the valve, and was withdrawn, leaving the free-floating balloon. The location in the fundus was verified radiographically. The balloon was left inflated for 10 days during which the women lost an average of 5.0 kg, was then removed gastroscopically, and a second balloon was later inserted for 10 days during which an average of 2.1 kg was lost. When the balloons were inflated, the patients noted reduced hunger, but the balloons were of limited durability, collapsing spontaneously in 7 to 21 days, during which they passed unnoticed in the stools.

Subsequently, Nieben and Harboe have developed the Ballobes™ intragastric balloon (DOT APS, Denmark 3390, Hundested), which is made of a more durable plastic material. Topical pharyngeal anesthesia is used, with no sedatives. The balloon is prepacked in a tube system, and a piston in the tube pushes the balloon out and into the stomach. Once in the stomach, the balloon is insufflated with 400 mL of room air, detached, and the tube system removed. Because the balloon is oval with rounded edges, if only 200 to 250 mL of air were inserted, it would pass into the intestine; >300 mL of air is necessary to avoid this, and the balloon is generally filled with 400 mL of air. After 3–4 months, the balloon is punctured, grasped with a foreign body forceps and removed with a gastroscope, and a new balloon can be inserted as required.

From November 1, 1985 to June 1, 1986 the Ballobes intragastric balloon was used in 202 patients in a cooperative study in centers in Denmark, Norway, Israel, Australia, France and Great Britain. Patients with a history of peptic ulcer were excluded from its use. In the first 16 weeks, 4% of balloons collapsed, and from 16–32 weeks, 31% collapsed, so that it is recommended that the balloon be removed in 3–4 months.[13] Modest weight losses of 0.5 to 1 kg per week were reported while the balloon was inflated. A diet and behavior modification program are combined. The group from Australia has noted that acute vomiting after insertion of the Ballobes balloon occurred exclusively in patients that harbor *Campylobacter pyloridis* in the stomach, so that presumably the balloon permits the bacterium to cause infection and gastritis.[14] Knut Kolle reported the use of the Ballobes balloon in 160 patients in Norway, with weight loss of 0.8 kg per week, but follow-up was short.[15]

Taylor in Manchester, England, reported the use of a pear-shaped silicone free-floating intragastric balloon (TIB, Mill-Rose Laboratories, Mentor, Ohio) in 31 obese patients for up to 6 months.[16] The valved silicone balloon was likewise passed through the mouth into

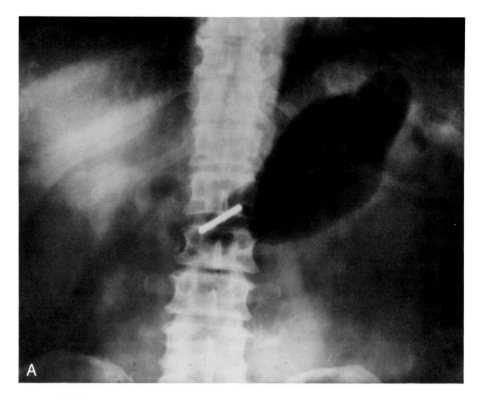

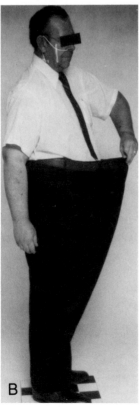

FIGURE 23.1A. Intragastric balloon consisting of a condom tied about lower part of a Keofeed tube used for inflations. **B.** The patient lost 44 kg in 5 months, regained on removal, lost again on reinsertions, but ultimately regained all lost weight.[10]

the stomach using an overtube (cover) and innertube (insufflation device) which permitted inflation with a 500 mL mixture of Dextran-40 and radiopaque medium. One-third of patients reported early satiety and one-half were aware of fluid movement on changing position. Patients lost 0.2 kg per week on an initial 800 kcal diet alone and 0.5 kg per week when combined with the balloon. Spontaneous deflation was associated with weight gain and occurred in 5 patients, resulting in uncomplicated passage of the balloon in the stool. Removal of the balloon was accomplished by endoscopy after puncture with a hooded needle or laceration with rat-tooth forceps.[17]

In dog studies, Taylor's group found that his device was not effective at 200 mL but was effective when inflated to 500 mL in reducing voluntary food intake.[18] They also found in dogs that prolonged inflation to 500 mL with this silicone balloon did not increase gastric acid secretion (likely due to adaptation) or produce gastric mucosal damage at 20 weeks (likely due to its smooth, rounded, pear-shaped configuration).[19]

In the USA, Bard (P.O. Box 5069, Billerica, Massachusetts) developed a spherical free-floating balloon, inserted and inflated with 400 mL of air through a narrow removable tube. An initial loss of 1% of body weight per week was observed, but because of a lack of documented long-term effectiveness of balloons, Bard removed the balloon from the market.[20]

McFarland and co-workers[21] developed a spherical silicone balloon. Following orogastric passage of the balloon, inflation with 600 mL of saline and radiopaque medium via a valve, and withdrawal of the fill-tube, the balloon was left free-floating. A diet was instituted. Weight loss occurred initially. However, there was adaptation by patients to the presence of the balloon, leading to regain of lost weight to initial or higher levels, despite the continued presence of the inflated intragastric balloon.

THE GARREN-EDWARDS GASTRIC BUBBLE

In the United States, the Food and Drug Administration (FDA) approved the use of the Garren-Edwards Gastric Bubble™ (American Edwards Laboratories, P.O. Box 1150, Santa Ana, California) in September 1985. The "bubble" was intended to be a temporary adjunct to a diet reinforced by a behavior modification and exercise program, which were to be continued for permanent success. The bubble is a polyurethane cylinder with a hollow central channel (Fig. 23.2). It is inflated with 210 mL of room air. The flat ends and size of the bubble allow this device to move freely about the gastric compartment, while resisting exit via the esophagus or the pylorus. The bubble is compressible, and the central hollow channel acts as a vent if antral impaction should occur.

An esophagogastroscopy is done first to confirm that the stomach is normal. The deflated bubble is compacted into the silicone-fluid-lubricated end of a modified introducer oro-gastric tube, and is passed per orum into the stomach. The bubble is then released from a lateral seam in the tube, while being inflated via an inflation cannula. The insufflation cannula and oro-gastric tube are then pulled back to the cardia, detached and removed, while the bubble remains free-floating in the stomach (Fig. 23.3). Gastroscopy is done to assure that the bubble is properly inflated and positioned.

For the first 5–7 days after implantation, a 500–700 calorie full liquid diet is prescribed, followed by an individualized 800–1000 calorie diet. Insertion of the Garren-Edwards Bubble is an outpatient procedure, performed with meperidine and diazepam sedation and topical anesthesia. Removal of the bubble is also an outpatient procedure, and is accom-

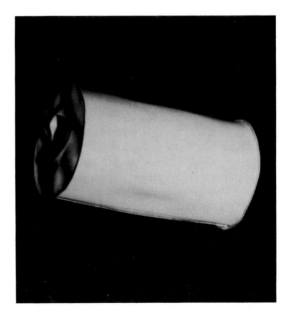

FIGURE 23.2. The gastric "bubble".

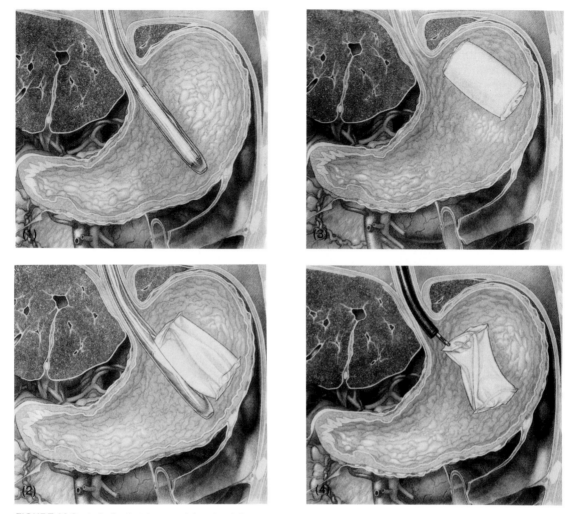

FIGURE 23.3. 1. A plastic tube containing the deflated bubble is inserted into the stomach. 2. The bubble is inflated and the tube is removed. 3. The bubble floats freely in the upper stomach to give a feeling of satiety. 4. After 3 months, an instrument is inserted through a viewing scope to deflate and remove the bubble.

plished by endoscopic puncture and deflation of the bubble, with subsequent retrieval per orum.

The Garren-Edwards bubble was originally considered to be a simple, safe, outpatient procedure. Contraindications were active peptic ulcer disease, a large hiatal hernia, or prior gastric or intestinal surgery. Dietary restriction of caffeine, heavy spices and alcohol, and postprandial administration of antacids or H2 blockers were intended to prevent mild gastritis due to the intragastric device. Aspirin, anti-inflammatory drugs and anticoagulants were contraindications to its use.

The bubble was originally introduced for treatment of obesity in patients weighing >20% above ideal weight. Initial satisfactory weight losses in multiple short-term studies of 4 to 12 weeks were reported.[22-24] However, intestinal obstructions due to impacted spontaneously-deflated balloons were reported.[25-31] The original FDA recommendation of implantation for 4 months was thus changed. It was now recommended that the bubble be removed after 3 months, because beyond 3 months, a significant increase in spontaneous deflation occurred. Deflated bubbles should be removed immediately, before they progress beyond the stomach. If necessary, another bubble can be inserted. If a bubble has passed beyond the stomach, close monitoring is mandatory. The recommendations for use of the bubble became limited to patients who were morbidly obese or who were not candidates for surgery because of serious complicating medical conditions.

The mechanism of action of the bubble was unclear,[30] and a decrease in between-meal hunger, an effect on stretch receptors in the proximal stomach, stimulation of satiety hormones or change in the gastric emptying rate have not been documented.

The American Edwards Company has requested that they be notified of complications.[32] The company estimates that from November 1985 to December 1986, 20,000 bubbles have been inserted, and has been notified of the complications shown in Table 23.1.

In March 1987, a comprehensive multidisciplinary workshop of 75 international experts found in controlled, prospective, double-blind, randomized and cross-over clinical trials comparing the bubble with sham insertion that there was no difference in weight loss of the 210 mL bubble over the diet and behavior modification program alone in the short-term treatment of obesity.[30,33-36] Almost two-thirds of the consensus workshop said that they did not believe that the gastric balloon was an effective adjunct to weight control. Gastritis was found in 30%, ulcers in 4% and deflations in 10% of patients. The consensus recommended that the procedure be limited to controlled clinical trials in centers with endoscopists skilled in balloon implantation and retrieval. It was also recommended that the bubble be made radiopaque.

PERSONAL EXPERIENCE

MATERIALS AND METHODS

From February to September 1986, 45 patients were followed after insertion of the Garren-Edwards Bubble. A total of 47 bubbles were inserted, and each bubble was in place for a maximum period of 4 months. The group consisted of 37 women and 8 men. Of the patients, 22 were morbidly obese (>45 kg above ideal weight as defined by the 1983 Metropolitan Life Insurance Tables) and 23 were >45 kg above ideal weight (ranging from 11.4 to 42.7 kg overweight). All patients were at least 20% above their ideal weight. The bubble was inserted using topical anesthesia and IV sedation, using the Gastric Bubble Kit. Despite the fact that the bubble had been tested for air-leaks prior to packaging, it was nevertheless inflated and rechecked prior to implantation. No leaks were found in the bubbles before insertion. All bubbles were loaded into the introducer just prior to implantation.

The large oro-gastric tube which serves as the introducer is somewhat rigid at the gastric end and can be difficult to introduce. Even with topical anesthesia, significant IV sedation was necessary. In the morbidly obese patient with reduced cardiac and pulmonary reserve, significant IV sedation can be life-threatening, especially because the airway is unprotected. For that reason, the intragastric bubble, when introduced into a morbidly obese patient, was always done in the presence of an anesthesiologist. Cardiac monitoring as well as monitoring of oxygen saturation were necessary, so as not to endanger the patient's life.

After insertion of the bubble the gastroscope was reinserted to check the inflation and position of the bubble. If at any time in the following months were was a question about the inflation status of the bubble, an upright film was obtained. Absence of the typical radiolucency of the bubble in the stomach led to endoscopic examination.

After insertion, all patients were enrolled in a behavior modification program, as previously arranged. They were instructed to take antacids 2 tablespoonsful after meals and at bed-time. The patients were given a multivitamin with minerals and a bulk-forming agent. They were advised to avoid foods containing heavy spices, caffeine or alcoholic beverages during the period of treatment.

RESULTS

Of the 45 patients treated with the intragastric bubble, follow-up was completed on 43 (2 patients lost to follow-up). Forty-one pa-

TABLE 23.1. CUSTOMER EXPERIENCE REPORTS TO AMERICAN EDWARDS LABORATORIES[30,32]

From Nov. 1985 to Dec. 1986, American Edwards estimates that 20,000 bubbles were inserted, and reports the following:

Incident Reported	No.
Insertion	
Pharyngeal perforation requiring surgery	1
Release in esophagus resulting in perforation requiring surgery	3
Partial release in esophagus (no surgery required)	4
Retrieval	
Esophageal tear requiring surgery	1
Aspiration pneumonia	1
Deflated bubble obstructing intestine	
Requiring surgery (20 had intestinal adhesions)	79
Death	1
Ulcers	53
Gastric perforation	1

tients were seen in the office, and 2 patients who passed a deflated balloon per rectum gave us their follow-up weight by telephone. Two patients refused to return for bubble removal, although they had no weight loss.

The 22 morbidly obese patients were an average of 65 kg overweight (203% of ideal weight). They lost an average of 9 kg per patient over an average of 9 months, representing a loss of 12.8% of excess weight. Two had a second bubble inserted. The group of moderately obese patients was an average of 29.5 kg overweight (148% of ideal weight) and lost an average of 6.5 kg (22.2% of excess weight) over 4 months. The overall weight loss for the entire group was 17.6% of excess body weight over 4 months.

Only 4 patients admitted to experiencing early satiety. Patients commonly complained that while following the diet as part of their behavior modification program, they were hungry most of the time. An upright film of the abdomen was obtained when a patient complained of hunger and, if the bubble was seen to be inflated, it was left in place. Five patients lost no weight or actually gained weight, and complained of gnawing "hunger" pains or epigastric pain and/or nausea, relieved by food intake; all were discovered to have mild to moderate gastritis. All patients had been successful with at least one weight loss program in the past (followed by weight gains); they felt that the gastric bubble added nothing to their efforts at weight loss.

Complications were seen in all but one patient (Table 23.2). Significant persistent pain occurred in 16 patients (36%) and intractable nausea occurred in 4 patients (9%), Complaints of pain or nausea were relieved by H2 blockers and/or sucralfate, in addition to the prescribed antacids.

Spontaneous deflation of the bubble occurred in 25 patients (56%), with 8 patients passing deflated balloons per rectum. Four

patients experienced mechanical small-bowel obstruction clinically. Obstruction progressed to signs of peritonitis in one patient, requiring emergency operative intervention. In the other three patients, the symptoms resolved and the deflated balloons passed per rectum. None of the patients in the series had had previous intestinal or gastric surgery. The syndrome of crampy abdominal pain, nausea, vomiting and abdominal distention together with radiologic evidence of small-bowel obstruction required hospitalization of all 3 patients and lasted several days. The remaining 16 patients with deflated bubbles had them removed gastroscopically.

Gastritis occurred in 26 patients (58%), who had inflamed, edematous, friable mucosa which bled easily during gastroscopy. All cases of gastritis were biopsied and documented histologically.

DISCUSSION

Significant weight loss did not occur; disappointment and frustration were frequent. We explained to all patients before insertion of the bubble that dietary management of obesity is the keystone of treatment and all patients understood that attendance in the behavior modification course was mandatory. Our patients expected that compliance with dietary restrictions would be easier with the bubble. This unfortunately did not turn out to be the case.

Lack of success of the gastric balloon was uniform. The group of patients who were morbidly obese did no better than the group of patients who were not morbidly obese. One young 4'11" registered nurse with a desire to lose 25 excess pounds was just as unsuccessful as some of the morbidly obese patients whose needs for weight control were more medically urgent.

A few patients did lose while the bubble was in place. One patient lost 15 kg (72% of excess weight) over 4 months and did, in fact, experience early satiety. She had no significant gastritis at the time of her bubble removal. Another patient who lost 26 kg over 4 months swore that this was due to her own efforts, that she was constantly hungry and that the bubble did not induce early satiety. She was unable to lose any further weight after the insertion of a second bubble and in fact gained 3.6 kg during the second 4 months. This patient who is 5'2" tall and orig-

TABLE 23.2. COMPLICATIONS

No complication—1 patient
Complications—
1) Persistent epigastric pain—16 patients
2) Persistent nausea/vomiting—4 patients
3) Endoscopically proven gastritis—26 patients
4) Spontaneous balloon deflation—25 patients
   a) Complete loss of bubble integrity—3 patients
   b) Passed per rectum—8 patients
   c) Discovered on endoscopy—13 patients
   d) Causing obstruction—4
      i) Treated medically—3
      ii) Treated surgically—1

inally weighed 143 kg is still trying to deal with her obesity.

A third patient who experienced a 23 kg weight loss over the first 4 months also did not have early satiety. Instead, this patient had anorexia. He was plagued by a constant feeling of severe nausea from the time the bubble was placed to the time of its removal. On endoscopy he was found to have severe gastritis. A second intragastric bubble was not placed. Three other patients had moderate weight loss (14–18 kg over 4 months), and only one of them experienced early satiety. None of the other patients achieved excellent weight loss.

Because of its supposed safety and ease of insertion, it has been suggested that use of an intragastric bubble might be considered in super-obese patients in whom there is a significant anesthesia risk for bariatric surgery The super-obese have markedly reduced functional reserve capacity and desaturate very quickly. This problem is often compounded by high output cardiac failure. Intravenous sedation in these patients in the absence of endotracheal intubation and ventilatory support seemed to us and our anesthesiologist to represent a potentially lethal combination. We were unwilling to subject these patients to this risk.

CONCLUSION

Following insertion of a balloon, the stomach enlarges to accommodate more intake with time. To maintain satiety, a balloon which can have its size adjusted and enlarged in a stepwise fashion by a nasal cannula appears to be necessary. For safety, a sturdy balloon with no sharp edges is required. However, gastric balloons appeared to add little to the weight loss of the behavior modification programs that these patients are required to follow. Furthermore, there is no effective mechanism to prevent the patients from regaining the lost weight.[37]

Morbidly obese patients can lose weight on behavioral and conservative treatments, but regain occurs (i.e. the yo-yo pattern). Maintenance of weight loss is the problem. However, the balloon may offer a temporary means of reducing caloric intake for some patients to turn them into a suitable risk for surgery.

ACKNOWLEDGMENT

We thank George S.M. Cowan, Jr., M.D., Associate Professor of Surgery, University of Tennessee, Memphis, for valuable information.

REFERENCES

1. Miller JD: Intragastric prosthesis for management of obesity. World J Surg 6:492–493, 1982.
2. Geliebter A, Westreich S, Kral JG, et al: Intragastric balloon reduces spontaneous food intake and induces weight loss. Fed Proc 42:664, 1983 (abstr 2177).
3. Yang Y, Kuwano H, Okudaira Y, et al: Use of intragastric balloons for weight reduction: an experimental study. Am J Surg 153:265–269, 1987.
4. DeBakey M, Ochsner A: Bezoars and concretions. A comprehensive review of the literature with an analysis of 303 collected cases and a presentation of 8 additional cases. Surgery 4:934–963, 1938 and Surgery 5:132–160, 1939.
5. Percival WL: "The balloon diet": a noninvasive treatment for morbid obesity. Preliminary report of 108 patients. Can J Surg 27:135–136, 1984.
6. 'Balloon' proves worth as weight loss device. The Medical Post, Maclean Hunter, Toronto, August 19th, 1986, p 22.
7. Holland S, Bach D, Duff J: Balloon therapy for obesity—when the balloon bursts. J Can Assoc Radiol 36:347–349, 1985.
8. Zakhary GS, Deitel M: Intragastric balloon for morbid obesity. J Am Coll Nutr 1:391–392, 1982 (abstr 21).
9. Bojm MA, Deitel M: An easy method for passing fine silicone nasogastric tubes. Am J Surg 143:385, 1982.
10. Deitel M, Bojm MA, Atin, MD, et al: Intestinal bypass and gastric partitioning for morbid obesity. Can J Surg 25:283–289, 1982.
11. Mathus L: Presentation, International Conference on Obesity, Jerusalem, Sept. 1986.
12. Nieben OG, Harboe H: Intragastric balloons as an artificial bezoar for treatment of obesity. Lancet 1:198–199, 1982.
13. Nieben OG, Harboe H: Gastric bubble. Fifth Annual Symposium, the Center for Surgical Treatment of Obesity, Universal Sheraton Hotel, Feb 12, 1987.
14. Lee A, Carrick J, Borody TJ: Campylobacter pyloridis infection as possible complication of weight loss therapy. Lancet 2:1343, 1986.
15. Kolle K: Second International Symposium on Obesity Surgery, Eilat, Sept 1986.
16. Taylor TV, Durrans D, Holt S: Safety and efficacy of the Taylor intragastric balloon (TIB) device in the treatment of gross obesity. Am J Gastroenterol 9:859, 1986 (abstr 58).
17. Durrans D, Taylor TV: The intragastric balloon, a new treatment for obesity. Clin Nutr 6:113–115, 1986.
18. Durrans D, Taylor TV, Holt S: Volume of gastric balloons for obesity treatment determines food intake. Am J Gastroenterol 82:943, 1987 (abstr 84).
19. Durrans D, Taylor TV, Holt S: The effect of the Taylor intragastric balloon device (TIB) on gastric mucosa and acid secretion. Am J Gastroenterol 82:943, 1987 (abstr 83).
20. Cowan GSM Jr, University of Tennessee, Memphis: Personal Communication.

21. McFarland R, Grundy A, Gazet J-C: The intragastric balloon: a novel idea proved ineffective. Br J Surg 74:137–139, 1987.

22. Garren L, Garren M, Garren R, et al: Gastric balloon implantation for weight loss in the morbidly obese. Am J Gastroenterol 80:860, 1985 (abstr).

23. Goldberg SJ, Kommor RH, Lutter DR: Preliminary experience using the Garren-Edwards gastric bubble for treatment of morbid obesity. Am J Gastroenterol 9:854, 1986 (abstr 36).

24. White SC, White MA: The Garren gastric bubble therapy for weight loss. Am J Gastroenterol 9:860, 1986 (abstr 61).

25. Bonefas E, Garth J, Sasso R: Small-bowel obstruction due to migration of intragastric balloon. Surgical Rounds Apr 1987, pp 84–85.

26. Fleisher A, Conti PS, McCray RS, et al.: Jejunal entrapment of a gastric balloon (letter). JAMA 257:930, 1987.

27. Boyle TM, Agus SG, Bauer JJ: Small intestinal obstruction secondary to obturation by a Garren gastric bubble. Am J Gastroenterol 82:51–53, 1987.

28. Kirby DF, Mills PR, Kellum JM, et al: Incomplete small bowel obstruction by the Garren-Edwards gastric bubble necessitating surgical intervention. Am J Gastroenterol 82:251–253, 1987.

29. Benjamin SB: Small bowel obstruction and the Garren-Edwards bubble: lessons to be learned? Gastrointest Endosc 33:183, 1987 (abstr).

30. Schapiro M, Benjamin S, Blackburn G, et al: Obesity and the gastric balloon: a comprehensive workshop. Gastrointest Endosc 33:323–327, 1987.

31. Fedotin MS, Ginzberg BW: Partial deployment of the Garren gastric bubble: a new complication. Am J Gastroenterol 82:470–471, 1987.

32. Access, American Edwards Laboratory Bulletin, Issue No. 87-1, Apr 25, 1987, p 2.

33. Benjamin SB, Maher K, Cattau EL Jr, et al: Double-blind controlled trial of the Garren-Edwards bubble: an adjunctive treatment for exogenous obesity. Gastroenterology 95:581–588, 1988.

34. Hogan RB, Johnston JH, Long BW, et al: The gastric bubble vs sham endoscopy: a prospective, randomized, controlled double-blinded comparison as an adjunct to a standard weight loss program. Gastrointest Endosc 33:172, 1987 (abstr).

35. Meshkinpour H, Hsu D, Farivar S: Effect of gastric bubble as a weight reduction device: a controlled, crossover study. Gastroenterology 95:589–592, 1988.

36. Stoltenberg PH, Piziak VK, Dietscher JE: Intragastric balloon therapy of obesity: a randomized double-blind trial. Gastroenterology 92:1655, 1987 (abstr).

37. Kral JG: Gastric balloons: a plea for sanity in the midst of balloonacy. Gastroenterology 95:213–215, 1988.

24

Jaw Wiring for Massive Obesity

MERVYN DEITEL
SUNDARAM V. ANAND

Maxillo-mandibular fixation is a standard procedure for the stabilization of mandibular fractures. Weight loss was observed in patients with wired jaws on a fractured jaw diet. Thus, maxillo-mandibular fixation has been applied to restrict caloric intake in patients with massive obesity.

GENERAL TECHNIQUES

Fixation can be achieved by either metal cap splinting or interdental wiring. Cap splints are made of silver alloy and are fixed to the teeth by cement; the upper and lower splints are held together by four to six rubber bands or wires.[1] Interdental wiring is simpler but requires healthy upper and lower dentition;[2,3] dental examination including X-rays of the teeth and jaws is done first, as correction of cavities and healthy periodontal tissue are necessary before fixation is applied. Interdental wiring can be performed with eyelets or continuous loops according to the principles for treatment of jaw fractures by the method of Obsweger.[4] The jaws can be fixed by rubber bands which the patient can remove or by stainless steel wires in patients who do not trust their capacity to resist the temptation to remove the fixation. Fixation of arch bars on the maxilla and mandible, with inter-arch bar wiring, is another method. Castelnuovo-Tedesco and associates[5] use Kazanjian-type buttons on the premolars to permit fixation with stainless steel wires, and alternate 2 months of wiring with 1 month of non-fixation, repeated to six months.

The procedures are carried out by oral, plastic or head and neck surgeons. All procedures are done on an outpatient basis and require usually no anesthesia or only local anesthesia. When wire fixation is employed, patients are instructed how to cut the wires to release the jaws in case of an emergency. They are also instructed in oral hygiene. Patients must be seen in follow-up every 2–3 weeks, and dental hygiene is monitored. Adjustment of fixation is done as indicated. If broken wires are not fixed, major stresses on the teeth ensue. The wires are removed if body weight reaches 10% of ideal or if a sustained plateau in weight loss occurs.

DIET

Patients are able to speak. However, they must take a liquid or blended diet, consumed through a straw. The diet consists of soups, juices, yoghurt, pureed baby food in bouillon, and a liquid supplement such as Meritene, Sustacal or Ensure. Professional dietary supervision is necessary to provide 3100–4200 kJ (750–1000 kcal) daily, including 60–65 g of protein. The diet must be supplemented by liquid vitamins and iron. Unfortunately, failure to adhere to the prescribed diet is frequent.[5] Furthermore, to maintain the weight loss, dietary counselling, exercise and behavior modification are mandatory.

RESULTS AND FOLLOW-UP

Rodgers et al[6] described 17 patients. Early weight loss occurred in all patients, but the median rate of loss fell from 9 kg/month to 1.5 kg/month over a 6-month period, with half the patients dropping out. In those who continued to 6 months, an average weight loss of 24 kg or 20% of body weight was found, but with marked variation. The plateau in weight loss after 4 months was associated with loss of enthusiasm, missed appointments, and later weight gain on limited follow-up.

Kark and Burke[2,7] reported a 2-year follow-up on 14 patients: 13 patients failed to maintain their initial weight loss, and 9 of these underwent a gastric reduction operation (gastric bypass) after unwiring. In a further follow-up of 17 patients to 4 years by this group, all but one patient who did not undergo gastric bypass regained significant weight.[3]

In another series[5] of 14 patients with initial enthusiasm, only one-third completed the study as weight loss slowed. Of this one-third, about two-thirds ultimately regained the weight.

A feeling of panic due to jaw immobilization is a common cause of dropping out.[8] Ross et al[9] used the Minnesota Multiphasic Personality Inventory (MMPI) panic fear scale to identify patients with a low fear panic tolerance. High scale scorers are described as fearful, emotionally labile, more sensitive individuals, who are unable to persist when faced with difficulty. In their study, 60 morbidly obese patients underwent jaw wiring, and the authors concluded that the MMPI panic fear scale can delineate those individuals who are likely to have negative reactions to jaw wiring. High scorers are unlikely to carry through to the conclusion of treatment. Males more frequently defaulted or cut their wires, but the male-female differences on the panic fear scale did not reach statistical significance.

PROBLEMS

The major hazard of jaw fixation is inability to vomit, with danger of aspiration. However, Kark states that vomiting is not a hazard in the conscious patient and can be effected satisfactorily.[7] The problems with jaw wiring are listed in Table 24.1. An adequate nasal passage is essential so that the patient can be sure of a patent airway. If the patient has a known hayfever history, jaw wiring should not coincide with the allergy season.

MAXILLO-MANDIBULAR FIXATION IN THE EDENTULOUS PATIENT

Goss and coworkers[10] have used jaw immobilization in 55 obese patients who were edentulous in one or both jaws. Dentures were secured directly to the maxilla by a single circum-palatal wire through the denture and nasal floor or by bilateral circum-zygomatic wires with an anterior nasal spine wire. Mandibular dentures were secured by bilateral circum-mandibular wires. Stainless steel 24-gauge wire was used. Wire eyelets of 26-gauge wire were used on the teeth, and the jaws were immobilized with interdental wires.

For those edentulous in one jaw, satisfactory results have been attained. For those edentulous in both jaws, however, pain from periosteal irritation and infection around the attachment wires are frequent. Circum-palatal wiring of the dentures is better than circum-zygomatic, as the latter carries the risk of infratemporal fossa infection. Circum-mandibular wiring has the risk of parapharyngeal infection.

General anesthesia is necessary for this technique because of pain. Because of the danger of post-anesthetic vomiting or of nosebleed from the circum-palatal wire, interdental wiring is not placed until anesthetic recovery is complete, to avoid aspiration. Patients are given a short course on an antibiotic, usually penicillin, to reduce risk of in-

TABLE 24.2. INDICATIONS FOR INTERDENTAL FIXATION FOR MASSIVE OBESITY

1. <45 kg overweight
2. >225 kg (500 lb), *before* undertaking gastric reduction surgery
3. Too great a risk to withstand a bariatric operation
4. For weight loss in highly motivated patients, followed by low energy diet
5. For weight loss to enable other operations, e.g., orthopedic

fection from oral bacteria from wires passed through tissues, especially in the diabetic obese. The authors note a high rate of regain of weight.[10]

INDICATIONS FOR JAW WIRING

The uses of jaw wiring are outlined in Table 24.2. However, experience with past bariatric operations has shown that if a treatment is not permanent, a procedure will usually fail. In long-term follow-up of patients who had received jaw wiring for obesity, Drenick and Hargis found that the average final weight was 3 kg higher than the initial weight.[11]

CONCLUSION

Jaw wiring has been used to initiate weight loss, followed by a low calorie diet, exercise and behavior modification. The patients must first be screened for a lack of neurotic symptoms. Geographic location must allow follow-up, dental hygiene and possible adjustment of fixation. Following early weight loss, unfortunately there is frequent regain.

TABLE 24.1. PROBLEMS WITH JAW WIRING

Bad breath
Difficulty maintaining oral hygiene
Dental infection
Panic
Danger of vomiting, e.g. with flu
Difficulty with upper respiratory infection, cankers
Local pain
Loosening of wires
High rate of weight regained

REFERENCES

1. Wood GD: Early results of treatment of the obese by diet regimen enforced by maxillo-mandibular fixation. J Oral Surg 35:461–466, 1977.
2. Kark, Burke M: Gastric reduction for morbid obesity: technique and indications. Br J Surg 66:756–761, 1979.
3. Fordyce GL, Garrow JS, Kark AE, et al: Jaw wiring and gastric bypass in treatment of severe obesity. Obesity/Bariatric Med 8:14–17, 1979.
4. Rowe NL, Killey HC: Fractures of the Facial Skeleton, 2nd edition. Edinburgh and London, E & S Livingstone, 1968.
5. Castelnuovo-Tedesco P, Buchanan DC, Hall HD: Jaw-wiring for obesity. Gen Hosp Psychiat 2:156–159, 1980.
6. Rodgers S, Burnet R, Goss A, et al: Jaw wiring in treatment of obesity. Lancet 1:1221–1222, 1977.
7. Kark AE: Jaw wiring. Am J Clin Nutr 33:420–424, 1980.

8. Björvell H, Hadell K, Jonsson B, et al: Long-term effects of jaw fixation in severe obesity. Int J Obesity 8:79–86, 1984.

9. Ross MW, Goss AN, Kalucy RS: The relationship of panic fear to anxiety and tension in jaw wiring for obesity. Br J Med Psychol 57:67–69, 1984.

10. Goss AN with the Adelaide Obesity Group: Treatment of massive obesity by prolonged jaw immobilization for edentulous patients. Int J Oral Surg 9:253–258, 1980.

11. Drenick EJ, Hargis HW: Jaw wiring for weight reduction. Obesity Bariatric Med 7:210–213, 1978.

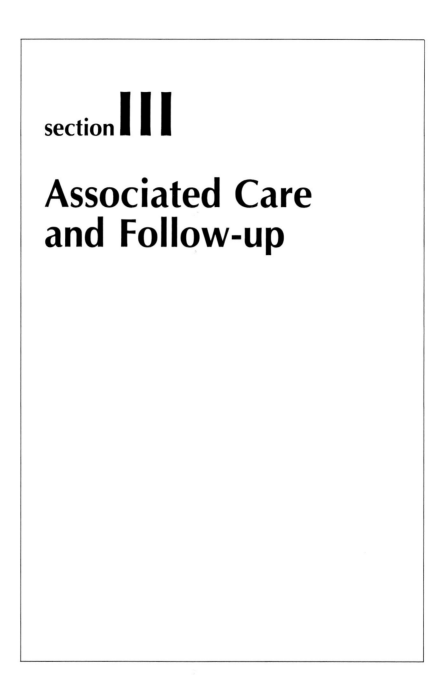

section **III**

Associated Care
and Follow-up

25

Anesthetic Management of the Morbidly Obese Patient Undergoing Abdominal Surgery: Epidural Anesthesia and Postoperative Epidural Analgesia

DOUGLAS E. CROWELL

Anesthesia in the massively obese may present many challenges which, if not met, will jeopardize the outcome of technically sound surgery. We have come to recognize that not all anesthetists at all times are able or wish to attempt thoracic epidural anesthesia in this group of patients (Fig. 25.1). As more members of our department of anesthesia have become involved in providing anesthetic care to morbidly obese patients, there has been a dilution of the interest and expertise in pursuing the use of epidural anesthesia and analgesia postoperatively—mainly due to block failure, patient choice, and an inability to provide the mandatory postoperative supervision of patients who receive epidural opiates for pain control. This usually younger group of patients tolerates narcotic relaxant anesthetic techniques for the shorter more commonly performed vertical banded gastroplasty. It is still this author's belief that the use of epidural peroperatively and epidural analgesia post-operatively is a superior method of anesthesia and patient management, and leads to more rapid recovery of patient activity and a reduction in postoperative pulmonary and thromboembolic complications.

The acceptance of the customary need of patients for a period of postoperative ventilation[1] should not be considered a deterrent when assessing these patients as candidates for surgery preoperatively. Irrespective of what technique is ultimately chosen, it is inevitable that a percentage of these patients will require postoperative ventilatory support as part of their management.[2,3]

Preoperative assessment often reveals respiratory failure based not only upon poor ventilatory mechanics but also upon underlying pulmonary parenchymal disease. One should be able to anticipate that postoperative upper abdominal pain and a poor effect from parenterally administered narcotics may pose a problem of balancing the need for analgesia and the patient's ability to tolerate even minimal degrees of narcotic-induced respiratory depression. The severity of this problem may be further demonstrated by the presence of orthopnea, tachypnea, shortness of breath with minimal exertion, a history of difficulty in staying awake, a reticence to give up smoking, productive cough, a reduction of the arterial pO_2 and a mild-to-moderate elevation of the arterial pCO_2.

Hypertension is frequent. Underlying coronary artery disease, in these usually sedentary patients, may not be clinically obvious. Antihypertensive treatment with diuretics requires a search for hypokalemia. Diuretics

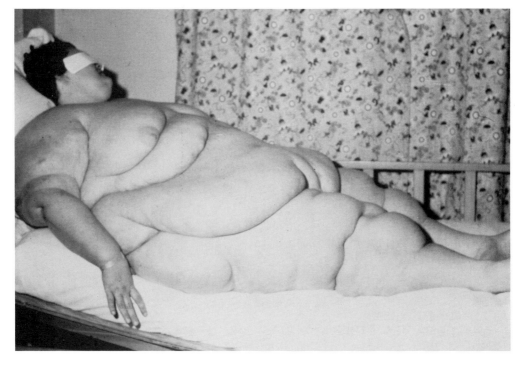

FIGURE 25.1 Patient who presents a problem for anesthetic management.

may also have been prescribed chronically to minimize fluid retention as part of a weight loss regimen.

Glucose tolerance is impaired[4,5] to a degree which parallels the severity of the obesity. Arthritis of the hips, knees and ankles is usual. Involvement of the back may preclude any consideration of some form of conduction anesthesia. Anti-arthritic medications, especially steroids and aspirin, may complicate the management of both anesthesia and surgery.

Other hurdles must be anticipated: the possibility of using an epidural should be discussed and consented to; what management might be possible if an epidural cannot be carried out; the likelihood of postoperative ventilation and admission to an intensive care unit; will a preoperative cutdown be necessary? Venipunctures in these patients should only be done by persons very skilled at preserving the few veins which may be visible. If it is likely that there may be problems intubating and ventilating if an intravenous induction is used, the patient should certainly be prepared to accept an awake intubation. This may be the only safe approach to the problem. An Allen's test for normal arterial palmar arch should be demonstrated before the radial artery is cannulated for monitoring purposes.

The operating-room facilities and staff must be prepared to manage such a patient (Fig. 25.2). Moving 150–250 kg of anesthesized patient is beyond the capabilities of most patient lifting systems. We utilize a heavy canvas sheet placed under the patient preoperatively, supported by sewn-in cross-supports and handles,[6] in addition to a patient roller,* and assisted by as many as 6 to 8 operating-room personnel at this very challenging time (Fig. 25.A and 25.3B).

Consideration should also be given to the width of the operating-room table. To add extra width at the hips and thighs, we have designed a plywood spacer 1.9 cm in thickness, which is placed under the mattress of the operating table and does not limit the use of clip-on armboards (Fig. 25.4); nor does it interfere with the use of surgical retractors which clamp onto the side-rails of the *standard* operating-room table (Fig. 25.5).[6] A support to the floor for the foot of the table may be necessary when patients are in the sitting position, as most operating-room tables can be tilted by these patients' weight. Consideration must also be given to the specifications of the hydraulic lifting system. Most operating tables do not go beyond 136–160 kg. No attempt should be made to raise the table beyond its basic height; for complete safety, the table should be positioned at the basic lowest height, when the patient is first moved there at the start of the procedure.

MONITORING

Most operating rooms will already be equipped with the basic required monitors. Invasive arterial monitoring of blood pressure may be necessary even if blood pressure can be measured by other techniques. The use of a thigh blood-pressure cuff[7,8] containing a bladder which completely encircles the arm and an automatic blood-pressure reading machine are very helpful and least invasive (Fig. 25.6). At times, it may be necessary to apply the thigh blood-pressure cuff on the forearm, using the radial artery at the wrist as the source of the Korotkoff sounds. One should also plan to monitor urinary output, electrocardiogram, body temperature and ventilation. Pulse oximetry has added a new dimension to patient safety, permitting constant assessment of lung and ventilator function peroperativey as well as postoperatively when discontinuance of assisted ventilation and/or extubation are being considered.

PREMEDICATION

The plan of anesthesia is shown in Table 25.1. For premedication, an intermediate-acting barbiturate is usually given orally 60 to 90 minutes before induction followed by meperidine 75–100 mg and is kept on the light side to avoid narcotic depression and to minimize any additive significant depression of cardiovascular dynamics by sympathetic blockade when epidural anesthesia is induced.

PROCEDURE

Preoperatively, the anesthetist must explain the procedure and answer the patient's questions about it, to ensure that he has indeed obtained informed consent. The back is examined. One of the interspaces between T-8 and T-12 usually is chosen for introduction of the block. Accentuation of the thoracic curve brings these interspaces closer to the skin and makes them easier to locate. Often

---

*David Patient-Roller, Chick Orthopedics, San Diego, California.

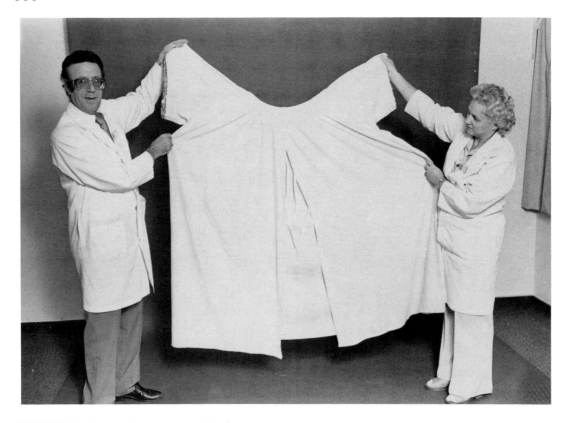

FIGURE 25.2. Gown made by sewing staff to fit patient.

it is impossible to palpate the spines in the massively obese, but the operator can locate the interspace after injecting a local anesthetic into the overlying skin, using a fine 5-cm needle. The extra-long (12-cm) Tuohy needle is usually necessary to identify the thoracic epidural space in patients who weigh more than 150 kg. The thoracic region is chosen as the block level to keep to a minimum the dose of local anesthetic needed to induce abdominal anesthesia during surgery, as well as analgesia postoperatively.

The anesthetist must plan ahead to anticipate the development of hypotension as the epidural block takes effect. This is more severe in the presence of dehydration. A suitable vasopressor should be prepared. Abuse of vasopressors will result in a loss of the benefits of sympathetic block. One must avoid elevation of the pulse rate/pressure product and increasing the O_2 demand.

With our abandonment of the jejunoileal bypass procedure in favor of gastric restrictive operations, a significantly higher conduction block must be induced if the sympathetic response to surgery is to be avoided, and if the patient is to be free of upper abdominal pain and the referred shoulder-tip pain often experienced postoperatively.

For the block, the patient assumes the sitting position with the legs extended, to minimize peripheral pooling of blood and to make it easier to place him supine if he faints during the placement of the block. The sitting position also allows a more accurate estimate of the mid-line when the dorsal spinous processes cannot be palpated (Fig. 25.7).

After it is tested to ensure that it will accommodate a patent epidural catheter, an appropriate length Tuohy needle is manipulated until the needle tip is gripped firmly by ligamentous structures. Entrance into the epidural space is marked by the usually definitive loss of resistance to saline injection through a 5-mL glass syringe. The operator must exercise extreme caution when using the long Tuohy needle; for example, he must adjust his grip on the needle when performing the 'loss of resistance' test. In addition, considerable experience is required to make an accurate visual assessment of needle depth, when anticipating entry into the epidural space.

A test dose of 4 to 6 mL of 2% lidocaine

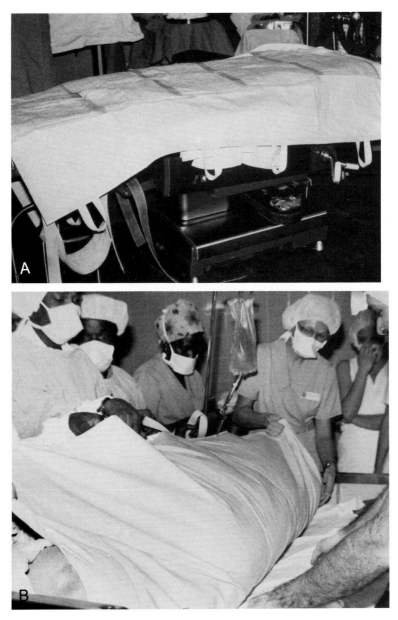

FIGURE 25.3. A. Sewing staff made a heavy canvas lifting sheet with handles along each side and at both ends. B. This enables operating-room staff to transfer patient onto the bed at the conclusion of the operation.

with 1,200,000 epinephine is instilled before introduction of the catheter, to help open the space for it. The operator should never attempt to introduce more catheter than is required to ensure its proper retention postoperatively, as the patient begins to move about in bed. The presence of an excess length of catheter increases the risk of entering a blood vessel or provoking bleeding into the space. At this stage, even minute amounts of bleeding will reduce the effectiveness of local anesthetics, because the plasma protein may block the absorption of the agent into nerve tissue or plug the minute holes in the catheter, thus rendering it totally useless. Attention to details at this stage is important, since the proper placement and function of the catheter at this time will dictate the success or failure of its use not only during the surgical procedure but also for the production of postoperative analgesia. Bromage[9] recommends at this stage that a 2-mL test dose of adrenalin-containing local be injected through the catheter to rule out inadvertent

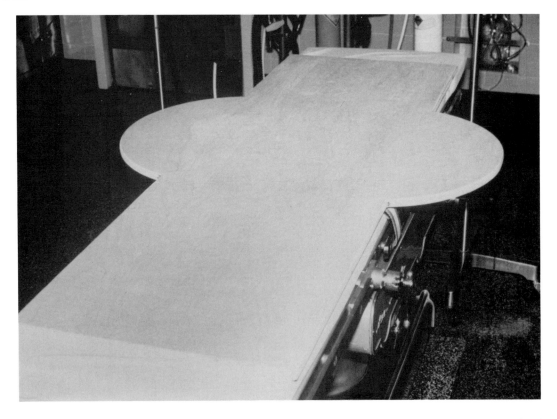

FIGURE 25.4 Maintenance department constructed an hour-glass-shaped board of ¾-inch plywood to go under the mattress of the operating table, to support the overlap of adipose tissue in the hip area.

cannulation of an epidural vein. Observation of a sudden increase in heart rate shown by the ECG monitor will confirm improper placement of the catheter and allow reinsertion at this more convenient time, and avoid any risks of further toxic reactions due to rapidly absorbed local anesthetic agents.

CHOICE OF DRUG

Response and extent of spread of regional agents in the epidural space in obese patients has been well documented by Bromage.[10] In the obese, customary doses of all agents in all concentrations diffuse more extensively than in patients of similar age but of average weight. This difference is even more marked in the presence of diabetes, in the final trimester of pregnancy, and in patients with overt arteriosclerosis. One should use an agent with which one is most familiar and which has a predictable duration of action. If the blockade is allowed to wear off under anesthesia, the patient will lose relaxation abruptly and it may be necessary to stop the surgical procedure until a short-acting muscle

relaxant takes effect. Movement by the patient with the *fixed* retractors in situ could result in injury to liver or spleen.

INDUCTION OF GENERAL ANESTHESIA

Except as previously noted when intubation difficulties are anticipated, patients are induced with incremental doses of 100–125 mg of sodium pentothal, establishing at the same time the arm-to-brain circulation time, and using this as an index to estimate the dose which may be required. In spite of their massive body weight, these patients rarely require a full 0.5 g of Pentothal® to induce a loss of consciousness. The majority of our patients then receive intubating doses of succinylcholine and are ventilated with 50% nitrous oxide and oxygen and 0.5–1% isofluorane (Forane®) during the establishment of the relaxant effect. We do not recommend the sole use of a longer acting nondepolarizing relaxant to assist in intubation in this group of patients.

In the light of our experience, we have de-

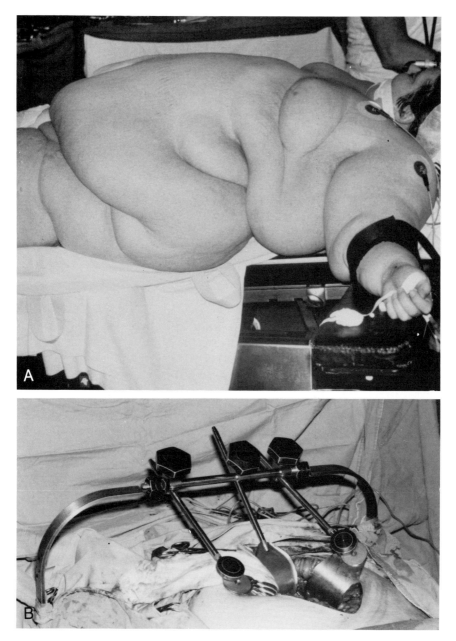

FIGURE 25.5. A. Operating-room table, showing access to side-rails with mounting-clamp. B. Polytract® retractor, using upper two bows only, with attached Gomez hand over the padded left lobe of liver.

termined that the course of anesthesia after intubation is smoother when a longer-acting relaxant is used in conjunction with enflurane (Ethrane®) or isofluorane (Forane®).

Only rarely is it difficult to establish an airway. Fat deposition in the neck appears to displace the trachea and larynx posteriorly and superiorly, and thus facilitates visualization of the vocal cords. This position of the larynx may explain why obese patients aspirate more easily.[11] For intubation, we rest the patient's head on a small pillow and use a curved MacIntosh blade to expose the vocal cords. Occasionally the laryngoscope blade must be inserted into the mouth before attaching the handle, if the patient has large folds of fat in the upper chest and neck. Insufflation of topical lidocaine spray helps the patient to tolerate the tracheal tube during light anesthesia. Throughout the procedure, ventilation is controlled to maintain the pCO_2 between 35 and 40 torr and the pO_2 at 85 to 95 torr (Fig. 25.8).

The majority of the obese patients will re-

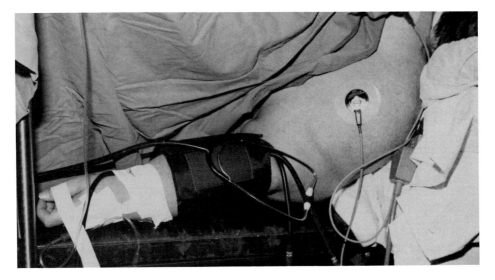

FIGURE 25.6. Thigh cuff on forearm to measure blood pressure. Stethoscope taped over radial artery.

quire 15 to 20 minutes of nitrous oxide anesthesia supplemented with 0.25 to 1% isofluorane before they will tolerate the tracheal tube. During this stabilization period, the operator gives a further 6 to 9 mL of 2% lidocaine through the epidural catheter, and passes a 32F Ewald tube or bougie orally into the stomach. An indwelling arterial line is often placed at this time percutaneously into a radial artery. In addition, a Foley catheter is inserted and urine volumes are recorded. The anesthetist must use caution when combining isofluorane and nitrous oxide in conjunction with epidural sympathetic block, because isofluorane can induce undesirable hypotension, even though some degree of hypotension is desirable. He will avoid halothane and other potentially hepatotoxic agents because

morbidly obese patients often have abnormal liver architecture.[3,12–14]

REAWAKENING

The isofluorane component of the anesthetic is discontinued so that reawakening is allowed to occur in the operating room under the direct supervision of the anesthetist. With the concurrent effect of the conduction block, the patient is allowed to resume spontaneous ventilation, after relaxant reversal has been accomplished, which is usually during or shortly after the fascia has been closed. Often, with isofluorane anesthesia, reawakening may be sudden and complete. The ability to cough effectively should be the main criterion for extubation. We measure tidal volumes with a Wright meter to help confirm the appropriate time to extubate. If an associated conduction block is not used during surgery, reawakening may likely occur in the recovery room after a period of ventilation. In addition, these patients tend to be more drowsy and less responsive and less able to maintain their own airway.

Supplementary humidified oxygen is administered, and the patients are moved to a semi-sitting position as vital signs allow. They are nursed in a full-size hospital bed to allow room for easier turning and physiotherapy. After an epidural block, the patients reawaken free of pain and with no reduction of tidal volume or inhibition of the cough reflex.

Arterial blood gases are analyzed in the recovery room to ensure that the patient's ven-

TABLE 25.1.   OUTLINE OF ANESTHESIA

Premedication (1 hour pre-op)	—Demerol® 75–100 mg —Atropine 0.4–0.6 mg
Induction	A—Continuous epidural with 2% Xylocaine® or ½% Marcaine® B—Pentothal® —Anectine®→Intubation
Maintenance	—Nitrous oxide (30–40%) —Ethrane®/Forane® analgesia —Oral intubation with controlled ventilation or hyperventilation —Sublimaze® or Demerol® analgesia
Intra-op	—Sympathetic block from epidural anesthesia with hyperventilation + Forane® or Ethrane®
Post-op	—Epidural morphine 1.5–3.0 mg prn, in 5–10 mL saline

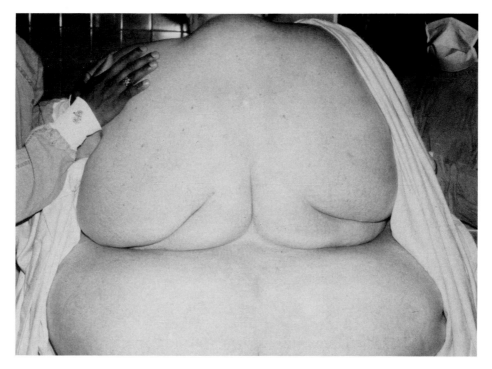

FIGURE 25.7. Sitting patient, positioned for the epidural block.

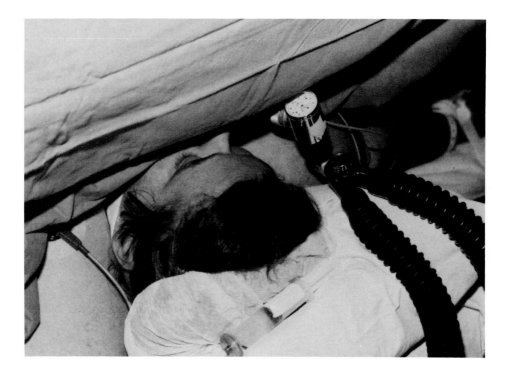

FIGURE 25.8. Wright respirometer directly attached to tracheal tube monitors exhaled gas volumes.

tilatory function is adequate. If the results are satisfactory, the arterial line is usually removed. The anesthetist must write appropriate orders for continuing epidural analgesia.

POSTOPERATIVE EPIDURAL ANALGESIA

The use of epidural morphine for producing analgesia has gained widespread popularity and acceptance.[15-22] This no doubt has been the result of the excellent quality and the long duration of pain relief using minimal doses of drug. We attempt to control pain with this technique for 36–48 hours postoperatively.

In contrast to parenterally administered narcotics, one usually observes an absence of central nervous system depression. One can see the maintenance of respiratory function, ability to cough, low incidence of postoperative atelectasis, the absence of abdominal splinting, the continuing stability of the vasomotor system, and the maintenance of an ability to move and turn oneself as required and dictated, as part of usual postoperative nursing care.

In terms of the price paid for this analgesia, one must be prepared to accept some sequelae (Table 25.2).[15,20,23-32] Furthermore, there is a potential for late respiratory depression if any doses of systemic narcotics are administered within 6–24 hours after the last epidural dose of drug.

Davies et al[28] have shown that when postured in the supine position, these patients are more likely to develop both early and late respiratory depression. Samii et al,[17] using intrathecal morphine, demonstrated that patents could tolerate 40 times the dose of morphine intrathecally if kept in the sitting position as compared to the supine position (0.5 mg vs. 20 mg). They reported that no respiratory depression was observed. Behar et al[21] noted that a decreasing respiratory rate and miosis may warn of impending early or late respiratory depression.

TABLE 25.2. REPORTED INCIDENCE OF SEQUELAE OF EPIDURAL MORPHINE

Urinary retention 10–56%*
Nausea and vomiting 17%
Pruritus 1–16%
Late respiratory depression 0.3–0.4%
Euphora/anxiety/hallucinations—occasional

*Patients usually have urinary catheter, so that retention is not a feature.

Others have clearly shown that the patient position (supine), the dose of morphine (8–10 mg), the volume of diluent (up to 10 mL of saline), thoracic catheter placement and increasing age all help to enhance the spread of epidural morphine rostrally.[9,10,15,22-25,31-34] This has been further substantiated by personal experience[35] with 34 morbidly obese patients who inadvertently received 30 mg of epidural morphine due to an error in the pharmacy preparation of the 3 mg morphine (preservative-free) in 10 mL saline (single-dose vials stored in nitrogen). Only four of the patients required treatment of early-onset respiratory depression. All four responded to intravenous naloxone. However, two still required reintubation and ventilation for the subsequent 24 to 30 hours. All morbidly obese patients are routinely nursed in the sitting position and this was the likely reason why this series of respiratory complications was so few.[17,33] There is general agreement in all reports that in spite of only rare occurrence of respiratory depression, patients receiving epidural morphine must be monitored in a special care area for at least 6–12 hours after the last dose of the drug. Our experience would substantiate this in view of one observation of respiratory depression coming only after the third dose of epidural morphine, given during a 48-hour period.

Urinary retention may require catheterization, but there have been reports of successful reversal using naloxone.[36] Pruritis, too, has been successfully relieved with naloxone. The use of morphine with preservatives (methylparaben) has been associated with a significantly higher incidence of itching (15 times).[25] This may be due to the rostral spread in the cerebrospinal fluid. The incidence of itching is increased in the face and neck. Experience has shown that intravenous naloxone given to effectively reverse the side-effects of epidural morphine, does not appear to alter the analgesic state,[37] as is seen when naloxone is administered to patients who have received morphine systemically.

Epidural morphine does not appear to affect endocrine, metabolic or renal response to surgery.[11] Indeed, it may decrease the postoperative negative nitrogen balance.[3]

Rawal et al[38] in a randomized study of 30 massively obese patients undergoing gastroplasty for weight reduction found that intramuscular morphine was only one-seventh as effective as epidural morphine in the production of analgesia. The group receiving epidural morphine demonstrated earlier ambulation, were more alert, were able to benefit more from physiotherapy, had fewer pulmonary complications and had shorter hospitalization. With respect to side-effects, there was no evidence of prolonged respiratory depression at the doses used. However, delayed respiratory depression, which responded to naloxone, occurred in 0.25–0.4% of patients in the large Swedish study.[16]

SITE OF ACTION

About 10% of epidural morphine is absorbed into the cerebrospinal fluid,[21,22] thus directly affecting the neuraxis. Yaksh[39] and Snyder[30,40] initially showed that the substantia gelatinosa contained opiate receptors. Behar and co-workers[21,27] first reported on the clinical effectiveness of epidurally administered morphine. These observations further substantiate the gate theory of pain control, proposed by Malzak and Wall.[41] It is not clear to date why systemic naloxone does not appear to reverse analgesia produced by narcotics acting at the cord level.[37]

DOSES

Preparations of morphine to be used epidurally must be preservative-free. Shelf-life can be extended if they are prepared and stored under nitrogen to retard the oxidation process.

The level of epidural catheter insertion will usually dictate the dose to be given. For lumbar use, we would recommend 3 mg of morphine in 10 mL of saline, but one-half this dose for an upper thoracic catheter placement. With failure to achieve analgesia, we repeat half the initial dose after 15–20 minutes, provided the patient is kept in a semi-sitting position.

Concurrent administration of other sedatives and narcotics will more than likely increase the chances of producing clinically significant respiratory depression.[23,31] In spite of its rare occurrence, both early and late respiratory depression may occur, and careful observation for 24 hours after the last dose is recommended.

Bromage[9] has commented on the practice of using minidose heparin, related to the risk of epidural space hematoma. He feels that with minidose heparin the use of an epidural catheter is not contraindicated. The concurrent administration of aspirin, which induces

platelet dysfuction, is of greater concern, and contraindicates the use of epidural anesthesia and epidural catheters.

Cullen et al[42,43] performed a randomized, double-blind study of *continuous* epidural infusion of opiates and bupivacaine, singly or in combination, compared with epidural saline solution and no epidural catheter (i.e. traditional systemic narcotics), for 72 hours immediately after major abdominal surgery. Continuous epidural was used to minimize the side-effects of bolus epidural bupivacaine and avoid hypotension. The group that received the combination of morphine and bupivacaine enjoyed superior pain relief, recovery of respiratory function and ambulation, followed very closely by the group that received epidural morphine alone. The other groups had considerably poorer pain relief and were indistinguishable from one another. The bupivacaine group required I.M. narcotics similar to the saline and control groups which showed peaks and valleys in the pain control. The pain levels of all five groups decreased to a low level during the 72-hr period, which reinforces the concept that 72 hours is an appropriate period for use of the epidural catheter after surgery. Respiratory depression was not noted at the doses of morphine given. However, runaway narcotic blocks with respiratory depression can be a complication, especially with continuous infusion techniques. Careful patient monitoring is mandatory.

PATIENT-CONTROLLED ANALGESIA AND OTHER MODALITIES

Narcotics given intravenously frequently and in very small amounts can maintain pain relief with minimal sedation, and avoid the peaks and valleys of serum concentrations found with I.M. narcotics given at 3–4 hr intervals. Some workers have given continuous I.V. infusion of morphine at 2 mg/hr in the morbidly obese, using an accurate pump.

In a number of centers, patient-controlled analgesia (PCA) is being used with a small computerized, programmable continuous-infusion pump.[44] By pressing a button on the PCA unit (Abbott), the patient controls his intravenous infusion of narcotic. In the morbidly obese, the pump is set to permit delivery of 2 mg of morphine sulfate which may be repeated at intervals of greater than 10 minutes to a predetermined amount—usually a total of 20 mg in any 4-hr period. The patient is instructed regarding the pump on the day before surgery. After the patient arrives on the floor from the recovery room, the PCA unit is attached securely to the I.V. pole for later ambulation and the door is safety-locked to make the unit tamper-proof. Prepackaged cartridges of Demerol or morphine are used. A peripheral vein can be used, but Headley prefers a subclavian venous cathether which he inserts at the end of gastric restrictive operations.[45] Patients are secure and mobile, the self-administered narcotic acts rapidly, and nursing time is saved. Headley found that 75% less narcotic was used over the postoperative course with PCA compared to I.M. The pump cannot overdose, as it shuts down if the 4-hr dose has been given.[46] The pump can be changed to a smaller dose (e.g. 10 mg morphine over 4 hr) for smaller patients (e.g. undergoing reversal of an intestinal bypass).

Other surgeons have decreased the need for postoperative narcotics by injecting about 20 mL of 0.25% bupivacaine HCl (Marcaine) into both sides of the incisional wound at the end of the operation.

SUMMARY

This chapter has outlined a method of managing anesthesia for the morbidly obese patient, using epidural blockade as the major component of anesthesia for surgery. Advantages of this technique are discussed. An attempt has been made to review opinion, and the results of the use of epidural opiates. General recommendations are offered for their clinical use at the present state of our knowledge and experience.

REFERENCES

1. Fox GS: Anaesthesia for intestinal short circuiting in the morbidly obese with reference to the pathophysiology of gross obesity. Can Anaesth Soc J 22:307–315, 1975.
2. Scott HW Jr, Law DH 4th, Sandstead HH, et al: Jejunoileal shunt in the surgical treatment of morbid obesity. Ann Surg 171:770–782, 1970.
3. Scott HW Jr, Dean R, Shull HJ, et al: Considerations in the use of jejunoileal bypass in patients with morbid obesity. Ann Surg 177:723–735, 1973.
4. Stein T, Vaughan R, Wise L: Glucose tolerance in the obese surgical patient. Surg Gynecol Obstet 148:380–384, 1979.
5. Sanderson I, Deitel M, Bojm MA: The handling of glucose and insulin response before and after weight loss with jejuno-ileal by-pass. JPEN 7:274–276, 1983.
6. French G: A nursing guide to gastric partitioning. Canadian Operating Room Nursing Journal 1:24–25, 1983.
7. King GE: Taking the blood pressure. JAMA 209:1902–1904, 1969.
8. Kirkendall WM, Burton AC, Epstein FH, et al: Recommendations for human blood pressure determination by sphygmomanometers. Circulation 36:980–988, 1967.
9. Bromage PR: Extradural and intrathecal opiates. Unpublished data—ASA refresher course lectures, Las Vegas, Nevada, Oct. 1982.
10. Bromage PR: Physiology and pharmacology of epidural anesthesia. Anesthesiology 28:592–622, 1967.
11. Vaughan RW, Bauer S, Wise L: Volume and pH of gastric juice in obese patients. Anesthesiology 43:686–689, 1975.
12. Deitel M, Bojm MA, Atin MD, et al: Intestinal bypass and gastric partitioning for morbid obesity: a comparison. Can J Surg 25:283–289, 1982.
13. Adler M, Schaffner F: Fatty liver hepatitis and cirrhosis in obese patients. Am J Med 67:811–816, 1979.
14. Kern WH, Heger AH, Payne JH, et al: Fatty metamorphosis of the liver in morbid obesity. Arch Pathol Lab Med 96:342–346, 1973.
15. Bromage PR: The price of intraspinal narcotic analgesia (editorial). Anesth Analg 60:461–463, 1981.
16. Gustafsson LL, Schildt B, Jacobsen K: Adverse effects of extradural and intrathecal opiates. Report of a nation wide survey in Sweden. Br J Anaesth 54:479–485, 1982.
17. Samii K, Feret J, Haraci A, et al: Selective spinal analgesia (correspondence). Lancet 1:1142, 1979.
18. Yaksh TL, Rudy TA: Analgesia mediated by direct spinal action of narcotics. Science 192:1357–1358, 1976.
19. Gjessing J, Tomlin PJ: Postoperative pain control with intrathecal morphine. Anaesthesia 36:268–276, 1981.
20. Mehnert JH, Dupont TJ, Rose DH: Intermittent epidural morphine instillation for the control of postoperative pain. Am J Surg 146:145–151, 1983.
21. Behar M, Magora F, Olshwang D, et al: Epidural morphine in the treatment of pain. Lancet 1:527–529, 1979.
22. Bromage PR, Camporesi E, Chestnut D: Epidural narcotics for postoperative analgesia. Anesth Analg 59:473–480, 1980.
23. McCaughey W, Graham JL: The respiratory depression of epidural morphine—time course and effect of posture. Anaesthesia 37:990–995, 1982.
24. Gustafsson LL, Feychting B, Klingstedt C: Late respiratory depression after concomitant use of morphine epidurally and parenterally. Lancet 1:892–893, 1981.
25. Reiz S, Westberg M: The side effects of epidural morphine. Lancet 2:203–204, 1980.
26. Christensen V: Respiratory depression after extradural morphine (correspondence). Br J Anaesth 52:841, 1980.
27. Sidi A, Davidson JT, Behar M, et al: Spinal narcotics and C.N.S. depression. Anaesthesia 36:1044–1047, 1981.
28. Davies GK, Tolhurst-Cleaver CL, James TL: CNS depression from intrathecal morphine (correspondence). Anesthesiology 52:280, 1980.

29. Knill R, Clement JL, Thompson WR: Epidural morphine causes delayed and prolonged ventilatory depression. Can Anaesth Soc J 28:537–542, 1981.

30. Snyder SH: Opiate receptors in the brain. N Engl J Med 296:766–771, 1977.

31. Bromage PR, Camporesi EM, Durant PAC, et al: Rostral spread of epidural morphine. Anesthesiology 56:431–436, 1982.

32. Bromage PR, Camporesi EM, Durant PAC, et al: Non-respiratory side effects of epidural morphine. Anesth Analg 61:490–495, 1982.

33. Hodgkinson R, Husain FJ: Obesity, gravity and spread of epidural analgesia. Anesth Analg 60:421–424, 1981.

34. Dichiro G: The movement of C.S.F. in human beings. Nature 204:290–291, 1964.

35. Crowell DE, Deitel M: Unpublished data.

36. Rawal N, Möllefors K, Axelsson K, et al: An experimental study of urodynamic effects of epidural morphine and of naloxone reversal. Anesth Analg 62:641–647, 1983.

37. Jones RDM, Jones JG: Intrathecal morphine-naloxone reverses respiratory depression but not analgesia. Br J Med 281:645—648, 1980.

38. Rawal N, Sjöstrand U, Christoffersson E, et al: Comparison of intramuscular and epidural morphine for postoperative analgesia in the grossly obese: influence on postoperative ambulation and pulmonary function. Anesth Analg 63:583–592, 1984.

39. Yaksh TL: Spinal opiate anesthesia—Characteristics and principles of action. Pain 11:293–346, 1981.

40. Snyder SH: Opiate receptors and internal opiates. Scientific American 236:44–56, 1977.

41. Melzak R, Wall PD: Pain mechanisms—a new therapy. Science 150:971–979, 1968.

42. Cullen ML, Staren ED, El-Ganzouri A, et al: Continuous epidural infusion for analgesia after major abdominal operations: a randomized, prospective, double-blind study. Surgery 98:718–728, 1985.

43. Staren ED, Cullen ML: Epidural catheter analgesia for the management of postoperative pain. Surg Gynecol Obstet 162:389–404, 1986.

44. Dahlstrom B, Tamsen H, Paalzow L, et al: Patient-controlled analgesic therapy i.v.; pharmacokinetics and analgesic plasma concentrations of morphine. Clin Pharmacokinet 7:266–279, 1982.

45. Headley WM, Mandel S, McEver JA: Intravenous patient controlled analgesia vs intramuscular narcotic injection: a comparative study of 114 vertical banded gastroplasty patients. Program, 3rd annual meeting, American Society for Bariatric Surgery, Iowa City, June 18–20, 1986, p 103.

46. English MJM: Patient-controlled analgesia—new treatment modality for the relief of postoperative pain. To-day's Therapeutic Trends 5:15–29, 1987.

26

The Nurses' Role in Bariatric Surgery

GLENNA FRENCH
JANET L. GALBRAITH
MERVYN DEITEL

PREOPERATIVE PHASE
OPERATIVE PHASE
POST-ANESTHETIC RECOVERY
  PHASE
POSTOPERATIVE PHASE
SUPPORT GROUPS

The nursing care of the morbidly obese patient presents a challenge that requires the cooperation of all the disciplines of the medical, nursing and support staff. Just the sheer added weight of these patients poses many problems that have to be carefully considered. Although we are safety conscious with any patient, just changing the position of a morbidly obese patient in bed or transporting him or her to radiology can mean a safety hazard to both staff and equipment. The use of proper body mechanics and careful planning is necessary to carry out the simplest procedure. The nurse in charge should always ensure that adequate personnel are available each time the patient has to be re-positioned or transported for various tests and procedures.

At St. Joseph's Health Centre, more than 1,300 patients have undergone bariatric operations, so that nursing staff have become quite familiar with problem solving in most situations. The criteria for selection of patients have been rigidly adhered to.[1,2] These patients are more knowledgeable than the average surgical patient, and because surgery is a "last resort" for them to lose weight, they are generally very willing to cooperate.

The operating-room nurse can play a special role in emotional support, as this nurse will often see the patients back for subsequent operations, e.g. abdominal lipectomies, reduction mammoplasties. The nurse reassures the patient that the entire ordeal will be worth it. It is a long process from the time these candidates are accepted for surgery, prepared, operated upon and proceed to recovery and weight loss.

The nursing team must never become complacent about the morbidly obese patient and bariatric surgery, even though they may take care of many such patients each week. The nurse must constantly be aware of possible complications and nursing interventions that may be necessary to prevent any potential hazards to both patients and staff.

PREOPERATIVE PHASE

An accurate measurement of weight should be determined. The usual standing scale only goes up to 160 kg. By a special added weight, the scale can be made to measure greater weights. The Acme Medical Scale will weigh up to 200 kg. The super-morbidly obese may be weighed by balancing themselves on two standing scales placed together side-by-side,

without shifting their weight; their weight will be equal to the sum of the two readings. The massively morbidly obese patients may be weighed on a laundry, purchasing department or morgue freight scale or a grain scale.

The preoperative phase for the morbidly obese patient consists of physical, psychological and educational preparation. The nurse, who spends the greatest portion of time with the patient, plays an important role in this preparation.

Preoperative teaching, specifically deep breathing and coughing exercises, cannot be stressed enough. Postoperative atelectasis and congestion can result from shallow respirations due to incisional pain, depressive analgesia, inactivity and the obesity. The patient must understand that prevention of respiratory complications is of utmost importance and requires frequent and effective chest physiotherapy. The patient will have been required to stop smoking completely, well before admission. Demonstrations of deep breathing and coughing exercises should include splinting (putting arm across abdomen to apply gentle pressure over operative area and provide support to the sensitive area during the vigorous movement which is caused while coughing) and the use of the incentive spirometer. This will act as visual proof to the patient of progress during recovery. By practicing preoperatively with the incentive spirometer, the patient is aware of the capabilities to strive for postoperatively.

The patient must also be instructed in the appropriate leg exercises for the purpose of maintaining proper limb circulation, to prevent stasis of blood which could lead to deep vein thrombosis. Teaching includes demonstrations of calf-pumping; this exercise of calf muscles involves moving the feet in an up and down motion, in order to extend and flex the muscles in the back of the leg, and moving the feet in a rotary motion.

The massively morbidly obese can wear their own clothes, but this can make them feel different to other patients. Thus, we have double-sized gowns made by the hospital sewing staff in pink, blue, yellow or white.[3] The morbidly obese require heavy duty beds, as the patient may exceed the load limit of the standard hospital bed.[4]*

These patients, who frequently perspire and have intertrigo, scrub the navel and sub-

*Burke Bariatric Bed, Box 1064, Mission, Kansas 66222; Magnum 800 Motorized Obesity Bed, 6900 Aragon Circle, Buena Park, California 90620.

abdominal and submammary skinfolds twice daily as indicated, with Hibitane, Hibiclens or Phisohex. We do not shave the pubis. They receive a Fleet enema the evening before surgery, and take a shower the night before surgery.

To provide an enlightened, smooth postoperative course, the nurse should spend time with the patient reinforcing the explanations of postoperative care given by the physician. The patient should be informed of the use and importance of the nasogastric tube, Foley catheter, epidural catheter if intended (see Chapter 25) and appropriate suction equipment. Epidural anesthesia (supplemented by general) and epidural analgesia for the first 2 days postoperatively are used in our institution for the super-morbidly obese, the past heavy smoker, the Pickwickian (alveolar hypoventilation) or the somnolent patient. The patient receiving analgesia epidurally does not develop respiratory depression, and can move himself with minimal assistance by the nurses. The patient should be aware of the routine for pain control (either parenteral or epidural means) and general postoperative care. The patient will be visited by the anesthetist, and this will be discussed.

The nurses endeavor to involve family members in the care of the patient. An atmosphere of understanding and cooperation aids the patients and their families during the hospitalization, and ensures a smooth working environment. Support for the patient is necessary from all members of the health team and when possible from other patients who have undergone similar surgery. These patients can offer each other significant emotional support that can come from someone who has had personal experience.

OPERATIVE PHASE

Surgical intervention should only proceed when the surgeon, anesthetist and nursing team are completely prepared and satisfied that all details have been taken care of, especially with regards to safety.

Occasionally, the extremely obese patients are not premedicated so that they are able to walk up to the operating-room. If the patient is very large, eg. >225 kg (500 lb), we have them come to the operating-room the day before surgery to ensure that they will fit on the operating-table. We had a ¾″ plywood board expecially made by the carpentry department to accommodate the vast adipose tissue on

the thighs and hips of the massively morbidly obese.[3] This board is placed under the mattress of the operating-table (Fig. 26.1). The operating-room table has to remain in the lowest position, as the hydraulics may be damaged if we attempted to raise it with such excess weight on the table. Other workers have placed the patient on two operating-tables side-by-side or used a wider obstetrics table. However, using our regular width table permits use of standard retractor systems.

If epidural anesthesia is to be used, arrangements are made for two nursing attendants to be on hand to support the patient and prevent him or her from falling during insertion of the epidural catheter. The greatest risk of falling occurs when the patient is sat up for the insertion of the epidural catheter and then lies down again.

Most surgical procedures require two nurses—a scrub nurse and a circulating nurse. For those patients undergoing bariatric

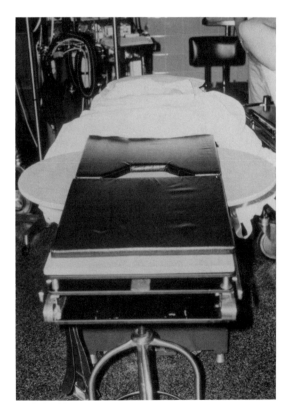

FIGURE 26.1. Board, widened for hips, is secured to operating-table with adhesive tape. Mattress of table is placed over the board. The canvas lifting-sheet with multiple loop-handles will be placed on top of the mattress (see also Chapter 25, Figs. 25.3A and 25.4). Foot of table is supported by adjustable sitting stool, for added security with these patients.

operations, the nurse in charge should ensure that a third nurse is present, especially at the beginning of the procedure, to assist with the catheterization of female patients and to provide general assistance to the surgeons, anesthetist and the other circulating nurse.

After the patient is anesthetized, the circulating nurses along with the surgical and anesthetic team check for correct positioning and proper body alignment before proceeding further. Any pressure points are well-padded with large superior pads, especially under the heels and elbows and any other area that the nurse notes could pose a problem.

At this point, a urinary catheter may be inserted. Because of the difficulty placing these large patients immediately postoperatively on a bedpan, we put urinary catheters in the female patients for monitoring. The Foley is removed 24–36 hours postoperatively, if the patient is doing well. The decision to catheterize the male patient is made by the surgeon, as, with the long narrow urethra and tighter prostatic urethra in males, postoperative urethral irritation may present a problem. Patients receiving epidural require a Foley catheter, because of the potential for associated urinary retention. The catheter is connected to a urinary drainage bag and placed where the anesthetist can see it easily. An electrosurgical cautery grounding pad is applied to the thigh for use of the cautery during the operation, and a large safety-strap is fastened just above the patient's knees as an added precaution.

Some surgeons use reverse-Trendelenburg position (legs down) during the operation to allow the viscera to fall inferiorly. If so, supporting blocks must be placed against the feet. However, this position leads to venous stasis. With an abdominal incision which is not excessively long and with pads holding the bowel inferiorly and with a properly applied retractor, the operation can be done with excellent exposure with the patient supine. We believe that the briefness of the operation is the reason for our almost non-existent incidence of deep vein thrombosis and pulmonary embolism. Tensor bandages or antiembolism stockings or reusable Venodyne boots may be used to prevent deep venous thrombosis. A lightweight portable intermittent compression (PIC)* device applies peristalsic compression from the foot to the knee.

*Taheri, 1275 Delaware Ave., Buffalo, NY 14209.

The surgical scrub and prep are very important in these patients, due to the huge folds of adipose tissue. The circulating nurse must ensure that all areas are cleaned, scrubbed and painted vigorously (Fig. 26.2). The second circulating nurse is often needed to do one side while the circulating nurse does the other. After the patient is draped and the vertical bars of the retractor positioned, surgical intervention can begin.

During surgery, the circulating nurse monitors blood loss, assists the anesthetist and anticipates the needs of the surgeon. As in any other major surgical procedure, all surgical instruments, cartridges, sponges, needles, gauze, retractor parts, etc. in the surgical field are counted. This is usually done quietly while the anesthetic is being initiated. One circulating nurse stays with the patient and assists the anesthetist, while the other circulating nurse can attend to the needs of the scrub nurse and ensure that all necessary supplies are ready and available.

A surgeon's preference card for bariatric operations should be compiled, so that the nurses can follow it as a guideline.

All parts of the retractor system (e.g. Gomez Poly-tract) are also counted, and periodically during the operation, the surgeon may ask for a sponge count. Because of the immense adiposity of these patients, absolute vigilance is mandatory in accounting for surgical sponges in these operations.

As the operation is completed and the surgeon begins to close the abdomen, the circulating nurse does a closing count, accounting for all surgical instruments, cartridges, sponges, needles, gauze, retractors, etc., and the surgeon is informed of the result. As skin is being closed, another count is done of the sponges and needles as an added safety measure.

Documentation is carried on throughout the surgical procedure by the circulating nurse on the Operative Record, listing the personnel involved, the times the anesthetic started and finished as well as the surgery times. Catheters and drains are recorded as well as the result of the surgical count. Both the circulating nurse and scrub nurse sign the Operative Record at the end of the procedure, to attest to the completion and result of the count. The circulating nurse also records any specimens taken during the procedure, e.g. liver biopsy, gastric rings from the circular stapling-gun, gallbladder, etc. (The surgeon during the operation has examined the gastric

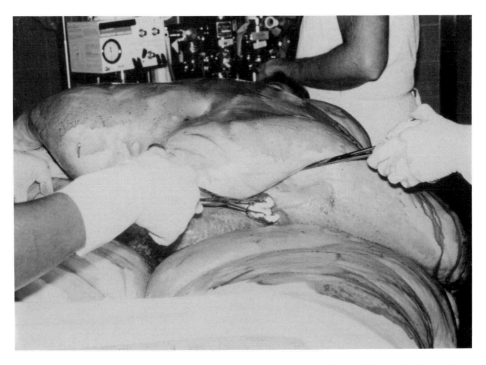

FIGURE 26.2. One circulating nurse is elevating folds of adipose tissue, so that patient can be thoroughly prepped by second nurse.

rings for completeness, to ensure that the circular staple-line is complete.)

The dressing is applied and the circulating nurse adheres the dressing with adhesive. Warm sheets and a clean gown are provided for the patient. As the patient is coming out of the anesthetic, it is again essential that adequate personnel are available in case the patient starts to move around on the operating-room table. When the anesthetist is ready, rather than a tight stretcher in the massively obese, the patient's bed is brought into the room and the patient can be transferred. On super-obese patients, we utilize a heavy canvas lifting-sheet with handles along each side and at both ends, which was made by our sewing-staff using a heavy-duty sewing machine[3] (Fig. 25.3A, Chapter 25).

Recovery-room staff are kept informed of any special requirements. The circulating nurse informs the control desk if the patient's own bed is required, so that we can place the massively obese patient on his or her own bed at the end of the procedure. Thus, we will only have to transfer the patient once and will have all the necessary personnel available at the end of the operation to provide for the safe transfer of the patient from the operating-

room table to the bed. If the patient is to receive postoperative epidural analgesia, the patient is monitored in the Acute Care Unit for a day or two. If there is no epidural, the patient will usually return from the recovery-room to his or her own room.

POST-ANESTHETIC RECOVERY PHASE

Routine monitoring of vital signs is carried out in the recovery-room. The patient is usually conscious and awake when arriving in the recovery-room, and is encouraged to follow breathing exercises which had been practiced preoperatively. The anesthetist is kept informed of the patient's progress in the recovery-room. Epidural morphine may be given by the anesthetist for pain control during the patient's stay in the recovery-room.

Careful documentation is kept on the recovery-room flow-sheet of all vital signs including blood pressure, pulse, quality and number of respirations per minute, temperature, coughing, deep breathing, etc. When the patient is ready to leave the recovery-room, extra personnel are required to transfer the patient to the appropriate unit.

POSTOPERATIVE PHASE

The patients who are transferred postoperatively to the Acute Care Unit usually receive epidural morphine for long-lasting pain control. It is necessary to move the patient gently so as not to disturb the catheter placement. Securing tape should be checked before each administration of analgesic. Our procedure for the administration of epidural analgesia involves first placing the patient in the supine position and secondly checking the vital signs prior to injection and then every 5 minutes for 20 minutes post-injection. The patients require frequent observation to monitor any change in condition which would warrant medical intervention.

Those patients who are maintained on parenteral analgesics should be given sufficient doses at regular intervals to ensure proper compliance with postoperative routines, especially exercises.

The head of the bed is usually kept elevated 30°, as this removes the weight of the massive abdominal adipose tissue against the diaphragm, and makes the work of breathing easier. Patients frequently have a flushed appearance and some fever on the day following surgery, and this could be related to absorption of crushed gastric tissue between staple-lines.[5,6] Elevated white blood cell counts of 20,000 (12,000–30,000) often occur on the day following surgery, and fall to normal over the ensuing days. The patient is encouraged to perform leg exercises, and is mobilized and given adequate hydration, in order to inhibit deep vein thrombosis. A trapeze over the bed is attached to strong secure overhead bars to aid patient movement. On the day after surgery, the patient advances to sitting up at the bedside for short periods three times daily. During this time, the patient may walk several steps from bed to chair, thus helping to strengthen the legs and maintain balance. Each day the activity level increases to such that the patient soon becomes independent.

Other immediate postoperative considerations which require monitoring include:
—Possible hemorrhage due to the surgical procedure which would be evident from the operative site, the nasogastric suction, or tachycardia and fall in blood pressure.
—Unexplained dyspnea, chest pain, tachycardia, fall in urine output, diaphoresis, fall in blood pressure and apprehension, which may indicate pulmonary embolus, atelectasis,

pneumonitis or, most importantly, leak (especially with shoulder-tip pain).
—Possible nausea and/or vomiting due to the anesthetic or an occluded nasogastric tube. Administration of an anti-emetic drug may resolve the problem, but under no circumstances may the nasogastric tube be irrigated or manipulated by the nurse. Unresolved problems should be referred to the attending physician for further orders.
—Possible low urinary output, for which appropriate nursing interventions (e.g. irrigating the catheter to check for patency) should be employed prior to alerting the physician.

Pink or deep amber urine occurs from 4 to 48 hours postoperatively in 30% of patients who have undergone gastric partitionings, due to the accumulation of uric acid dihydrate crystals.[5] These patients have high-normal serum uric acid levels preoperatively. Postoperatively, serum uric acid decreases, as urinary uric acid increases and adsorbs urinary pigments, producing amber urine and a pink coating where uric acid precipitates on the plastic urinary tubing (see Chapter 14). This is a transient occurrence, causing no problem.

Many surgeons have found a universally-sized abdominal binder* with Velcro closures, which is very easily applied and removed by the patient, to be effective in postoperative mobilization. The patients are instructed in application and removal of the binder prior to surgery. However, other surgeons have found that postoperative binders in the upper abdomen may constrict the lower costal margin and foster splinting and atelectasis.

Ideally, the epidural catheter should be removed by the anesthetist in order to check the tubing for its completeness and for any flaws. After the catheter has been removed, a small strip dressing is placed over the insertion site and is checked frequently for any leakage. It is advisable that the patient remain in an acute care facility which provides frequent monitoring of vital signs for at least 12 hours following the administration of epidural morphine.[7]

After leaving the Acute Care Unit, postoperative activity is essentially no different than for other patients undergoing major abdominal surgery. Activity levels should be increased steadily each day, and barring complications (e.g. wound infection), the patient

---

*Texas Orthopedic Abdominal Binder, P.O. Box 12877, Houston, Texas 77217

should be educated regarding nutrition and preparation for discharge.

Because the nurse is the primary care-giver, it is important for him or her to reinforce the physician's orders for the diet as well as the teaching given by the dietician. These patients should be supervised when commencing oral fluids to ensure that they only ingest the amounts which are ordered. By our routine, the patients begin with sips of room-temperature water (up to 150 mL/hr) taken from a 30-mL plastic medicine cup. The diet is restricted to full fluids for 4 weeks to optimize staple-line healing.[8] The diet is progressed (Fig. 26.3), with patient education to ensure that the patient comprehends fully and adjusts to requirements. After gastric restrictive operations, a minority of patients have diarrhea initially, due to temporary neuropraxia of the vagus or the effect of fruit juices. However, they may then tend towards constipation, because of lack of roughage in the diet, but the majority of patients settle out with normal bowel habits.

After the biliopancreatic bypass, the patients initially take four to five small meals per day because of small gastric capacity. However, by 12 weeks these patients take three fairly normal-sized nutritious meals per day because the gastric pouch has enlarged. Biliopancreatic bypass patients are advised to avoid large amounts of sugared juices which produce dumping, keep sugar intake to a very modest level, and avoid lactose because of gas problems (see Chapter 11). They avoid ASA and irritating anti-arthritic medications, and take multivitamins and Tums as directed or a calcium salt.

The question is often asked as to when intimate relations may be resumed. Any time is fine as long as common sense is used.

SUPPORT GROUPS

Bariatric surgery support groups (spontaneous or organized) have arisen for the various operations, and have regular meetings or reunions to share experience. Some groups have modest membership dues, association offices, a charter, newsletter and national liaisons. Support groups offer preoperative contact and information sheets, booklets with diagrams and models of the stomach. By meeting other patients or persons interested in the surgery, the group assists in fully informing the patient regarding treatment and changes in eating patterns.

Support groups can emphasize the patient's role in preventing postoperative complications, and assist the patient in behavioral changes, provide emotional support and develop closeness. Nutritional counselling, helpful books and recipes are shared, with blended foods for the post-gastroplasty patients, increasing dietary compliance and avoiding bingeing and purging. These patients must consume adequate protein, and nutritional supplements may be necessary with hair loss. Guest speakers, e.g. plastic surgeons, psychologists, nutritionists or exercise specialists may be invited.

Family members and friends are encouraged to attend, and marital support is if necessary provided. A customized structured fitness program can be organized. The therapeutic support group can act as an agent for the surgeon. Furthermore, in the surgeon's office, a good medical assistant, office nurse or receptionist can play a vital role in preventing litigation.

The goal of nutritional education is to ensure that the patient understands the dietary restrictions that must be adhered to for a lifetime. Effective education and support will assist in successful and healthy weight loss.

Post-Gastroplasty Instructions

1. **For 4 weeks from the day of the operation, eat liquids:** e.g. tea, juice, jello, junket, milk (e.g. 2%), coffee, juices, soups, yogurt, puddings, soft custards, water, etc. Nothing too cold or too hot. With pop, allow the bubbles to disappear—i.e. flat. Soft ice-cream.

   Liquid vitamin (e.g. Paramettes or Pardec) two teaspoons daily, *or* suck or chew two chewable vitamins daily e.g. Flintstones. *No* large pills!

2. **Second 4 weeks:** tiny *blended*, minced, pureed, or baby foods—taken slowly, with fluids. Cereals. Mashed potatoes. Hamburger in small amounts.

3. **Thereafter:** very soft foods, chewed well, taken slowly. Will not be able to tolerate red meat, unless blended well and taken very slowly in tiny amounts.

If unable to keep an appointment, phone Doctor's secretary and change to another date.

If repeated vomiting, dry feeling, dark urine, pain, weakness, or any problem, phone or see Dr. _____ (and your own family doctor *if urgent*).

FIGURE 26.3. Form given to vertical banded gastroplasty patients prior to admission to hospital, for future programming.

REFERENCES

1. Deitel M: Selection of patients for gastric partitioning. Can J Surg 27:237, 1984.

2. Deitel M: Morbid obesity—the problem, and indications for surgery. J Am Coll Nutr 6:416, 1987.
3. French G: A nursing guide to gastric partitioning. Canadian Operating Room Nursing Journal 1:24–25, 1983.
4. Kawasaki G, Benz LA, Reeder L, et al: Solving the very problems of the morbidly obese. Nursing 80, pp 40–43, Nov. 1980.
5. Deitel M, Thompson DA, Saldanha CF, et al.: "Pink urine" in morbidly obese patients following gastric partitioning. Can Med Assoc J 130:1007–1011, 1984.
6. Deitel M, Jones BA, Petrov I, et al: Vertical banded gastroplasty: results in 233 patients. Can J Surg 29:322–324, 1986.
7. Mehnert JH, Dupont TJ, Rose DH: Intermittent epidural morphine instillation for the control of postoperative pain. Am J Surg 146:145–151, 1983.
8. Ellison EC, Martin EW, Jr, Laschinger J, et al: Prevention of early failure of stapled gastric partitions in treatment of morbid obesity. Arch Surg 115:528–533, 1980.

27

Informed Consent in Bariatric Surgery

GEORGE S. M. COWAN, JR.

REQUIREMENTS OF INFORMED
   CONSENT
  1. Relevant Information
    a. Appropriate Presentation
      Method
    b. Nature of the Proposed
      Procedure
    c. Options
    d. Possible Pain and Suffering
    e. Recuperation
    f&g. Risks and Possible
      Complications
    h. Potential Benefits
  2. Patient Comprehension
  3. Document Consent
  4. Patient Competency and
    Psychiatric Status
  5. Patient Autonomy
COMMENT

Informed consent means sufficient understanding by a patient, or the patient's surrogate, to sign consent for the patient's medical or surgical treatment. Informed consent allows the patient to exercise freedom of choice in the receipt of medical or surgical care. Potential medical-legal liability exists when it is not "properly" done or documented, although there are no specifically required methods to satisfy the doctrine of informed consent.[1] Those caring for the patient also have an ethical and moral obligation to try to meet the requirements for obtaining informed consent for their patients' care. The purely elective nature of most bariatric surgery, when taken in perspective with its known serious complications, reinforces the need to carefully and compulsively approach the legal, ethical and moral aspects of informed consent.

REQUIREMENTS OF INFORMED CONSENT

Although it has been stated that fully informed consent is seemingly impossible,[2] it does not relieve the bariatric surgeon from assuring, as reasonably as possible, that the patent's consent to surgery fulfills the requirements of informed consent. The elemental requirements of informed consent are that the patient: 1) has adequate, relevant information disclosed via the surgeon; 2) comprehends this information; 3) documents consent; 4) is competent; and 5) has active, autonomous participation in the decision-making process. Adherence to these requirements is intended to maximize good, and minimize harm, to the patient[3] as well as uphold and embody the ethical principle of respect of persons.[2]

An investment of time is required for this type of informed consent. Increased retention and comprehension of the material has been shown to correlate with longer time spent in patient education. The methods used, by necessity, depend upon the individual surgeon's approach, available time, and graphic, audiovisual and personnel resources. These may include extensive personal interviews with each patient and the patient's relatives or significant others, audiovisual materials seen by these parties, written materials and explanations by the surgeon, dietitians, nurses and others.

1. RELEVANT INFORMATION

Relevant patient information includes: (a) appropriate presentation method; (b) nature of the proposed procedure(s); (c) options; (d) possible pain and suffering; (e) recuperation; (f) the risks; (g) possible complications; and (h) potential benefits. This implies that the surgeon has a current knowledge of past and present literature and maintains a well-balanced flexibility of thought and opinion.[4]

A. APPROPRIATE PRESENTATION METHOD. Such information is best provided by the surgeon directly to the patient in simple lay language, allowing ample time for discussion with expressed openness to questions. Witnesses should be present. The surgeon's attitude, as well as the means of verbal and nonverbal expression, should be sympathetic towards the patient.[2]

The disclosure should be tailored to the patient's ability to comprehend in a positive, sympathetic fashion. Since patient autonomy is so essential to informed consent, the requirement to uphold and embody respect for the patient as an individual is also inseparable from the consent process. From an experimental point of view, an impatient, negative, condescending or disrespectful attitude, or a confused approach to the subject, can be readily detected by most of these generally sensitive individuals and can damage the physician-patient relationship.

In the program at The University of Tennessee, Memphis, in order to be as complete as reasonably possible, Appendix A is read and signed by the patient and witnessed. It lists most complications, including material ones.

B. NATURE OF THE PROPOSED PROCEDURE. After the bariatric surgeon has described the surgical approach selected, it is wise to address the possibility of need for additional concurrent surgery. Time, financial, physical and technique constraints limit the surgeon's ability to pre-operatively detect all intra-abdominal pathology which may be found. It is advisable to document whether the patient will permit any additional or unplanned surgery. In the handwritten section describing the proposed procedure, we usually write: "Exploratory laparotomy, vertical banded gastroplasty, live biopsy and/or any other procedure(s) necessary in Dr. Cowan's judgment." If additional procedures are planned or another type of bariatric procedure is to be done, appropriate changes are made in this section. We stress to the patient that the "other procedure(s) necessary" phase includes only the procedure(s) that the surgeon will, at the time of surgery, find necessary in the exercise of his judgment just as other surgeons would do. Common examples such as ventral herniorrhaphy and cholecystectomy are given.

C. OPTIONS. The patient has many options to exercise towards achieving weight-loss goals. These include no surgery, non-prescription medications or diets, hypnosis, acupuncture, dental wiring, physician-supervised weight-loss programs, intragastric balloon placement and the different bariatric surgical procedures currently available. Bariatric patients have familiarity with most of the options but, at some point in their pre-operative counselling, it is advisable to review these.

D. POSSIBLE PAIN AND SUFFERING. Most prospective bariatric surgery patients, like other patients, know that a certain amount of pain and discomfort will be experienced for a few days postoperatively, despite pain medications. Postoperative "suffering" may also be experienced by the known limitations or consequences of the bariatric procedure such as nausea, vomiting, diarrhea, catheters and other tubes, small food portions, and taste alterations. These may be described to the patient as a part of patient counselling but, in any event, are contained in the patient required reading material in Appendix A.

E. RECUPERATION. Most of our patients return to work 4 to 6 weeks postoperatively. They are usually informed of this in addition to many of the restrictions imposed during convalescence. While this information is unlikely to impact upon the patient's decision concerning bariatric surgery, it can be important in anticipating the need to make certain arrangements pre-operatively to cover postoperative limitations. The implications for the patient may include timing of the procedure, length of sick leave needed, a job that requires heavy lifting, time and travel to the surgeon's follow-up appointments, shopping for special diet foods, travel plans, home help, etc. We have tried to minimize postoperative "surprises" by our earlier counselling, while realizing that, as hard as one may try, it is not possible to anticipate everything in every circumstance.

F AND G. RISKS AND POSSIBLE COMPLICATIONS. The number of possible complications and risks is too large and impractical to verbally present in detail. However, the material risks and probabilities of complications need to be described to the patient. Wherever reasonable, risk information should include local experience.[5] Material risks include any risks of a serious nature, even if infrequent, together with those which are more common, severe or not, and their likely outcome.[1,6] Any information concerning proposed treatment, which might lead the patient to reject operative care, is material.[7] The patient should also be told about the possible consequences of not having the proposed bariatric operation.[6] Certain possible risks are not presently known, such as those occurring 15, 20 or more years after vertical banded gastroplasty and, therefore, are not material. In this regard, it is unreasonable to expect the surgeon to state other than the fact that this or any of the other currently performed bariatric surgical procedures are still relatively new and their long-term results, including complications, are unknown at this time.

H. POTENTIAL BENEFITS. The main benefits expected from bariatric surgery are psychosocial and medical. We emphasize that no patient is guaranteed to lose a single pound or derive any psychosocial or medical benefit as a result of the procedure; however, we inform the patient that many patients do meet realistic weight-loss goals and experience psychosocial benefits together with amelioration of medical problems associated with morbid obesity. Since bariatric patients, by the time they seek surgical help, have tried and failed most options, they fear repeated failure following surgery, and some strongly press for guarantee of success. We provide no guarantees, express or implied. It is unwise to compromise regarding this point.

2. PATIENT COMPREHENSION

The patient needs, as part of the informed consent process, to receive all information in language that can be understood by the average lay person.[8] Despite the time and effort expended to provide adequate information, it is difficult to be assured, or to prove, that the patient has received and understands all appropriate information sufficient to meet the requirements for informed consent. Educational level, ability to concentrate or retain information, and regional language differences are among the difficulties that can impair communication.

3. DOCUMENT CONSENT

In order to document understanding of informed consent, we have, for two years, been administering a 20-question true/false written examination (Fig. 27.1) to each patient the evening before surgery. A similar examination, adapted for gastric bypass and bilio-pancreatic bypass (Figs. 27.2 and 27.3), is provided for those who primarily perform these procedures. Our education of the patient in preparation for this exam usually starts with the first visit, a 1½ to 2 hour informal lecture-discussion by the surgeon with the patient and others. These group presentations contain definitions of obesity, morbid obesity and super-obesity, a discussion of morbidity and mortality, psychosocial problems, and medical and non-medical management, as well as a historical description of surgical management up to present-day practice. Drawings illustrate intestinal bypass, gastric bypass, vertical banded gastroplasty and other procedures. Finally, the risks and possible complications of the surgery are presented, including those which are relatively common, as well as the less common but more devastating (e.g., intra-abdominal leaks, abscess, organ failure and death). A frank and open

OBESITY SURGERY PATIENT EXAMINATION (GASTROPLASTY)

This examination is given to indicate to your surgeon that you understand the information he has discussed with you. If you answer any question incorrectly, it will alert him to review this area with you and re-test you on it until he is satisfied that you satisfactorily understand the material/concept(s) involved. Where you re-take the exam using this same sheet, please initial and date your change in answer.

All questions are true/false. Please circle the answer you choose as correct.

True/False 1. There are other operations for morbid obesity available than vertical banded gastroplasty.

True/False 2. Staple lines NEVER leak & result in infection or communication between the stomach or intestines and the skin.

True/False 3. Clots in the legs or pelvis may happen from obesity surgery. These clots can loosen and go to the lungs, causing such sensations as breathlessness and chest pain.

True/False 4. A few months after obesity surgery, the patient is able to eat or drink ANYTHING he/she wants in any amount.

True/False 5. The obesity surgery patient is GUARANTEED to permanently lose weight from this surgery.

True/False 6. Diabetes, high blood pressure, back pain and similar ailments ALWAYS get better after obesity surgery.

True/False 7. There is a possibility I could require intensive care, short or long-term, in hospital after obesity surgery.

True/False 8. Re-operation is sometimes necessary due to bleeding, hernias, ulceration, bursting of "stitches" or staples, leakage, blockage of the intestines or stomach and other causes.

True/False 9. This operation for obesity will commit me to periodic physician follow-ups for life, severe eating restrictions and additional operations if needed.

True/False 10. After obesity surgery, the patient is committed to taking vitamin-mineral supplements and having periodic nutritional assessments/studies made for life.

True/False 11. After this surgery, I will never be able to swallow whole (uncrushed or unchewed) pills or tablets again.

True/False 12. Obesity surgery is not a very serious or risky procedure.

True/False 13. Sometimes patients vomit a lot after obesity surgery.

True/False 14. After I recover from the obesity surgery and go home, I should just be patient with any medical problem I may have and not call my surgeon for at least two or three days.

True/False 15. No patient ever gets dangerously depressed after obesity surgery.

True/False 16. Patients are usually quite miserable for the first 48 hours after obesity surgery.

True/False 17. I have been told that I am guaranteed to lose weight after this gastroplasty surgery.

True/False 18. It is absolutely necessary that I take prescribed vitamins after surgery for life.

True/False 19. In the United States, approximately one in two hundred patients who have their stomachs stapled die.

True/False 20. For ten weeks after the obesity surgery, the only solid foods which patients may eat are finely puréed or purée-like (e.g. scrambled eggs) foods.

This is to certify that I took this test myself without any help in the actual answers to questions during the exam.

Date: Signature of Person Examined:

Examiner's Signature:

FIGURE 27.1. Patient examination prior to vertical banded gastroplasty.

OBESITY SURGERY PATIENT EXAMINATION (GASTRIC BY-PASS)

This examination is given to indicate to your surgeon that you understand the information he has discussed with you. If you answer any question incorrectly, it will alert him to review this area with you and re-test you on it until he is satisfied that you satisfactorily understand the material/concept(s) involved. Where you re-take the exam using this same sheet, please initial and date your change in answer.

All questions are true/false. Please circle the answer you choose as correct.

True/False   1. There are other operations for morbid obesity available than gastric bypass.

True/False   2. Staple or suture lines NEVER leak & result in infection or communication between the stomach or intestines and the skin.

True/False   3. Clots in the legs or pelvis may happen from obesity surgery. These clots can loosen and go to the lungs causing such sensations as breathlessness and chest pain.

True/False   4. A few months after obesity surgery, the patient doesn't need to worry about dieting and can eat whatever he/she wants.

True/False   5. The obesity surgery patient is GUARANTEED to permanently lose weight from this surgery.

True/False   6. Diabetes, high blood pressure, back pain and similar ailments ALWAYS get better after obesity surgery.

True/False   7. There is a possibility I could require intensive care, short or long-term, in hospital after obesity surgery.

True/False   8. Re-operation is sometimes necessary due to bleeding, hernias, ulceration, bursting of "stitches" or staples, leakage, blockage of the intestines or stomach and other causes.

True/False   9. This operation for obesity will commit me to periodic physician follow-ups for life.

True/False 10. After obesity surgery, the patient is committed to taking vitamin-mineral supplements and having periodic nutritional assessments/studies made for life: this may include periodic vitamin injections.

True/False 11. After this surgery, I will probably have diarrhea especially after eating too much, too fast or the wrong kind(s) of food.

True/False 12. Obesity surgery is not a very serious or risky procedure.

True/False 13. Sometimes patients vomit after obesity surgery.

True/False 14. After I recover from the obesity surgery and go home, I should just be patient with any medical problem I may have and not call my surgeon for at least two or three days.

True/False 15. No patient ever gets dangerously depressed after obesity surgery.

True/False 16. Patients can be quite miserable for the first 48 hours after obesity surgery.

True/False 17. I have been told that I am guaranteed to lose weight after this obesity surgery.

True/False 18. It is absolutely necessary that I take prescribed vitamins after surgery for life.

True/False 19. In the United States, approximately one in two hundred patients who have their stomachs stapled die.

True/False 20. For five weeks after the obesity surgery, the only solid foods which patients may eat are finely puréed or purée-like (e.g. scrambled eggs) foods.

This is to certify that I took this test myself without any help in the actual answers to questions during the exam.

Date: Signature of Person Examined:

Examiner's Signature:

FIGURE 27.2. Examination modified for gastric bypass patients.

approach to questions is used throughout the session. At a later office visit for history and physical examination, the patient is given further opportunity to ask questions and discuss the subject. If the patient is accepted for surgery, further post-admission instruction by nurses, clinical dietitians, psychiatrist, anesthesia personnel and surgeon is provided. A booklet describing the usual expected events of the pre-operative work-up, operation, recovery room, possible intensive care unit stay, postoperative management and convalescence is provided on admission. A fairly detailed diet booklet is also provided, which the dietitian closely reviews pre- and postoperatively with the patient.

Each patient's written examination is accompanied by a 3-page review of much of the material previously covered, especially addressing possible complications (Appendix A). The patient is instructed to read this review and then take the examination, unassisted, the afternoon or evening before surgery. A staff nurse witnesses and signs both documents together with the patient. The surgeon, before the patient signs the surgical

This examination is given to indicate to your surgeon that you understand the information he has discussed with you. If you answer any question incorrectly, it will alert him to review this area with you and re-test you on it until he is satisfied that you satisfactorily understand the material/concept(s) involved. Where you re-take the exam using this same sheet, please initial and date your change in answer.

All questions are true/false. Please circle the answer you choose as correct.

True/False 1. It is important to eat high protein foods such as eggs, cheese, fish and chicken the first year following obesity surgery since malnutrition can occur.

True/False 2. There are no other operations or programs for morbid obesity available than bilio-pancreatic by-pass.

True/False 3. Staple or suture lines NEVER leak & result in infection or communication between the stomach or intestines and the skin.

True/False 4. Clots in the legs or pelvis may happen from obesity surgery. These clots can loosen and go to the lungs causing such sensations as breathlessness and chest pain.

True/False 5. Patients with bilio-pancreatic by-pass often experience more frequent, soft, strongly-smelling bowel movements.

True/False 6. The obesity surgery patient is GUARANTEED to permanently lose weight from this surgery.

True/False 7. Diabetes, high blood pressure, back pain, and similar ailments ALWAYS get better after obesity surgery.

True/False 8. There is a possibility I could require intensive care, short or long-term, in hospital after obesity surgery.

True/False 9. Re-operation is sometimes necessary due to bleeding, hernias, ulceration, bursting of "stitches" or staples, leakage, blockage of the intestines or stomach and other causes.

True/False 10. This operation for obesity will commit me to periodic physician follow-ups for life.

True/False 11. After obesity surgery, the patient is committed to taking vitamin-mineral supplements and having periodic nutritional assessments/studies made for life; this may include periodic vitamin injections.

True/False 12. If not already removed, the gall bladder is usually taken out at the time of bilio-pancreatic surgery since there is such a high-rate of gall bladder disease in these patients.

True/False 13. Obesity surgery is not a very serious or risky procedure.

True/False 14. Patients don't vomit after obesity surgery.

True/False 15. After I recover from the obesity surgery and go home, I should just be patient with any medical problem I may have and not call my surgeon for at least two or three days.

True/False 16. No patient ever gets dangerously depressed after obesity surgery.

True/False 17. Patients can be quite miserable for the first 48 hours after obesity surgery.

True/False 18. It is not necessary that I take prescribed vitamins and mineral supplements after surgery for life.

True/False 19. In the United States, approximately one in two hundred patients who have obesity surgery die.

True/False 20. In the first year or more after obesity surgery, significant protein, iron, vitamin, body salt, or body fluid abnormalities may occur in some patients.

This is to certify that I took this test myself without any help in the actual answers to questions during the exam.

Signature of person examined: _____

Date: _____

Examiner's signature: _____

FIGURE 27.3. Examination modified for bilio-pancreatic bypass patients.

consent form, identifies any incorrect answers, and reviews those in detail with the patient until the patient understands better. The patient then re-answers the incorrectly answered questions, initialing each corrected answer. The results of these first and second examinations are recorded in the patient's chart. The 3-page review and the examination become a permanent part of the medical record.

The examination is intended to alert the surgeon to areas in which the patient needs further instruction as well as to document a properly obtained informed consent. The questions are designed to test important areas in which they have or have not been able to retain or to understand the material presented. They contain information such as "one in 200 patients dies as a result of obesity surgery." In light of this statistic alone, one would expect that no competent individual, after due consideration, would sign a bariatric surgical consent form without actually wanting to have such surgery. Many patients remark upon this question and we discuss it relative to other risks the patient may face; no patient in our center has refused or deferred surgery as a result of these questions. Other questions are potentially intimidating to reasonably demonstrate that the patient is positively stimulated to exercise autonomy; complications of pulmonary embolism, deep venous thrombosis, staple leak, re-operation, bleeding, as well as death, are all contained within the examination. Since the patient may claim that the surgery was presented as an easy or inconsequential procedure, one question contains the statement "Obesity surgery is an easy procedure." A "false" answer indicates that the patient understands the serious nature of the bariatric surgery proposed. Other questions are posed, including the need for lifetime follow-up and additional risks and restrictions of the bariatric surgery postoperatively. Once the patient has successfully completed the examination and has had it signed and witnessed, permanent evidence exists that the surgeon has obtained what we consider to be reasonably acceptable informed consent. The examination records that the patient understands the nature and implications of the procedure(s) beyond the usual operative permit, and documents patient *understanding* of the risks, complications, benefits and alternatives to bariatric surgery. This must strengthen the surgeon's response to any situation in which the patient might claim inadequately informed consent. It has not, however, been tested in court.

In the administration of 50 of these examinations to patients in our bariatric surgery program, only three patients had more than three incorrect answers. Nearly 25% of patients had 100% of the answers correct when given the exam for the first time. The worst examination result was six out of 20 incorrect answers. As a result of discussions during post-exam counselling of these patients, most of the incorrect answers were due to improper reading of the question or answering the exception rather than the rule by over-interpretation. The double-negatives were purposely designed to require, and to demonstrate, thought on the patient's part rather than test purely rote memory.

The results of the examinations, obviously, depend upon the amount and relevancy of the information given to the patient prior to this testing. Since we provide pre-operative patient education similar to that of many bariatric surgeons, most bariatric surgery patients would be expected to score similarly the evening before surgery. We recommend that these, or similar, tests of understanding be used following the pre-operative education of the patient, prior to obtaining signed surgical consent. The examination can be modified easily for use with other bariatric surgical procedures.

Many consent forms are written at the college level of comprehension.[9] Use of simple lay terms, clear sentence structure, brevity and comprehension level of the sixth grade should characterize operative consent forms and other material for patient review.

4. PATIENT COMPETENCY AND PSYCHIATRIC STATUS

Competency revolves around whether the patient has adequate capacity to choose from the options available. The President's Commission for the Study of Ethical Problems in Medicine and Biomedical and Behavioral Research defines such decision-making capacity as: ". . . [having] sufficiently stable and developed personal values and goals, an ability to communicate and understand information adequately, and an ability to reason and deliberate sufficiently well about the choices."[10] We obtain a psychiatric consultation for each patient pre-operatively. Many bariatric surgeons feel such consultations have limited or no utility. The psychiatrist we use, while interviewing the patient, documents the patient's competency, realistic views of the procedure and its outcome, as well as determines that there is no specific psychiatric contraindication to the surgery. In our practice, we attempt to identify, before admission, any adult patients who might be mentally incompetent. However, there have been a number of instances where the psychiatrist has determined that the patient has had an almost magic feeling that, after the surgery, everything would be automatically wonderful, that they would rapidly become thin and their dreams would come true. The psychiatrist examining such patients, among other things, seeks out such feelings, attempts to divest the patient of them, records these events and informs the surgeon. We also use a licensed clinical psychologist in lieu of a psychiatrist and feel this is an acceptable alternative.

5. PATIENT AUTONOMY

Patient autonomy means the right of involvement and voluntariness in the choice of medical treatment on the patient's part, without being coerced or otherwise unduly influenced by others, particularly those responsible for medical-care delivery. It is exercised by the patient with regard to handling any request for informed consent to perform a given procedure or treatment. The medical-care team shows respect for the patient by assuring that patients participate in decisions affecting their lives so long as they have the capacity, or competence, to do so.[2,11] Sometimes the surgeon may encourage or facilitate interaction with others, especially family members, who can help the patient make a rational choice for or against bariatric surgery.[12] He may also advise the patient and relatives of his reasoned opinion. Some feel he may even use acceptable persuasion,[2] although this must be approached with considerable caution and is best witnessed and well-annotated in the medical record.

Most morbidly obese patients have been aware of bariatric surgery for years before seeking surgical help. The years prior to their exploring the surgical option are often characterized by repeated failures to lose weight or maintain weight loss by multiple, different methods. Many of our patients have shelves full of diet books, have tried many mail-order weight-loss offers, attended weight-loss groups, and tried physician-supervised diets, plus other methods. Some have had an earlier form of bariatric surgery which has failed. Therefore, their decisions may be said to revolve around the experience of the problems with their obesity, as well as many prior failures to achieve or maintain weight loss. Although they seek help, many are doing so in desperation. Their psychosocial or medical problems may be unacceptable or deteriorating, and they have finally decided to seek surgical assistance. Some patients are so desperate that, once having independently decided upon bariatric surgery and a surgeon, they only want the results and have less concern for the choice of surgical procedure or other vital information. They may be trying to relinquish their autonomy as regards surgery. This needs to be recognized and discouraged. The bariatric surgeon should resist accepting this type of decision-making authority.[2] This type of patient must be involved in the entire body of material information required for properly informed consent. Lack of communication of all material information on this subject to the patient can have a strong negative effect on that individual's autonomy.[13] The legal implications should be obvious. Fully informed, autonomous decision-making is at least as important for the elective bariatric surgery patient, who has to live with the results of the surgery, as it is for the surgeon.

COMMENT

It is important to obtain and document the proper informed consent for treatment. Acute situations, emergencies, very ill or elderly patients can present considerable barriers to meeting the informed consent requirements.[14] However, their obvious need and the often non-elective nature of circumstances are, for the most part, well removed from that of most bariatric surgery. The chronic nature of obesity, the electiveness of bariatric surgery, the relative youth of the patient population and patient competence in all but rare exceptions, permit us the opportunity to come somewhat closer to the ideal of providing our patients with the basics necessary to give an informed consent for their bariatric surgery.

If the surgeon has covered a complication which the patient later develops as a result of bariatric surgery, but there is no record of informed consent, the patient cannot recollect ever receiving the information, or if such information is claimed not to have been understood, liability can exist. The examination technique presented, while as yet not legally tested, is a logical approach to documenting the patient's receipt and understanding of information as well as the surgeon's positive ethical and moral intent not only to provide but test it as well.

Use of the examination technique with patients who are to receive different bariatric surgical procedures, such as bilio-pancreatic bypass, have required modification of a number of the questions (Fig. 27.3). The questions, as they presently stand, have evolved by relatively minor periodic alterations since the start of our examination method. The examinations themselves, therefore, are not to be regarded as static entities, but rather as tools for documenting informed consent which are still being developed as bariatric surgery itself continues to evolve. They can be expanded to other forms of surgery as well.

The pre-operative examination does not test intelligent decision-making. It merely documents that the patient has been informed concerning the subject matter of the examination questions and understands that material. The doctrine of informed consent "encourages . . . but does not require, patients to make informed or intelligent decisions about medical care."[14] Variables, including personal values and subjective preferences important to the patient, are thus allowed to influence, or even control, the patient's decision-making activities. How the individual patient arrives at a decision for or against bariatric surgery, as long as it is autonomously made, is the patient's own responsibility. The bariatric surgeon is, therefore, not to be held accountable for the mechanisms by which the competent patient makes any decision for or against a given surgical procedure, as long as the elements of informed consent have been reasonably met.

Many hospital consent forms seldom include all the essential elements of informed consent and rarely provide any indication that the patient signing the form understands what the consent means.[15] The generally acceptable consent form is one which is designed particularly for the contemplated procedure(s), written in non-medical and non-legal language, and kept as short as possible, and describes the procedure, its risks and probabilities, options and their likely consequences.[1,16]

The standard of patient disclosure which we use and have described is the "layman's standard." In essence, this standard legally requires, in an increasing number of states, that the physician must disclose what any reasonable man would have expected to disclose. Its legal origin is in the case of *Canterbury v. Spence*,[17] tried in 1972.[2] Our use of this standard also seeks to incorporate the earlier professional standard of disclosure, which is still applicable in many states. It requires that the physician must disclose what is standard for other physicians to disclose in the individual's community. However, it must be noted that the British courts recently rejected the layman's standard in favor of the professional standard.[7]

There is no reason to expect the evolution of informed consent to remain in its present state.[13] Even now, some would require physicians to elicit the patient's values and preferences.[12] The use of computer logic for diagnostics and problem-solving and other tasks, second opinions, economic pressures, further advances in audiovisual technology, ever increasing public awareness, legal decisions, changes in societal ethics and other sources will, to some degree, impact upon informed consent in the future.[16] Hopefully, they will be constructive and work to the benefit of the patient and physician alike, much as is intended by the written examination we have described.

APPENDIX A

FACT SHEET

RECORD OF HAVING BEEN INFORMED OF THE FOLLOWING FACTS ABOUT OBESITY SURGERY

Obesity surgery is quite major surgery and is done only for strict reasons in morbidly obese patients, with very few exceptions. Your surgeon reserves the right to interpret these reasons and accept or reject patients for surgery based upon his clinical judgment of them.

There are many operations available for morbidly obese patients including stomach stapling (gastroplasty), putting a band around the stomach (gastric banding), cutting certain nerves to the stomach (vagus nerves), teeth wiring, balloon(s) in the stomach, etc. Continuing to try to lose weight by dieting and not having surgery is also possible.

Many patients have done well, but there is no guarantee of any benefit from this surgery. For each potential benefit, such as improvements in diabetes, high blood pressure or less back pain, etc., there have been failures. Some obese patients have problems with breathing while they sleep. The breathing problems may not always get better after losing weight.

It is hoped that the weight loss one year after surgery will be at least $\frac{1}{3}$ or $\frac{1}{2}$ of the patient's extra weight. This happens in many patients, but some don't lose weight or they may gain their weight back afterwards. While obesity surgery usually works, it only helps with weight loss and is not anything "magic" or guaranteed. The patient must cooperate and make changes in lifestyle with regular small meals for life, cut out snacks, drink almost all non-calorie liquids, eat slowly and make other changes in eating and drinking habits.

Almost every surgeon who performs obesity surgery has complications some time or another. Every patient has a real risk for one or more complications. There are no guarantees that a serious complication will not occur in any case. The more frequent or serious complications that can occur are:

Infection of the wound, body cavity (abdomen

or chest especially), lungs (pneumonia, for example) can occur.

Inflammation or infection of these organs can occur: pancreas (pancreatitis), stomach (gastritis, stomach ulcer), esophagus (esophagitis with chest pain, burning, etc.), liver (hepatitis), gallbladder (cholecystitis, gallstones), kidney (pyelonephritis, kidney failure, nephritis), bladder (cystitis), duodenum (duodenitis, duodenal ulcer).

The spleen may be injured during surgery and need to be removed. This can seriously increase the risks of infection in the patient's body.

Organ failure such as of the heart, kidney, liver, lungs has occurred after obesity surgery.

Clots in the lower limbs, pelvis or elsewhere in the body can form and travel to the lungs, causing difficulties with breathing or even death. These clots can also result in temporary or permanent swelling or ulceration, especially of the legs.

Fluids from the stomach or intestines can leak into the body cavity, other organs or through the skin. They may continue to drain into a bag for a long time.

Changes in taste and food preferences often occur. Many patients have difficulties eating certain foods such as red meats which they may have liked before surgery. Sometimes after surgery, certain cravings for some foods may occur in some patients.

Food or liquids may not be able to pass through the pouch, lower stomach or intestines, which may need stretching (dilating) by instruments or endoscopies (which have their own risk). Tubes for nourishment fluids may have to be placed into the stomach, intestines or veins, if the patient is unable to eat or drink enough by mouth. Operation may be necessary.

Vomiting or diarrhea can frequently occur after this type of surgery and may make it a problem to eat certain types or quantities of food. This can be, in one sense, a benefit of this surgery, because it prevents eating or drinking of certain food(s) for fear of diarrhea or vomiting.

Bleeding from the stomach, hernia, breakdown of the surgical stitches, need to re-operate for these or other reasons, complications of anesthesia, psychiatric problems such as depression requiring psychiatric care and admission to a psychiatric ward, and even death are all possible as a result of surgery. Across the United States, approximately one in 200 patients dies after obesity surgery.

Persistent vomiting, nausea, swelling of the abdomen, heartburn, etc., can occur and may make the patient think seriously of having the operation undone in certain instances.

The stomach pouch or its outlet may get bigger or the staple-lines open up, so that, in time, the patient can eat more at a mealtime or even gain back to the original or greater weight.

Re-operation may be necessary, and no patient should have obesity surgery performed who is not prepared to accept the need for re-operation if it should become necessary.

Admission to an intensive care unit may be necessary to observe the patient closely or to treat any of the problems that can arise from surgery.

Over the months and years, any type of nutrition problem or infection may occur, including lack of vitamin(s), protein, calories, mineral(s), etc. Signs of this can include weakness, paralysis, confusion, rashes, anemia, hair loss, bone and joint problems, wounds that heal poorly, tongue soreness, night blindness, numbness, etc. After obesity surgery, taking extra vitamins and minerals and being followed by the obesity surgeon, or a physician well experienced in this area, is necessary for life. The patient may need to have vitamin injections every month or so for life. Food may stick in the stomach pouch and may need to be taken out with a special tube.

Due to possible problems in the future, obesity surgery patients need to be followed by a physician experienced in this area for life.

The patient's weight loss goal, no weight lost or even further gain of weight may occur any time after surgery.

With weight loss, the skin on the arms, legs, neck, abdomen, face and elsewhere may become wrinkled, sag, droop or hang as large folds. It may become quite annoying, embarrassing or develop rashes or infections and odors. As a result, the patient may feel a need for further surgery. If this happens, the surgeon will be available to discuss this and any other matter.

As soon as any problem arises, medical help must be obtained soon—the patient has the duty to call for help quickly and without delay.

All of the currently performed types of surgery for obesity are still relatively new. Therefore, the long-term results of such surgery, including weight loss or possible complications, are unknown at this time.

I have read the above, which has been described to me by my surgeon. I understand this material, the risks, possible complications, other choices and the possible benefits of obesity surgery, as well as the operation which my surgeon recommends for my case.

By signing this statement, I am showing that I have read and accept the above and that I understand it. I have been encouraged to ask all the questions I want; they have been answered well, and I understand the answers.

_____   _____
Signed (patient)   Signed (person present)

Date:

REFERENCES

1. Plumeri PA: The gastroenterologist and the doctrine of informed consent. J Clin Gastroenterol 5:185–187, 1983.

2. Liebert VW: Informed consent: an imperative impossibility. Am Surg 48:225–229, 1982.

3. Mahler DM, Veatch RM, Sidel VW: Ethical issues in informed consent. JAMA 247:481–485, 1982.

4. Buchwald H: True informed consent in surgical treatment of morbid obesity. Am J Clin Nutr 33:482–494, 1980.

5. Brody H: The meaning of informed consent. Michigan Med 557–558, 1984.

6. Brown FC: Some comments about informed consent. Can J Surg 27:131–132, 1984.

7. Annas GJ: Why the British courts rejected the American doctrine of informed consent. Am J Public Health 74:1286–1288, 1984.

8. Levine RJ: Informed consent in research and practice. Arch Intern Med 143:1229–1231, 1983.

9. Riecken HW, Ravich R: Informed consent to biomedical research in Veterans Administration hospitals. JAMA 248:344–348, 1982.

10. President's Commission for the Study of Ethical Problems in Medicine and Biomedical and Behavioral Research: Making Health Care Decisions, vol one. Washington, US Government Printing Office, 1983, p 45.

11. Drane JF: Competency to give informed consent. JAMA 252:925–927, 1984.

12. Hollander RD: Changes in the concept of informed consent in medical encounters. J Med Education 59:783–788, 1984.

13. Beasley AD, Graber GC: The range of autonomy: informed consent in medicine. Theoretical Medicine 5:31–41,1984.

14. Lidz CW, Meisel A, Zerubavel E: Informed Consent—A Study of Informed Decision Making Authority. The Guilford Press, 1984, p 10.

15. Dedeker K: Informed consent vs. consent forms. Minnesota Med 66:575–576, 1983.

16. Fletcher JC: The evolution of the ethics of informed consent. Progress in Clinical & Biological Research 128:187–228, 1983.

17. *Canterbury v. Spence*, 484 F. 2d 772 (D.C. Cir 1972).

28

Metabolic Complications Following Gastric Restrictive Procedures

D. MICHAEL GRACE

Rapid weight loss, whether induced by gastroplasty or diet, is associated with a variety of nutritional problems and deficiency states. Metabolic problems after gastric restriction procedures are most apt to occur when patients have inadequate knowledge or teaching about nutrition, when cooperation by the patient is poor, when follow-up by surgeon or dietician is inadequate, when the gastric stoma is too small, or when too much bowel is bypassed in combination with gastroplasty procedures. This chapter is an attempt to analyze some of the metabolic problems that can occur. It must be stressed that prevention of the problems by adequate patient selection and follow-up is the key to management. Vomiting, when severe, must be investigated and managed. It should be considered to be due to obstruction until proven otherwise.

Creation of a small gastric stoma reduces total caloric intake, especially early after operation. The quality of food is also altered considerably. Meat, especially red meat, is difficult to eat, and raw vegetables which are a source of vitamins and bulk in the normal diet are not well tolerated. Gut physiology may be altered by bypassing the duodenum or other portion of small bowel. Deficiency states may therefore occur early as a result of altered eating habits or late as a result of altered physiology.

Appropriate patient selection for gastric restrictive procedures is important but difficult. Patients who are uncooperative or of limited intelligence should probably be excluded and those with a history of emotional problems should also be excluded or followed very carefully. Careful dietary advice from surgeon, family doctor and dietician is essential to reduce nutritional and metabolic complications. The problems associated with jejunoileal bypass often showed up late and are still turning up. Procedures such as gastric bypass or biliopancreatic bypass may also carry late problems such as anemia or calcium deficiency. No surgeon should be in the field of obesity surgery unless he or she is prepared to follow patients indefinitely, although that is difficult because of the mobility of North American society and the emotional nature of some morbidly obese patients. Some of the complications of gastric restrictive procedures are summarized in Table 28.1.

OPERATIVE PROCEDURE AND COMPLICATIONS

To be successful, gastric restrictive procedures must create a pouch less than 50 mL,

TABLE 28.1. METABOLIC COMPLICATIONS OF GASTRIC RESTRICTIVE PROCEDURES

1. All procedures
   Vomiting
   Excessive weight loss
   Protein/calorie malnutrition
   Impaired immunocompetence
   Vitamin deficiency, especially thiamine with neuropathy and encephalopathy
   Hair loss
   Gallstone formation

2. Gastric bypass
   Anemia
   Iron, B_{12} and folate deficiency
   Dumping
   ? Calcium deficiency

3. Biliopancreatic bypass
   Malabsorption
   Iron, B_{12} and folate deficiency
   Deficiency of fat-soluble vitamins
   Metabolic bone disease

a secure partition usually by two applications of a double staple-line and a secure stoma less than 1.2 cm in diameter. In my personal experience with more than 150 gastric bypass procedures and 300 vertical banded gastroplasties, the weight loss has been similar although published series favor gastric bypass. Early benefits in terms of weight loss achieved by bypassing the duodenum may be balanced by later dilatation of the sutured stoma and weight gain. The altered physiology of gastric bypass fosters iron, B_{12} and folate deficiency with anemia, especially late after operation.[1] However, anemia can occur after gastroplasty, and deficiencies of protein or various vitamins can occur with either operation. Calcium deficiency may occur late after gastric bypass but especially after biliopancreatic bypass. Because biliopancreatic bypass causes gastric restriction as well as shortening of the small bowel and entry of bile and pancreatic juice into the terminal ileum, there is more marked weight loss than following other gastric restrictive procedures and more impairment in absorption of fat and fat-soluble substances.

NUTRITION, CALORIC INTAKE AND WEIGHT LOSS

Table 28.2 summarizes the type of weight loss and change in eating pattern that occur after gastric restrictive procedures. The changes in weight are taken from my own unpublished data and the changes in eating pattern from the data of Coughlin.[2] Similar results have been described by others.[3] The

TABLE 28.2. METABOLIC CHANGES AFTER GASTROPLASTY OR GASTRIC BYPASS*

	Preop.	3 Months	6 Months	1 Year
Weight (kg)	135	112	101	90
Weight loss (%)		17	25	33
Excess weight loss (%)		35	50	60–70
Intake (kcal)	2800–4000	500	900	1100
Protein (g/day)	164	19	38	60
Fat (g/day)	177	19	43	44
Carbohydrate (g/day)	433	56	98	113
Electrolytes				
Sodium	Normal	High normal	High normal	High normal
Potassium	Normal	Low normal	Normal	Normal
Chloride	Normal	High normal	High normal	High normal
Proteins				
Albumin	Normal	Low normal	Normal	Normal
Transferrin	Normal	Low normal	Normal	Normal
Lipids				
Triglycerides	High	Normal	Normal	Normal
Cholesterol	High	Normal	Normal	Normal
Glucose	High	Normal	Normal	Normal
Liver Function				
Bilirubin	Normal	Normal	High normal	High normal
Alkaline phosphatase	Normal	Normal	Normal	High normal
LDH	High	High	Normal	Normal
SGOT	High normal	High normal	Normal	Normal
Hemoglobin	Normal	Low normal	Low normal	Mild anemia
(gastric bypass)				(up to 50%)
Iron	Normal	Low normal	Low normal	Low (in 50%)
B_{12}	Normal	Low normal	Low normal	Low (in 50%)
Folate	Normal	Normal	Normal	Normal (but low in 18%)
Hemoglobin	Normal	Normal	Normal	Normal
(gastroplasty)				

*From Grace, unpublished data, Coughlin et al[2] and Amaral et al.[1,4]

rest of the table is modified from the excellent data of Amaral and his colleagues in Providence.[1,4] These results will be discussed in more detail later. Articles on starvation state "save for exceptional individuals, human beings do not survive weight losses greater than 35 to 40%"[5] and yet our patients commonly lose this much and more in the first postoperative year. Morbidly obese individuals, although by no means rare, are exceptional in having a tremendous store of energy in the form of fat. The energy equivalent of this excess weight is about 7,000 kcal per kilogram.[6] Although there is a rapid decrease in carbohydrate stores soon after operation,[7] this fat is soon called upon as a source of calories. Nutritional competence can be maintained with an intake as low as 600 to 900 kcal per day, as long as protein intake is adequate and suitable vitamin supplementation is provided.[8,9]

Morbidly obese patients tend to be less educated and from lower socioeconomic classes than the normal weight population.[10] They have less knowledge of nutrition than normal weight patients having other operative procedures "although this knowledge does not correlate with weight loss."[11] Some unsophisticated patients may need careful explanation of postoperative diets to avoid quantitative and qualitative deficiencies. Close follow-up is essential because compliance decreases with time. There is marked variation in postoperative weight loss depending on the procedure, pouch and stoma size and motivation of the patient. In general, weight loss is better for the younger, smaller patients and when follow-up is close.[12] Older patients tend to lose more slowly.[13] Individual variations in resting energy expenditure and energy requirements may also contribute to the marked variation in weight loss.[14] It is important that each surgeon record and follow the weights of each patient to compare the weight loss with other patients who had the same procedure and with weight loss charts from the literature. Excessive weight loss, often accompanied by vomiting, must be recognized, investigated and treated.

PROTEIN AND BODY CELL MASS

Halverson[9] has reviewed some of the metabolic problems of gastric restrictive operations. Acute starvation depletes carbohydrate stores; then the body adapts to enable it to derive calories from lipid.[7] Protein mass is preserved and fat stores depleted. Extremely low protein intake is common soon after gastroplasty or gastric bypass,[2] although total caloric and protein intake increase with time. At least 40 to 60 grams of protein per day should be provided, since lower intake may be accompanied by signs of malnutrition such as low serum transferrin or albumin.[8] Since red meat is poorly tolerated, protein must be obtained from such sources as milk, cheese, fish and chicken, although milk may not be tolerated by some. Protein intake must be emphasized preoperatively and in regular postoperative visits. Rapid weight loss is mainly due to the use of fat for energy while lean body mass is spared.[15] Most studies show some loss of body cell mass within the first 3 months after gastroplasty,[16,17] but this returns to near normal values 12 to 18 months after operation. Stoma size may be critical in the preservation of body cell mass.[18] With small stomas significant vomiting, malnutrition and loss of body cell mass may occur, although the decrease in body cell mass may reflect the smaller muscle mass required to carry a patient who has lost considerable weight.[19] As Halverson emphasizes,[9] even in patients who are doing well there is a real threat of protein malnutrition that requires close follow-up and intake of an adequate diet.

LIPIDS

Lipids provide a significant source of energy in the normal diet and after gastroplasty or gastric bypass.[2] There is a massive reduction in endogenous lipid after extreme weight loss.[17] This lipid source contributes about 7000 kcal per kilogram.[6] Fatty acid deficiencies have not been reported after gastroplasty. The changes in lipid metabolism are beneficial rather than harmful. Moderate decreases in serum cholesterol and triglycerides occur, especially after gastric bypass,[20-22] although the changes are less marked than after jejunoileal bypass.[23] At the same time there is an increase in high density lipoprotein (HDL) and a decrease in low density lipoprotein (LDL),[22,23] which implies improvement in cardiac disease risk factors.[21] Biliopancreatic bypass procedures are followed by even more marked reductions in triglycerides and cholesterol.[24]

Fatty changes in the liver are common in non-alcoholic obese patients and are more severe in the morbidly obese.[25,26] Severe damage is uncommon but such changes may be accompanied by a reduction in serum albumin and an increase in alkaline phosphatase.[4,27] Weight loss after gastric bypass has been associated with a marked decrease in hepatic lipid[28] and improvement in liver function,[4] although alcoholic hyaline has been described in the liver after gastric bypass,[29] possibly as a complication of malnutrition. This picture cleared after parenteral nutrition and reversal of the gastroplasty. The increase in cholesterol excretion and contribution to gallstone formation after gastroplasty is described later in this chapter.

CARBOHYDRATES AND DIABETES

As in the case of lipids, the effects of gastroplasty or gastric bypass on carbohydrate metabolism are mainly beneficial rather than harmful. Carbohydrates form the major source of calories before and after gastric restriction procedures.[2] High calorie soft drinks are easily ingested after such operations and may be a major source of calories. Patients must be advised on the importance of switching to low calorie soft drinks or fluids. For the confirmed sweet-eater, gastric bypass may be advantageous, because dumping, normally an undesirable side-effect, restricts sugar ingestion.[30] Weight loss alone, without operation, is enough to reduce plasma glucose and increase glucose tolerance in the obese diabetic.[31] Gastric stapling procedures have the same effect, often beginning very early after operation, and adult onset obese diabetics can often discontinue insulin entirely.[32,33] Insulin resistance also decreases. Since these changes occur very early after operation, decreased oral intake may be as important as weight loss. I have carried out a gastric bypass on an obese adult onset diabetic woman who had needed insulin for 15 years. With moderate weight loss she was able to discontinue insulin 2 months after operation and there has been late improvement in peripheral neuropathy. The combination of this type II diabetes and morbid obesity is an additional indication for gastroplasty. Even in non-diabetic morbidly obese patients, a significant reduction in plasma glucose occurs.[4]

VITAMIN DEFICIENCY AND NEUROPATHIES

Prolonged low calorie diets may be associated with vitamin deficiencies and neuropathies,[34] and Wernicke's encephalopathy has occurred during prolonged starvation in an attempt to lose weight.[35] Acute reductions in vitamins A and C may be more marked in obese patients after gastric bypass than in normal weight patients having other operations,[36] but this does not seem to be of clinical significance. Deficiencies of vitamins A and K have been observed after gastric bypass without major clinical problems.[9]

Deficiency of the water-soluble B complex vitamins, especially thiamine,[37] a few weeks or months after gastroplasty may produce severe symptoms including encephalopathy,[38–40] with confusion, ataxia or coma, acute visual loss,[41] peripheral neuropathy,[42–44] and death.[44] Rapid vitamin, especially thiamine, replacement by the intravenous and intramuscular route is important, with oral replacement when possible. Recovery may be complete but ataxia and gait disturbance may persist.[42,45] The key however is prevention. This problem occurs within 3 months of gastroplasty and is associated with rapid weight loss (often 30 to 40 kg), excessive vomiting, inadequate vitamin intake due to poor advice or poor compliance and inadequate follow-up by family doctor, surgeon or dietician. The problem of Wernicke's encephalopathy has been reviewed by Reuler.[46] This condition is due to a deficiency of thiamine (vitamin B_1) which most commonly occurs in alcoholics on an inadequate diet. Prolonged intravenous feeding, severe vomiting or fasting may result in thiamine deficiency with the classical clinical symptoms of ocular abnormalities, ataxia and confusion. Onset may be gradual or sudden. The normal daily requirement of thiamine is 1.4 mg for an adult. Patients with poor nutrition should receive prophylactic thiamine, even if there are no clinical signs of Wernicke's encephalopathy. Acute Wernicke's encephalopathy and coma can occur acutely after beginning intravenous therapy in high-risk patients.[46] Some symptoms may resolve with as little as 2 or 3 mg of thiamine, but the usual initial dose is 100 mg by the intravenous or intramuscular route. Treatment should be based on clinical grounds,

although an assay is available based on erythrocyte transketolase activity.[46]

Neuropathies can also occur for mechanical rather than nutritional reasons. Obese patients are subject to postoperative ulnar and peroneal nerve palsies even though they are protected by an extra cushion of subcutaneous fat. We have seen an unusual pattern of severe hip pain after gastroplasty in very obese patients.[47] This appears to be due to compression of the lateral cutaneous nerve of the thigh by retractors fixed to the operating-room table. Mild thiamine deficiency may be more frequent after gastroplasty procedures than has been recognized so far. Deficiencies of vitamin B_{12} and folate will be reviewed under the heading of anemia, and vitamin D deficiency is reviewed under calcium.

ANEMIA

Morbidly obese patients are subject to the usual causes of anemia before and after gastroplasty. Excessive menstrual bleeding in younger females may be a factor contributing to iron deficiency. Anemia is most commonly reported as a complication of gastric bypass,[1] which is not surprising in view of the frequent development of anemia after partial gastrectomy.[48] Hines found anemia in about 50% of 292 patients from 1 to 20 years after partial gastrectomy.[48] The major cause of the anemia was iron deficiency in 63%, B_{12} deficiency in 33% and folate deficiency in 4%. However, many of the patients with iron or vitamin B_{12} deficiency also had folate deficiency. In the entire group, nearly 50% had a degree of iron deficiency, 26% folate deficiency and 20% vitamin B_{12} deficiency. Iron deficiency was explained by bypass of the duodenum, B_{12} deficiency by the gastrectomy with loss of intrinsic factor, and folate deficiency by a degree of malabsorption.

Gastric bypass bypasses the duodenum, where iron is normally absorbed. A degree of malabsorption might be anticipated with mild folate deficiency. However, the distal stomach is intact, although excluded, so vitamin B_{12} deficiency would not be expected. In fact, a deficiency of all three occurs after gastric bypass, as reported in an excellent study of 150 consecutive patients by Amaral and colleagues.[1] Anemia developed in 37% of the patients at a mean of 20 months after the operation, and women were more commonly affected than men. Iron deficiency occurred in 47%, vitamin B_{12} deficiency in 40% and RBC folate deficiency in 18%. Microcytic anemia developed in 18%, normocytic anemia in 12% and macrocytic anemia in 7%. Poor nutrition was thought to be a major factor in these results, related to small meals and intolerance to meat and dairy products. Although patients had been advised to take vitamins, compliance may have been poor since iron and folate levels were corrected by the oral route. Amaral reports that 95% of the B_{12}-deficient patients had a normal Schilling test, although others have reported abnormal Schilling tests and intrinsic factor deficiency after gastric bypass.[49,50] Folate deficiency is associated with alcoholism, pregnancy and malabsorption.[51] Amaral's patients were not pregnant and apparently not alcoholic. Malabsorption of a significant degree seemed excluded by the rapid response to oral folic acid. Other studies have not reported as much anemia as found in this study. However, anemia appears to be a common problem after gastric bypass. Vitamin and iron supplementation as well as lifetime follow-up are essential for these patients.

CALCIUM, MAGNESIUM AND ZINC

Deficiency of fat-soluble vitamins and metabolic bone disease were reported after jejunoileal bypass for morbid obesity,[52–54] likely as a consequence of malabsorption. The frequency of the problem has been disputed and may be related to the length of ileum in continuity.[55] Similar problems may occur as the result of malabsorption induced by biliopancreatic bypass. Vitamin D deficiency and metabolic bone disease may occur in patients with gross obesity who have not had any surgical treatment.[56] Osteomalacia is a known complication of gastrectomy, but it was reported to be relatively rare and responsive to vitamin D.[57] More recent reports indicate that as many as 25% of patients develop osteomalacia with bone pain and tenderness and increase in serum alkaline phosphatase on longterm follow-up after gastrectomy.[58] Malabsorption may be the explanation. In the absence of Paget's disease or disease of the liver and biliary tract, an increase in alkaline phosphatase usually indicates osteomalacia which is associated with an abnormal calcium infusion test and decreased plasma vitamin D activity.[59] Osteomalacia is important because of an increased risk of fractures. Treatment and prevention are possible with vitamin D.[59] So far vitamin D deficiency and osteomalacia have

not been reported after gastric bypass, and serum calcium remained normal in the study of Amaral and colleagues.[4] However, they reported that 34% of patients developed elevated alkaline phosphatase postoperatively and this remained elevated in 15%. They suggest the possibility of subclinical bone disease and recommend calcium and vitamin D supplements. Further studies including bone biopsies and longterm follow-up are necessary in this area. Since many gastroplasty patients are middle-aged females, osteoporosis is a risk which could be affected by calcium intake, changes in sex hormone levels and effect of decreased weight on weight-bearing bones.

Magnesium levels have been reported to be decreased 7 to 17 years after gastrectomy[60] and in some patients after gastric bypass.[9] No abnormality of magnesium was noted on shorter follow-up after gastric bypass for obesity.[4] Zinc deficiency can occur during prolonged starvation or parenteral nutrition and is associated with diarrhea, dermatitis and alopecia.[61] This problem has not been reported after gastroplasty, but could occur in patients with severe persistent vomiting and contribute to hair loss. A decrease in serum zinc and associated immunologic problems have been reported in untreated obese adolescents.[62]

ELECTROLYTES

No significant electrolyte abnormalities have been identified in the obese before or after operation, although Amaral[4] observed mild hypernatremia up to 18 months after gastric bypass, possibly as a result of dehydration from reduced fluid intake. The serum chloride also increased slightly after operation, and a small number of patients developed hypokalemia. In this study there was no change in serum creatinine. Halverson and associates[28] reported a higher frequency of hypokalemia in the first few months after gastric bypass. A variety of electrolyte abnormalities as well as dehydration may develop in patients with stomal obstruction and severe vomiting.

URIC ACID

Elevated uric acid is common in morbidly obese patients.[4] These values return to normal in most patients in the first year after gastric bypass, and in those with normal preoperative values a significant decrease also occurs. It may be possible to stop medication for gout after gastric bypass.[4]

MALNUTRITION AND IMMUNE RESPONSE

The degree of weight loss tolerated by our patients, especially active young men, is often astonishing. I have seen patients ranging from 300 to 400 lb (136 to 182 kg) lose as much as 50% of their preoperative weight in the first year after gastric bypass or vertical banded gastroplasty without apparent clinical or biochemical side-effects. On the other hand, some patients with severe vomiting and weight loss of 20% of body weight in the first 3 postoperative months may become anergic and face major complications if they require revision procedures or emergency surgery.[63] Such a patient with massive acute weight loss developed protein-calorie malnutrition with anergy and recurrent infections which resolved after parenteral nutrition.[64] Other factors which might have contributed to the patient's immunodeficiency were considered, including lack of vitamin A, pyridoxine, iron and zinc and the effects of infection and obesity on the immune response.

Most patients with weight loss of about 25% of body weight appear to have no significant change in skin-test responsiveness 6 months after gastric bypass.[63] A variety of other methods which might be used to assess malnutrition have been adapted from papers by Linn,[65] Dempsey,[66] and Pettigrew[67] and are listed in Table 28.3. Because of the massive depot of calories in the form of fat in these patients, percentage of weight loss may not mean as much as it does in patients of normal weight with acute or chronic illness. Skin-fold thickness is difficult to assess in obese patients even after significant weight loss. Physical examination of obese patients is also difficult, and hair loss in the early months after gastroplasty is common and usually not associated with other signs of malnutrition. This problem is discussed later.

Serum albumin does drop slightly but significantly for a few months after gastric bypass as do transferrin and blood urea nitrogen.[4] However, these are not associated with clinical problems in most patients. A reduction in albumin may be the most useful simple laboratory test in determining the presence of malnutrition in surgical patients.[67,68]

Lack of skin-test responsiveness to five standard antigens is termed anergy and is

TABLE 28.3. ASSESSMENT OF MALNUTRITION*

Clinical History
  Inadequate intake
  Excessive losses—vomiting, diarrhea, etc.
  Increased metabolic need—infection, pregnancy, etc.
  Catabolic medications—steroids, etc.

Anthropometric Data
  Percent weight loss
  Percent of ideal weight
  Skin-fold thickness

Exercise Data
  Exercise tolerance
  Grip strength

Physical Examination
  Cachexia
  Hair loss
  Hepatomegaly, ascites
  Muscle atrophy
  Edema
  Skin changes

Laboratory Tests
  Serum albumin
  Serum transferrin
  Hemoglobin
  Lymphocyte count
  Skin-testing

Special Tests
  K^{40} whole body counting
  Ratio of exchangeable sodium to potassium

*From Linn[65] and Dempsey et al.[66]

predictive of postoperative sepsis in surgical patients.[68,69] The relative roles of malnutrition and sepsis in producing anergy are still not clear. Malnutrition in developing countries is associated with impaired immune responsiveness.[70] Protein malnutrition in experimental animals is associated with susceptibility to infection when anergy occurs, but for reasons that are not clear some protein-deficient animals retain normal immunologic tests and resist infection.[71] In humans, anergy may be the result rather than the cause of sepsis and be corrected by abscess drainage or control of sepsis.[72] Obese patients may have some impairment of immune responsiveness even without operation,[62,73,74] but the meaning is not clear since postoperative infections and complications are relatively rare in many large series. Significant weight loss after gastric bypass seems to produce no change in skin-test responsiveness,[63] although immunosuppression may occur during the first 7 to 10 days after a wide variety of operations.[75] The recent partial biliopancreatic bypass caused no significant change in immunologic tests, while the earlier total biliopancreatic bypass which caused protein malabsorption was associated with severe immunosuppression which correlated with low serum albumin.[76]

Other methods of assessing malnutrition are more difficult. Blackburn[17] used total body potassium to show that body cell mass dropped in the first 3 months after gastric bypass but returned to near normal after 12 months. MacLean and co-workers[19] used a multiple isotope dilution test to determine total exchangeable sodium to potassium ratios which predicted malnutrition. Using a variety of gastroplasty procedures, often with a small stoma and high reoperation rate, the frequency of malnutrition was high. However, patients fed a 750 kcal balanced diet with supplemental vitamins did not develop malnutrition in spite of severe weight loss. After considering a wide variety of laboratory tests for assessment of malnutrition, several authors have concluded that careful clinical examination and good judgement are the best methods of determining malnutrition.[67,77] Patients with severe vomiting and rapid weight loss after gastroplasty need careful assessment and nutritional support prior to revision gastroplasty or elective surgery.

For patients who are malnourished, the best route for provision of protein, calories and vitamins is by mouth if possible. If the gastroplasty stoma is small, resulting in vomiting, it may be possible to pass a small feeding tube with the help of radiologists. Some have used routine placement of a gastrostomy[19] or jejunostomy[78] as a means of nutritional support when stomal obstruction occurs. These methods can cause extra complications, and most surgeons consider them unnecessary for routine gastroplasties. However, a gastrostomy can be very helpful for decompression and feeding after revision gastroplasty. I have fed one patient by gastrostomy for nearly one year after a particularly difficult revision gastroplasty. The stenotic stoma could not be dilated on repeated attempts but eventually it opened on its own. Good nutrition but adequate weight loss resulted from 750 kcal per day. When necessary, parenteral nutrition can help avoid postoperative complications.[79,80] It can be provided by peripheral intravenous or central venous routes, although venous access may be difficult in the morbidly obese.

In summary, malnutrition is relatively rare after gastroplasty and gastric bypass procedures despite substantial weight loss. For those with severe vomiting and low serum albumin, restoration of nutrition by the easiest route possible is essential before revision gastroplasty or elective surgery. Careful and regular follow-up and good dietary advice may help to avoid or allow early detection of most problems.

SPECIAL PROBLEMS

1. GALLSTONES

The development of gallstones after gastroplasty may be related to rapid weight loss with mobilization of fat and liberation of cholesterol and resulting increase in cholesterol saturation in the bile.[81,82] This is therefore a metabolic complication. Amaral[83] has reviewed the subject and found that anywhere from 14 to 45% of morbidly obese patients had a cholecystectomy prior to gastroplasty with an average of about 30%. Lithogenic bile[84,85] and poor gallbladder emptying[86] could be factors. Anywhere from 3 to 33% of patients may return for cholecystectomy during the first few years after gastric bypass. It is known that dieting and rapid weight loss alone may result in increased hepatic secretion of cholesterol and lithogenic bile.[87,88] Hepatic cholesterol secretion decreases when weight stabilizes. These results may explain why gallstones often occur early during rapid weight loss after gastroplasty. After gastric bypass, gallbladder stasis due to limited oral intake and bypass of the duodenum with lack of stimulation of cholecystokinin secretion could also be factors.[89] Stones which form may dissolve spontaneously when weight stabilizes or be prevented with chenodeoxycholic acid.[82] A variety of abdominal operations have been associated with the development of sludge in the gallbladder in the early postoperative course, although it often dissolves with time.[90] Routine cholecystectomy has been recommended at the time of gastroplasty because of the high frequency of developing symptomatic gallstones.[83] Acute cholecystitis or common duct stones were quite common. When routine cholecystectomy was performed, unsuspected cholesterolosis or gallstones were often found. Most would still not recommend routine cholecystectomy but careful preoperative ultrasound and operative palpation of the gallbladder are recommended, although it is still possible to miss small stones in large patients. Careful assessment for gallstones is recommended if postoperative epigastric or right upper quadrant pain develops.

2. HAIR LOSS

It is a common observation that hair loss occurs during the first 6 months after gastroplasty. The frequency may be as high as 50 to 75%.[4,91] Possible explanations include lack of protein, vitamin A or zinc.[2] This problem has also been observed during crash diets[92] and has been termed "telogen effluvium."[93] It may occur after a variety of events such as childbirth, prolonged surgery or anesthesia, severe febrile illness, acute physical or emotional trauma or as a result of various drugs.[92] The cause may simply be severe caloric restriction which affects the hair matrix where there is normally high cell turnover. Hair loss rarely results in baldness and seems unrelated to other postoperative complications. It is well tolerated as long as patients are warned that it may occur and reassured if it does occur.

3. PREGNANCY

Deitel has reviewed obstetric and gynecologic changes later in this book. We have found that there are substantial changes in sex hormones after gastroplasty and weight loss, with return of regular periods in many women.[94,95] The result is a return of ovulation with an increased chance of pregnancy. Pregnancy early after gastroplasty may be particularly hazardous to mother and child because of rapid weight loss and poor nutrition at this time. Women, even those with infertility problems, must be warned about the possibility of pregnancy and take appropriate precautions during the first year after gastroplasty. Pregnancy after this time has been uncomplicated in our experience and an extra benefit of weight loss to the previously infertile and obese woman.

4. CHILDREN

In general, children should not have a gastroplasty or gastric bypass because of potential effects on growth and development.[20] Most patients should be 18 or older to be considered for gastroplasty, although the rare younger child with extreme and persistent obesity may be a candidate. The exception may be children with the Prader-Willi syndrome,[96] which is associated with continuous hunger, severe obesity, short stature, cryptorchidism, mental retardation, and short lifespan.[20,96] Gastroplasty may control weight gain and prolong life.

5. GUT HORMONES

The system of gut hormones is complex, expanding and of great physiologic interest, but so far they have been of little practical importance in surgical practice. Studies of gut hormones after jejunoileal bypass showed no change in cholecystokinin[97] although it has been postulated to be important in appetite regulation. Other gut hormones were altered, depending on the portion of bowel bypassed.[98] After gastroplasty, basal gastrin and pancreatic polypeptide (PP) were unchanged but PP response to a meal was decreased.[99] Gastrointestinal polypeptide response to a meal may also be decreased after gastroplasty.[100] Other studies have confirmed a decrease in PP response to meals after gastric bypass, while fasting enteroglucagon was unchanged but increased after meals.[101] The significance of these changes is uncertain. Study of peptide hormones may help to clarify eventually some of the complex mechanisms involved in regulation of appetite (see Chapter 4).

6. THE LIVER IN OBESITY

The presence of excessive fat in the livers of the morbidly obese and the correction of this problem by weight loss has been reviewed under lipids.

7. DUMPING

Late dumping due to hypoglycemia occurs in some patients with a gastric bypass following ingestion of sugar. This may be more severe a few months after operation as the gastroenterostomy stoma enlarges. It may be a beneficial side-effect in discouraging intake of sweet foods.[30] This problem is reviewed under carbohydrates.

8. PINK URINE

Deitel and associates[102] have observed that some patients pass pink urine early after gastroplasty for morbid obesity. This appears to be due to uric acid crystals in urinary sediment. Many patients have an increased preoperative uric acid which drops early after gastroplasty with an increase in urinary uric acid. The pink urine was related to high urine osmolality and low urinary pH. This problem resolves in a few days and does not produce symptoms.

9. TOLERANCE TO COLD

Many formerly obese patients complain of poor cold tolerance after profound weight loss. This is a particular problem for those of us who live in Canada. There may be metabolic reasons for this observation but loss of insulation is the likely explanation. Wilmore[103] refers to lipid as "endogenous thermal underwear." Improved heat tolerance after profound weight loss may be an advantage in warm climates.

SUMMARY

Most metabolic changes after gastroplasty or gastric bypass are beneficial rather than harmful. For most patients, the postoperative course is surprisingly uneventful in spite of profound weight loss. Problems are usually prevented by careful patient selection and instruction and close postoperative follow-up. Severe vomiting requires prompt assessment and treatment. All gastroplasty patients require adequate protein intake and vitamin supplementation. Gastric bypass is particularly likely to be followed by iron, vitamin B_{12} and folate deficiency and resultant anemia. Late skeletal changes may also follow gastric bypass. Longterm surveillance of all gastroplasty patients is strongly recommended.

REFERENCES

1. Amaral JF, Thompson WR, Caldwell MD, et al: Prospective hematologic evaluation of gastric exclusion surgery for morbid obesity. Ann Surg 201:186–192, 1985.
2. Coughlin K, Bell RM, Bivins BA, et al: Preoperative and postoperative assessment of nutrient intakes in patients who have undergone gastric bypass surgery. Arch Surg 118:813–816, 1983.
3. Brown EK, Settle EA, van Rij AM: Food intake patterns of gastric bypass patients. J Am Diet Assoc 80:437–443, 1982.
4. Amaral JF, Thompson WR, Caldwell MD, et al.: Prospective metabolic evaluation of 150 consecutive patients who underwent gastric exclusion. Am J Surg 147:468–476, 1984.
5. Levenson SM, Crowley LV, Seifter E: Starvation. In Ballinger WF, Collins JA, Drucker WR (eds): Manual of Surgical Nutrition. Philadelphia, WB Saunders, 1975.
6. Garrow JS: Treat Obesity Seriously. London, Churchill Livingstone, 1981.
7. Cahill GF: Starvation in man. N Engl J Med 282:668–675, 1970.
8. Millikan WJ, Henderson JM, Warren WD, et al: Maintenance of nutritional competence after gastric partitioning for morbid obesity. Am J Surg 146:619–625, 1983.
9. Halverson JD: Metabolic sequelae of gastric restrictive operations. Proc Am Soc Bar Surg 1:113–121, 1984.
10. Millar WJ, Wigle DT: Socioeconomic disparities in risk factors for cardiovascular disease. Can Med Assoc J 134:127–132, 1986.
11. Hall JC, Veale B, Horne K, et al: The nutritional knowledge scores of morbidly obese patients selected for gastric bypass surgery. Int J Obesity 8:123–128, 1984.
12. Halverson JD, Koehler RE: Gastric bypass: analysis of weight loss and factors determining success. Surgery 90:446–455, 1981.
13. Printen KJ, Mason EE: Gastric bypass for morbid obesity in patients more than fifty years of age. Surg Gynecol Obstet 144:192–194, 1977.
14. Feurer JD, Crosby LO, Buzby GP, et al: Resting energy expenditure in morbid obesity. Ann Surg 197:17–21, 1983.
15. Tsoi CM, Westenskow DR, Moody FG: Weight loss and metabolic changes in morbidly obese patients after gastric partitioning operation. Surgery 96:545–548, 1984.
16. Bothe A Jr, Bistrian BR, Greenberg I, et al: Energy regulation in morbid obesity by multidisciplinary therapy. Surg Clin North Am 59:1017–1031, 1979.
17. Palombo JD, Malestaskos CJ, Reinhold RW, et al: Composition of weight loss in morbidly obese patients after gastric bypass. J Surg Res 30:435–442, 1981.
18. MacLean LD, Rhode BM, Shizgal HM: Gastroplasty for obesity. Surg Gynecol Obstet 153:200–208, 1981.
19. MacLean LD, Rhode BM, Shizgal HM: Nutrition following gastric operations for morbid obesity. Ann Surg 198:347–355, 1983.
20. Mason EE: Surgical Treatment of Obesity. Philadelphia, WB Saunders, 1981.
21. Gleysteen JJ, Barboriak JJ: Improvement in heart disease risk factors after gastric bypass. Arch Surg 118:681–684, 1983.
22. Gonen B, Halverson JD, Schonfeld G: Lipoprotein levels in morbidly obese patients with massive surgically-induced weight loss. Metabolism 32:492–496, 1983.
23. Rucker RD, Goldenberg F, Varco RL, et al: Lipid effects of obesity operations. J Surg Res 30:229–235, 1981.
24. Gianetta E, Friedman D, Adami GF, et al: Effect of biliopancreatic bypass on hypercholesterolemia and hypertriglyceridemia. Proc Am Soc Bar Surg 2:138–142, 1985.
25. Andersen T, Gluud C: Liver morphology in morbid obesity: a literature study. Int J Obesity 8:97–106, 1984.
26. Braillon A, Capron JP, Herve MA, et al: Liver in obesity. Gut 26:133–139, 1985.
27. Anderson T, Christoffersen P, Gluud C: The liver in consecutive patients with morbid obesity: a clinical, morphological, and biochemical study. Int J Obesity 8:107–115, 1984.

28. Halverson JD, Zuckerman GR, Koehler RE, et al: Gastric bypass for morbid obesity: a medical-surgical assessment. Ann Surg 194:152–160, 1981.

29. Hamilton DL, Vest TK, Brown BS, et al: Liver injury with alcoholic-like hyalin after gastroplasty for morbid obesity. Gastroenterology 85:722–726, 1983.

30. Sugerman HJ, Starkey JV, Birkenhauer R: A randomized prospective trial of gastric bypass vs vertical banded gastroplasty for morbid obesity and their effects on sweets vs non-sweets eaters. Ann Surg 205:613–624, 1987.

31. Hughes TA, Gwynne JT, Switzer BR, et al: Effects of caloric restriction and weight loss on glycemic control, insulin release and resistance and atherosclerotic risk in obese patients with type II diabetes mellitus. Am J Med 77:7–17, 1984.

32. Halverson JD, Kramer J, Cave A, et al: Altered glucose tolerance, insulin response, and insulin sensitivity after massive weight reduction subsequent to gastric bypass. Surgery 92:235–240, 1982.

33. Herbst CA, Hughes TA, Gwynne JT, et al: Gastric bariatric operation in insulin-treated adults. Surgery 95:209–214, 1984.

34. Denny-Brown D: Neurologic conditions resulting from prolonged and severe dietary restriction. Medicine (Baltimore) 26:41–113, 1947.

35. Drenick EJ, Joven CB, Swendseid ME: Occurrence of acute Wernicke's encephalopathy following prolonged starvation for the treatment of obesity. N Engl J Med 274:937–939, 1966.

36. Nanji AA, Freeman JB: Gastric bypass surgery in mobidly obese patients markedly decreases serum levels of vitamins A and C and iron in the perioperative period. Int J Obesity 9:177–179, 1985.

37. Villar H, Ranne RD: Neurological deficit following gastric partitioning: possible role of thiamine. JPEN 8:575–578, 1984.

38. Haid RW, Gutmann L, Crosby TW: Wernicke-Korsakoff encephalopathy after gastric plication. JAMA 247:2566–2567, 1982.

39. Rothrock JF, Smith MS: Wernicke's disease complicating surgical therapy for morbid obesity. J Clin Neuro Ophthalmol 1:195–199, 1981.

40. MacLean JB: Wernicke's encephalopathy after gastric plication (letter). JAMA 248:1311, 1982.

41. Gardner TW, Rao K, Poticha S, et al: Acute visual loss after gastroplasty. Am J Ophthalmol 93:658–660, 1982.

42. Maryniak O: Severe peripheral neuropathy following gastric bypass for morbid obesity. Can Med Assoc J 131:119–120, 1984.

43. Printen KJ, Mason EE: Peripheral neuropathy following gastric bypass for the treatment of morbid obesity. Obesity/Bariatric Med 6:185–187, 1977.

44. Feit H, Glasberg M, Ireton C, et al: Peripheral neuropathy and starvation after gastric partitioning for morbid obesity. Ann Intern Med 96:453–455, 1982.

45. Oczkowski WJ, Kertesz A: Wernicke's encephalopathy after gastroplasty for morbid obesity. Neurology 35:99–101, 1985.

46. Reuler JB: Wernicke's encephalopathy. N Engl J Med 312:1035–1039, 1985.

47. Grace DM: Meralgia paresthetica as a cause of severe hip pain after gastroplasty for morbid obesity. Can J Surg. 30:64–65, 1987.

48. Hines JD, Hoffbrand AV, Mollin DL: The hematological complications following partial gastrectomy: a study of 292 patients. Am J Med 43:555–569 1967.

49. Crowley LV, Olson RW: Megaloblastic anemia after gastric bypass for obesity. Am J Gastroenterol 78:406–410, 1983.

50. Marcuard SP, Sinar DR, Mulheim HD, et al: Absence of intrinsic factor after gastric bypass for morbid obesity (abstract). Gastroenterology 90:1533, 1986.

51. Antonenko DR: Vitamins and minerals. In Kirkpatrick JR (ed): Nutrition and Metabolism in the Surgical Patient. Mount Kisco, NY, Futura, 1983.

52. Rogers EL, Douglass W, Russell RM, et al: Deficiency of fat-soluble vitamins after jejunoileal bypass surgery for morbid obesity. Am J Clin Nutr 33:1208–1214, 1980.

53. Compston JE, Laker MF, Woodhead JS, et al: Bone disease after jejunoileal bypass for obesity. Lancet 2:1–4, 1978.

54. Parfitt AM, Miller MJ, Frame B, et al: Metabolic bone disease after intestinal bypass for treatment of obesity. Ann Intern Med 89:193–199, 1978.

55. Sellin JH, Meredith SC, Kelly S, et al: Prospective evaluation of metabolic bone disease after jejunoileal bypass. Gastroenterology 87:123–129, 1984.

56. Compston JE, Vedi S, Ledger JE, et al: Vitamin D status and bone histomorphometry in gross obesity. Am J Clin Nutr 34:2359–2363,1981.

57. Morgan DB, Paterson CR, Woods CG, et al: Osteomalacia after gastrectomy: a response to very small doses of vitamin D. Lancet 2:1089–1091, 1965.

58. Eddy RL: Metabolic bone disease after gastrectomy. Am J Med 50:442–450, 1971.

59. Thompson GR, Watts JM, Neale G, et al: Detection of vitamin D deficiency after partial gastrectomy. Lancet 1:623–626, 1966.

60. Tougaard L, Ricker H, Rodbro P, et al: Bone composition and vitamin D after Polya gastrectomy. Acta Med Scand 202:47–50, 1977.

61. Kay RG, Tasman-Jones C, Pybus J, et al: A syndrome of acute zinc deficiency during total parenteral alimentation in man. Ann Surg 183:331–340, 1976.

62. Chandra RK, Kutty KM: Immunocompetence in obesity. Acta Paediatr Scand 69:25–30, 1980.

63. Grace DM, Harle IA, Rycroft KM, et al: Immune response after gastric bypass and weight loss. Can J Surg 29:284–286, 1986.

64. Bromberg-Schneider S, Erikson N, Gebel HM, et al: Cutaneous anergy and marrow suppression as complications of gastroplasty for morbid obesity. Surgery 94:109–111, 1983.

65. Linn BS: A protein energy malnutrition scale (PEMS). Ann Surg 200:747–752, 1984.

66. Dempsey DT, Buzby GP, Mullen JL: Patient assessment for nutritional support. In Kirkpatrick JR (ed): Nutrition and Metabolism in the Surgical Patient. Mount Kisco, NY, Futura, 1983.

67. Pettigrew RA, Hill GL: Indicators of surgical risk and clinical judgement. Br J Surg 73:47–51, 1986.

68. Christou NV, Rode H, Larsen D: The walk-in anergic patient. Ann Surg 199:438–444, 1984.

69. Christou NV, Meakins JL, MacLean LD: The predictive role of delayed hypersensitivity in preoperative patients. Surg Gynecol Obstet 152:297–301, 1981.

70. Gross RL, Newberne PM: Role of nutrition in immunologic functions. Physiol Rev 60:188–302, 1980.

71. Ing AF, Meakins JL, McLean APH, et al: Determinants of susceptibility to sepsis and mortality: malnutrition vs. anergy. J Surg Res 32:249–255, 1982.

72. Pietsch JB, Meakins JL, MacLean LD: The delayed hypersensitivity response in clinical surgery. Surgery 85:496–503, 1979.

73. Krishnan EC, Frost L, Aarons S, et al: Study of function and maturation of monocytes in morbidly obese individuals. J Surg Res 33:89–97, 1982.

74. Kolterman OG, Olefsky JM, Kurahara C, et al: A defect in cell-mediated immune function in insulin-resistant diabetic and obese subjects. J Lab Clin Med 96:535–543, 1980.

75. Riboli EB, Terrizzi A, Arnulfo G, et al: Immunosuppressive effect of surgery evaluated by the multitest cell-mediated immunity system. Can J Surg 27:60–63, 1984.

76. Adami GF, Civalleri D, Gianetta E, et al: In vitro evaluation of immunological status after biliopancreatic bypass for obesity. Int J Obesity 9:171–175, 1985.

77. Ottow TR, Bruining HA, Jeekel J: Clinical judgement versus delayed hypersensitivity skin testing for the prediction of postoperative sepsis and mortality. Surg Gynecol Obstet 159:475–477, 1984.

78. Freeman JB, Burchett H: Failure rate with gastric partitioning for morbid obesity. Am J Surg 145:113–117, 1983.

79. Starker PM, LaSala PA, Askanazi J: The influence of preoperative total parenteral nutrition upon morbidity and mortality. Surg Gynecol Obstet 162:569–574, 1986.

80. Ferrara J, Fabri PJ, Carey LC: Total parenteral nutrition in the treatment of complications following surgery for morbid obesity. JPEN 6:140–142, 1982.

81. Deitel M, Petrov I: Incidence of symptomatic gallstones after bariatric surgery. Surg Gynecol Obstet 164:549–552, 1987.

82. Whiting MJ, Hall JC, Iannos J, et al: The cholesterol saturation of bile and its reduction by chenodeoxycholic acid in massively obese patients. Int J Obesity 8:681–688, 1984.

83. Amaral JF, Thompson WR: Gallbladder disease in the morbidly obese. Am J Surg 149:551–557, 1985.

84. Freeman JB, Meyer PD, Printen KJ, et al: Analysis of gallbladder bile in morbid obesity. Am J Surg 129:163–166, 1975.

85. Mabee TM, Meyer P, DenBesten L, et al: The mechanism of increased gallstone formation in obese human subjects. Surgery 79:460–468, 1976.

86. Vezina WC, Paradis RL, Grace DM, et al: Increased volume and impaired emptying of the gallbladder in morbid obesity: a mechanical explanation for the increased risk of cholelithiasis. Proc Am Soc Bar Surg. 3:119–136, 1986.

87. Bennion LJ, Grundy SM: Effects of obesity and caloric intake on biliary lipid metabolism in man. J Clin Invest 56:996–1011, 1975.

88. Schreibman P, Pertsemlidis G, Liu CK, et al: Lithogenic bile: a consequence of weight reduction. J Clin Invest 53:72A, 1975.

89. Wattchow DA, Hall JC, Whiting MJ, et al: Prevalence and treatment of gallstones after gastric bypass surgery for morbid obesity. Br Med J 286:763, 1983.

90. Bolondi L, Gaiani S, Testa S, et al: Gallbladder sludge formation during prolonged fasting after gastrointestinal tract surgery. Gut 26:734–738, 1985.

91. Knecht BH: Experience with gastric bypass for massive obesity. Am Surg 44:496–504, 1978.

92. Goette DK, Odom RB: Alopecia in crash dieters. JAMA 235:2622–2623, 1976.

93. Kligman AM: Pathologic dynamics of human hair loss. I. Telogen effluvium. Arch Dermatol 83:175–198, 1961.

94. Grace DM, Nisker JA, Hammond GL: Changes in menstrual cycle pattern and sex hormone binding after gastroplasty. Proc Am Soc Bar Surg 2:59–60, 1985.

95. Grace DM: Endocrine changes in obesity, correction by weight loss. Bariatric Surgery 4(3):4–5, 1986.

96. Touquet VLR, Ward MWN, Clark CG: Obesity surgery in a patient with Prader-Willi syndrome. Br J Surg 70:180–186, 1983.

97. Burhol PG, Jenssen TG, Jorde R, et al: Plasma cholecystokinin (CCK) befre and after a jejunoileal bypass operation in obese patients with reference to appetite regulation. Int J Obesity 8:233–236, 1984.

98. Sarson DL, Scopinaro N, Bloom SR: Gut hormone changes after jejunoileal (JIB) or biliopancreatic (BPB) bypass surgery for morbid obesity. Int J Obesity 5:471–480, 1981.

99. Shulkes A, Allen RDM, Hardy KJ: Meal stimulated gastrin and pancreatic polypeptide levels before and after partial gastric transection for morbid obesity. Aust NZ J Med 12:27–30, 1982.

100. Amland PF, Jorde R, Giercksky KE, et al: Diurnal GIP, PP and insulin levels in morbid obesity before and after stapled gastric partitioning with gastro-gastrostomy. Int J Obesity 8:117–122, 1984.

101. Mervyn S, Stein D, Straus EW: Pancreatic polypeptide, pancreatic glucagon and entroglucagon in morbid obesity following gastric bypass operation. Int J Obesity 10:37–42, 1986.

102. Deitel M, Thompson DA, Saldanha CF, et al: "Pink urine" in morbidly obese patients following gastric partitioning. Can Med Assoc J 130:1007–1011, 1984.

103. Wilmore DW: Fat metabolism. In Ballinger WF, Collins JA, Drucker WR, et al (eds): Manual of Surgical Nutrition. Philadelphia, WB Saunders, 1975.

29

Psychological Sequelae of Surgical Procedures for Obesity

PAULINE S. POWERS
ALEXANDER S. ROSEMURGY

INTRODUCTION

METHODOLOGICAL ISSUES

The psychological impact of the various bariatric procedures has been addressed in several studies, but interpretation of the results has been hampered by serious conceptual and methodological problems. One major problem has been that different surgical procedures have been studied, including the gastric bypass, the horizontal gastroplasty, the currently fashionable vertical banded gastroplasty and the now outmoded jejunoileal bypass. It seems likely that these radically different procedures (and perhaps modifications of the major types) might have very different effects on psychological, psychosocial, and behavioral functioning.

A second important problem is related to the issue of drop-outs; in every treatment thus far devised for obesity, the drop-out rate has been high, usually over 30 to 40%. Although many follow-up studies of bariatric surgery do not report the percent of patients who are lost to follow-up (in itself a serious methodological flaw), most of those that do have found a significant drop-out rate. In a four-year postoperative follow-up of 119 patients who had horizontal gastroplasty, Freeman and Burchett[1] found a 31% drop-out rate. In a later report from the same team,[2] 8 of 56 patients (14.3%) who had vertical banded gastroplasty had been lost to follow-up by 18 months postoperatively. Although it cannot be certain that the patients lost to follow-up have failed to lose significant weight, it is the most likely and most conservative explanation. In a study of patients who had the jejunoileal bypass, reported by Castelnuovo-Tedesco et al,[3] patients who did not return for follow-up had a less successful outcome than those who did return for follow-up. Freeman and Burchett[1] provide "circumstantial evidence" that patients who drop out fail to lose clinically significant amounts of weight. If the patients who are lost to follow-up have failed to lose weight, this may have significant psychological ramifications. As a group, the morbidly obese have experienced repeated failures and generally have internalized the censorious attitudes society has toward obese individuals who fail to lose weight; another failure at a weight loss attempt undoubtedly further lowers self-esteem.

Mason, at the University of Iowa, the orig-inator of the gastric bypass procedure, who is now studying the vertical banded gastroplasty, states that only 8% of their patients have been lost to follow-up.[4] However, the experience and dedication of the team led by Mason should not be underestimated: not only are the criteria for selection of patients much more rigorous[5] than at most other centers, but the perseverance in studying long-term outcome and the scientific acumen of this group outstrip most other centers.

CONCEPTUAL ISSUES

There are three general trends in the study of psychological factors in bariatric surgery. The first, and perhaps most important, has been an attempt to identify psychological, social or behavioral traits that might predict a successful outcome, in terms of both clinically significant weight loss and the absence of surgical, medical or psychiatric complications. The second general area of research has been an attempt to identify both positive and negative changes in psychosocial functioning post-surgery, including the emergence or suppression of major psychiatric syndromes (such as the affective disorders or various psychotic conditions) and changes in personality characteristics, self-esteem, body image, and marital and family relationships. A third general theme of the psychological studies is the evaluation of changes in eating and exercise patterns. Since compliance with post-surgical dietary constraints is crucial for successful weight loss and weight maintenance, an improved understanding of the physiological and psychological parameters which mediate eating and exercise patterns is necessary.

PREDICTIVE PSYCHOLOGICAL FACTORS

Clear-cut psychiatric contraindications to bariatric surgery are few but include alcoholism and currently active psychotic conditions (schizophrenia, psychotic depression and mania). There is also general agreement that patients with grossly unrealistic expectations of the surgery or with very chaotic lifestyles should be excluded. However, the more subtle psychological criteria for identifying patients likely to succeed have yet to be widely studied.

Mason,[5] Solow[6] and Wise et al[7] have suggested that the major predictor of an unto-ward psychiatric outcome is an unsuccessful weight loss; it is unclear in these studies if the unsuccessful weight loss and psychiatric complications are related to each other or to a third unknown variable. Leon and colleagues[8] found that amongst patients who have failed to lose a significant amount of weight following the jejunoileal bypass, a large proportion had severe psychological and medical problems; in the entire study, one-eighth of the patients had had severe psychological complications. This study leaves unanswered the question of whether the medical and psychological complications were etiologically related.

An interesting study by Valley[9] addresses this issue of the relationship between medical and psychiatric complications. She studied 57 morbidly obese patients prior to surgery and one year postoperatively. Preoperatively, patients had a psychiatric evaluation including evaluation of the quality of their social support system; an MMPI (Minnesota Multiphasic Personality Inventory) was also administered. This study found that both medical and psychological complications were highly correlated with a history of preoperative in-patient psychiatric hospitalization. Of the 41 patients with no in-patient psychiatric history, 33 had no complications; there were 6 medical and 4 psychiatric complications among the remaining 8 patients. In contrast, 2 of the 16 patients with a prior history of psychiatric hospitalization had no complications; among the other 14 patients there were 12 medical complications and 9 psychiatric complications. In addition, elevated scores on the MMPI (T score above 70) were significantly correlated with complications. Poor social support and negative life events were also correlated with complications. In all, 44% of the variance in medical complications and 31% of the variance in psychiatric complications were accounted for by in-patient psychiatic history, elevated MMPI scores, poor preoperative social support systems and negative postoperative life events. This author proposes that the key to the development of both medical and psychological complications is related to the extent of preoperative psychopathology. The major flaw of this study is that follow-up was only one year.

Olsson et al[10] studied 29 obese subjects preoperatively and for 18 months postoperatively. Preoperatively, patients were interviewed and given two personality tests: the Meta Contrast Technique and the Rod and Frame Test. Neither of these tests is in wide clinical use and we know of no other study of morbid obese patients using these tests. The authors found that less successful patients had more signs of denial and sensitivity and social phobia than patients who lost more weight and maintained the loss at 18 months. Furthermore, the less successful patients were younger and had higher levels of alcohol consumption.

In another attempt to identify factors that might predict successful outcome, Duckro et al[11] studied 199 female candidates for the gastric bypass procedure. The MMPI was administered and three psychologically similar sub-groups were identified. The first sub-group was essentially similar to the normal population. The second sub-group had neurotic traits with high scores on the Depression and Social Introversion scales and slightly elevated scores on the Hysteria and Hypochondriacal scales of the MMPI. The third sub-group had elevated scores on the Psychopathy, Schizophrenia, and Hypomanic scales; this group would be expected to be angry and express anger directly or indirectly and blame emotional stresses on others. The usefulness of these three profiles in predicting outcome has yet to be determined but does represent an improvement over some other studies in several ways. First, the authors assume that the morbidly obese represent a psychologically heterogeneous group and, second, there were a large number of subjects studied preoperatively.

In summary, attempts to identify psychological factors associated with poor weight loss or medical or psychological complications are still in the beginning phases. In addition to the currently agreed upon psychiatric contraindications (acute psychosis or alcoholism), patients with a prior history of in-patient psychiatric care or inadequate social support systems should probably not have the surgery. Elevated scores on the MMPI and unrealistic expectations of the surgery (especially related to anticipated social and psychological consequences of weight loss) are both relative contraindications to the surgery. These patients should be referred for preoperative psychotherapy, probably of lengthy duration. More subtle psychological contraindications to the surgery have yet to be firmly established.

EFFECTS ON PSYCHOSOCIAL FUNCTIONING

The second group of studies of psychosocial aspects of bariatric surgery focus on the positive and negative changes after surgery. These include development of major psychiatric disorders, personality changes, changes in self-esteem, body image and work capacity and effects on marriages.

MAJOR PSYCHIATRIC DISORDERS

Although there is the general impression that relatively few patients develop major psychiatric disorders after either intestinal[12] or gastric bypass surgery or gastroplasty,[13] there are some reasons to question this conclusion. Since different centers use different psychological exclusion criteria and provide widely variable psychiatric follow-up (from none to life-long), comparison of studies is difficult. Furthermore, the nature of the psychiatric assessment at follow-up varies from anecdotal or self-report by mail questionnaire[14] to careful, lengthy postoperative evaluation,[15] using strict DSM III criteria.[16]

Solow and colleagues[12] studied 29 patients following intestinal bypass and state that none developed substitute psychiatric symptoms. On the other hand, Abram and colleagues[17] found that 24% of the patients they studied following intestinal bypass developed psychiatric problems, including an increase in neurotic symptoms and personal problems or a psychosis. In a study of 21 patients who had had the intestinal bypass, Rigden and Hagen[18] found that half had significant postoperative psychological problems as judged by need for postoperative psychiatric care, antidepressants or self-report of increased unhappiness following the surgery. In this study, 20% of the patients had had psychiatric care prior to surgery.

Studies of psychiatric sequelae of gastric bypass have generally found a very low incidence of major psychiatric disorders postoperatively.[15,19] In a report by Bull et al[13] of 114 gastric surgery patients (either gastric bypass or gastroplasty), they imply that there is no increase in need for psychiatric treatment postoperatively because the vast majority of patients reported no formal contact with psychiatry, either on an in-patient or out-patient basis. However, patients were not formally evaluated by a clinician and consequently it may be that psychiatric treatment was needed but not sought. In the preliminary analysis of 40 patients followed up to one and one-half years at the University of South Florida who have undergone gastroplasty, five have failed to return for either surgical or psychiatric fol-

low-up and more than one-third have failed to return for formal psychiatric follow-up. Of those who have returned, two have required psychiatric in-patient hospitalization for depression and several more have required outpatient psychiatric intervention.

PERSONALITY AND SELF-ESTEEM CHANGES AFTER SURGERY

Several studies have assessed possible changes in personality after surgery. The most common psychological test used has been the MMPI. Bull et al[13] compared a group of 50 patients prior to gastric surgery to 19 "obese" controls and 34 normal-weight controls. The MMPI scores of all three groups were within clinically normal limits (i.e. less than 70 T Scores), although the gastric surgery patients had significantly lower self-esteem scores and slightly higher scores on the Hypochondriasis, Psychopathic deviate and Schizophrenia scales compared to normal-weight controls. The MMPI was readministered to the gastric surgery patients during the follow-up period at one year or longer; no significant changes were found between the average pre- and postoperative MMPI scores.

Leon and her colleagues[8] studied personality changes in 48 patients (42 females and 6 males) who had the jejunoileal bypass procedures, by administering the MMPI preoperatively and at 1 year postoperatively. They also administered the Semantic Differential Test preoperatively and at 3 months, 6 months and 1 year; this test includes a portion in which the patient is asked to rate "My Personality Right Now" by choosing a rating between 0 and 10 (10, the most positive) for certain dimensions (e.g. "shy-outgoing" or "hateful-lovable"). The mean preoperative MMPI scores were within the clinically normal range, although there were elevations on the Paranoia, Hysteria, and Depression scales (the so-called Pa-Hy-D configuration). At the one-year follow-up, 35 of 48 original subjects were given the MMPI again and there were statistically significant improvements on the Social Interversion scale, the ES scale (a measure of self-esteem) and the Depression scale. Two special sub-scales of the MMPI, the MacAndrews Addiction Scale (MAC) and the Overcontrolled Hostility Scale, were also scored on the pre- and postoperative MMPI and no differences were found; the MAC at both time-periods was just below the addiction cut-off score of 24; the preoperative score was 23.58 and the postoperative score was 23.87. The mean Semantic Differential ratings showed significant changes, all in a positive direction. For example, there were improvements in the ratings of the unpopular-popular" scale, the "weak-powerful" scale and the "inactive-active" scale.

Gentry and colleagues[20] studied the self-esteem of 33 morbidly obese patients using the Clinical Analysis Questionnaire (which includes some of the MMPI scales), an index of self-esteem and an optimism/pessimism scale. Patients were followed for 2 years. On the Clinical Analysis Questionnaire, the profile preoperatively was no different than the general population and there were no statistical differences between mean sub-scales pre- and postoperatively. All patients demonstrated low self-esteem on the self-esteem index prior to surgery, and there was no improvement at follow-up despite marked weight loss in most patients. Despite this finding, patients had high levels of optimism, although the level of optimism did not correlate with weight loss.

BODY IMAGE CHANGES

Since the classic studies of Stunkard and colleagues,[21,22] it has been known that many patients with severe obesity often have disturbances in body image and that those patients whose obesity is the most refractory to treatment are the most likely to have these disturbances. Body image is analogous to an inner mental blueprint of one's appearance and the associated attitudes toward that appearance. All the senses contribute to the perceptual aspect of body image but the tactile and kinesthetic senses seem to be the most important. Early interpersonal experiences, especially within the family, contribute to the development of body image. Cultural attitudes toward size and shape are important, particularly in the adolescent years. Stunkard has postulated that the body image is "imprinted" in adolescence and becomes relatively impervious to change after the teenage years. Since many morbidly obese patients have been obese since childhood and through their adolescent years and frequently have been castigated by their peers, the general culture and often their own families because of their obesity, it is not surprising that body image disturbances are so common among this group. The traditional method of dieting has generally not been associated with improvement of body image among the morbidly obese. The question of whether bariatric surgery and subsequent larger more clinically significant weight losses are associated with an improvement in body image has been studied by only a few groups of researchers.

Leon et al[8] studied both the perceptual and attitudinal aspects of body image preoperatively and for one year during a follow-up of 48 patients after jejunoileal bypass; 13 of the original 48 patients were lost to follow-up. They used a Semantic Differential scale entitled "My Body Right Now" to assess possible changes in the attitudinal aspect of body image. The test consists of 16 word pairs such as "fat-thin," "ugly-beautiful," "massive-fragile," "flabby-firm;" the patient chooses from a scale of 1–10 that best describes himself or herself on each word pair. The test was administered preoperatively and at 3 months, 6 months and one year following surgery. Thirteen of the 16 ratings changed after surgery in a more positive attitude. This group of investigators also used the Body Perception Test (BPT) to assess the perceptual aspects of body image preoperatively, at 6 months and one year postoperatively. The BPT, devised by Slade and Russell,[23] is a black wooden screen on which two metal rods can be moved back and forth by the experimenter. The subject is asked to indicate the distance between the rods which is equivalent to the widths of various body parts including face (from temple to temple), chest (armpit to armpit), waist, hips at the widest point, arm length, foot width, and body depth (the greatest depth from front to back of the body below the waist). Following these estimates, the actual sizes of these parts are determined by measurement with a caliper. At all time periods, there was a tendency to overestimate all body dimensions except foot and arm and there was no improvement at either follow-up evaluation.

EFFECTS ON MARRIAGE AND EMPLOYMENT

There are conflicting reports on the effects of surgery on marital adjustment. Neill and colleagues[24] followed 14 patients following jejunoileal bypass and reported that 9 had a poor marital outcome. One of the defects of this study was that it was retrospective in that patients were not evaluated preoperatively. Rand et al[25] studied consecutive married patients prior to jejunoileal bypass and initially evaluated their marriages 3 years postoperatively. Eight of 29 patients reported marital deterioration and six of these marriages eventually ended in divorce; 13 patients reported improvement in their marriage and eight described no change. The same group[26] studied 14 married patients and 13 of their spouses 5 years postoperatively; these married patients had rated their marriages good at the 3-year follow-up. They found that 13 patients and 11 spouses reported more positive attitudes and 12 patients and their spouses noted greater self-confidence; 11 patients and 8 spouses reported improved sexual relationships.

Williams and Jarvie[14] followed 92 patients who had had a vertical banded gastroplasty by sending them mail questionnaires at 6 months, 12 months and 18 months post-surgery. Eighty patients (87%) responded. Among the respondents, 20% reported their marriages greatly improved and 30% reported their marriages improved somewhat; 48% reported no change and 2% reported the marriage was somewhat worse postoperatively. Similarly, 60% of patients reported either great improvement or some improvement in sexual relationships and 5% reported sexual relationships were somewhat worse. Thus, in larger studies than initially reported by Neill et al,[24] deleterious effects on the marriage were relatively uncommon.

Several studies have documented improvements in occupational functioning following bariatric surgery. It is well known that patients with morbid obesity are frequently discriminated against in employment even when physical health is not an issue. Hall et al[27] followed 30 gastric bypass patients from 13 to 41 months postoperatively and found that no patients had lost work since the operation and 5 had become employed (3 part-time and 2 full-time). In the mail questionnaire follow-up reported by Williams and Jarvie[14] of 80 respondents who had a vertical banded gastroplasty, 28% reported a greatly improved work outlook and 30% reported a somewhat improved work outlook.

EFFECTS ON EATING PATTERNS

Several studies have examined changes in eating behavior following bariatric surgery. Several theories regarding the etiology of obesity have implicated abnormal eating behavior including "an obese eating style," "the binge-eating syndrome" and "emotional eating." Although the majority of these eating patterns have been demonstrated to occur in the normal-weight population as well as among obese patients, alterations in these eating patterns might be necessary for weight loss to be maintained even if the eating pattern did not cause the original obesity.

IMPROVEMENT IN EATING BEHAVIOR

Mills and Stunkard[28] reported changes in eating patterns following jejunoileal bypass. Patients ate less food at each meal, snacked less, ate fewer meals, had fewer binges, had reduced craving for sweets, had less difficulty stopping eating and were more likely to eat breakfast than prior to surgery. Furthermore, patients were less likely to eat during times of emotional stress. Bray and colleagues[29] also documented that after the jejunoileal bypass patients drank significantly less liquid than prior to surgery and drank it more slowly. This "normalization" of eating patterns was even more striking in that it seemed to occur without voluntary effort on the part of the patient.

In the report by Gentry et al,[20] there was a similar "normalization" of eating patterns among 30 patients who had gastric bypass. After surgery, 60% of these patients had less interest in food, ate smaller amounts, and ate more slowly; 76% no longer experienced hunger, 80% no longer ate when they were not hungry and 56% had decreased snacking. All patients reported bingeing prior to surgery, and after surgery 92% no longer binged. Patients still ate in association with both positive and negative feelings, but less food was consumed at these times.

In contradistinction to these studies, Bull et al[13] did not find alterations in all eating habits studied following gastric surgery in 114 patients. There were no changes postoperatively in snacking, meal frequency, number of night snacks or "eating unaware" (a term meaning eating without noticing that one was doing so). During the follow-up varying from 3 months to one year, there was a decrease in quantity of food eaten per meal, in the number of night binges, and there was less difficulty stopping eating. Although generally there was little change in eating behavior in response to emotional stimuli, there was a decrease in "eating in response to loneliness" at follow-up.

IATROGENIC BULIMIA

Some recent reports have found that a relatively large number of patients vomit after eating following the gastric procedures. Although it is to be expected that vomiting might occur a few times after surgery while patients learn what foods and amounts can be tolerated, there are probably some patients who are vomiting to be able to eat and yet continue weight loss. Hall et al[27] reported that 12 of 30 patients overate and vomited following gastric bypass. One of these 12 overate and induced vomiting by placing her fingers down her throat. In the report by Williams and Jarvie,[14] they have divided the vertical banded gastroplasty patients they evaluated postoperatively into two groups: vomiters and non-vomiters. Although there are insufficient data about vomiting at follow-up in gastric surgery patients to draw firm conclusions, it is clear that this is a phenomenon which should be investigated. The physiological consequences of vomiting are well known and have been studied in normal-weight bulimia. If there is a sub-group of "iatrogenic bulimic" patients, further investigation into possible predisposing, preoperative personality traits or attitudes needs to be undertaken.

CONCLUSION

In conclusion, much remains to be known about the psychological, behavioral and social consequences of bariatric surgery. In particular, the currently popular vertical banded gastroplasty needs to be better understood. Reasonable guidelines have been proposed by Makarewicz et al[2] and others for evaluating the effectiveness of various procedures in terms of maintenance of weight loss. These include reporting the original number of patients who have had the surgery, the patients lost to follow-up, the initial weight and weight at various points during follow-up expressed as a percentage of weight lost and lengthy follow-up periods.

Psychiatric evaluation should include a preoperative assessment of the presence or absence of any DSM III[16] Axis I diagnoses (such as schizophrenia or affective disorders) or Axis II diagnoses (e.g., personality disorders). Patients should be assessed for body image disturbances and the quality and extent of their social support system should be considered. The patient's expectations of the procedure should be evaluated and candidates with unrealistic expectations excluded. Postsurgically, patients should be followed by the same psychiatric team and changes in any parameters noted.

REFERENCES

1. Freeman JB, Burchett H: Failure rate with gastric partitioning for morbid obesity. Am J Surg 145:113–119, 1983.
2. Makarewicz PA, Freeman JB, Burchett H, et al: Vertical banded gastroplasty: assessment of efficacy. Surgery 98:700–707, 1985.
3. Castelnuovo-Tedesco P, Weinberg J, Buchanan DC, et al: Long-term outcome of jejuno-ileal bypass surgery for superobesity; a psychiatric assessment. Am J Psychiatry 139:1248–1252, 1982.
4. Mason EE: Vertical banded gastroplasty: assessment of efficacy. Surgery 98:700–707, 1985 (discussion, p 705).
5. Mason EE: Surgical Treatment of Obesity. Major Problems in Clinical Surgery, vol XXVI. Philadelphia, WB Saunders, 1981, pp 386–417.
6. Solow C: Psychosocial aspects of intestinal bypass surgery for massive obesity: current status. Am J Clin Nutr 30:103–108, 1977.
7. Wise TN, Melisaratos N, Gordon J, et al: Psychosocial sequelae of ileal bypass. Psychosomatics 21:855–859, 1980.
8. Leon GR, Eckert ED, Teed D, et al: Changes in body image and other psychological factors after intestinal bypass surgery for massive obesity. J Behav Med 2:39–54, 1979.
9. Valley V: Preoperative psychological assessment in determining outcome from gastric stapling for morbid obesity. Can J Surg 27:129–130, 1984.
10. Olsson S-A, Ryder O, Davidsson A, et al: Weight reduction after gastroplasty: The predictive value of surgical, metabolic and psychological variables. Int J Obesity 8:245–258, 1984.
11. Duckro PN, Leavitt JN, Beal DG, et al: Psychological status among female candidates for surgical treatment of obesity. Int J Obesity 7:477–485, 1983.
12. Solow C, Silberfarb PM, Swift K: Psychosocial effects of intestinal bypass surgery for severe obesity. N Engl J Med 290:300–305, 1974.
13. Bull RH, Engels WD, Engelsmann F, et al: Behavioral changes following gastric surgery for morbid obesity: a prospective, controlled study. J Psychosom Res 27:457–467, 1983.
14. Williams RC, Jarvie GJ: Psychological sequelae of bariatric surgery: assessment of psychosocial effects of vertical banded gastroplasty patients. Presented at Southeastern Psychological Association, March 1986.
15. Halmi KA, Stunkard AJ, Mason EE: Emotional responses to weight reduction by three methods: gastric bypass, jejunoileal bypass, diet. Am J Clin Nutr 33:446–451, 1980.
16. Diagnostic and Statistical Manual, Third Edition (DSM III). Washington, DC, American Psychiatric Association, 1980.
17. Abram HS, Meixel SA, Webb WW, et al: Psycholog-

ical adaption to jejunoileal bypass for morbid obesity. J Nerv Ment Dis 162:151–157, 1976.

18. Rigden SR, Hagen DQ: Psychiatric aspects of intestinal bypass surgery for obesity. Am Fam Physician 68–71, 1976.

19. Mason EE: Psychological aspects in surgical treatment of obesity. Major Problems in Clinical Surgery, vol XXVI. Philadelphia, WB Saunders, 1981, pp 365–385.

20. Gentry K, Halverson JD, Heisler S: Psychologic assessment of morbidly obese patients undergoing gastric bypass: A comparison of preoperative and postoperative adjustment. Surgery 95:215–220, 1984.

21. Stunkard A, Mendelson M: Obesity and the body image. I. Characteristics of disturbances in the body image of some obese persons. Am J Psychiatry 123:1296–1300, 1967.

22. Stunkard A, Burt V: Obesity and the body image. II. Age at onset of disturbances in the body image. Am J Psychiatry 123:1443–1447, 1967.

23. Slade PD, Russell GFM: Awareness of body dimensions in anorexia nervosa: cross-sectional and longitudinal studies. Psychol Med 3:188–199, 1973.

24. Neill JR, Marshall JR, Yale CE: Marital changes after intestinal bypass surgery. JAMA 240:447–450, 1978.

25. Rand C, Kuldau J, Robbins L: Surgery for obesity and marriage quality. JAMA 247:1419–1422, 1982.

26. Rand C, Kowalske K, Kuldau J: Characteristics of marital improvement following obesity surgery. Psychosomatics 25:221–226, 1984.

27. Hall J, Horne K, O'Brien PE, et al: Patient well-being after gastric bypass surgery for morbid obesity. Aust NZ J Surg 53:321–324, 1983.

28. Mills MJ, Stunkard AJ: Behavioral changes following surgery for obesity. Am J Psychiatry 133:527–531, 1976.

29. Bray GA, Zachary B, Dahms WT, et al: Eating patterns of massively obese individuals. J Am Diet Assoc 72:24–27, 1978.

30

Gynecologic-Obstetric Abnormalities of Morbid Obesity, and the Changes after Loss of Massive Excess Weight

MERVYN DEITEL
ELAINE STONE
TOAN B. TO

ACKNOWLEDGEMENT

The authors thank Donald J.A. Sutherland, M.D., F.R.C.P.(C), Associate Professor, Departments of Laboratories and Medicine (Endocrinology), University of Toronto Sunnybrook Medical Centre, for biochemical determinations.

Obesity is associated with various gynecologic-obstetric abnormalities, most of which are secondary to complex metabolic and endocrinologic disturbances resulting in sex hormonal changes. After adequate weight loss, these disturbances and changes normalize, with resulting correction of the clinical abnormalities.

CLINICAL FEATURES ASSOCIATED WITH OBESITY

In females, obesity is associated with an increased risk of developing irregular menses, hirsutism, urinary stress incontinence, infertility, obstetric complications and gynecologic malignancies.

IRREGULAR MENSES

In a study of 109 morbidly obese females (≥45 kg overweight), 40% had irregular menses. After loss of ≥50% of excess weight, this incidence dropped to 5%.[1] Furthermore, obese women have a high incidence of amenorrhea compared to normal weight women.[2] In one study of women who had amenorrhea or functional uterine bleeding, 29 of 60 (48%) of the former and 11 of 19 (58%) of the latter were classified as overweight (≥20% above ideal weight); in contrast, only 13% of 201 women without menstrual disorders were overweight.[2] The amenorrhea and menstrual irregularities tend to disappear with weight loss.[3]

HIRSUTISM

In our study of morbidly obese females, an incidence of facial hirsutism of 32% was found; this decreased slowly to 20% over 2 to 5 years after loss of ≥50% excess weight following bariatric operations.[1] Hartz reported a positive correlation between the incidence of hirsutism and percent overweight.[4]

URINARY STRESS INCONTINENCE

Urinary stress incontinence was a common finding in morbidly obese women, with an incidence of 61% in our study.[1] Usually, no cause such as cysto-urethrocele was found on physical examination. High intra-abdominal pressure increases the intra-vesical pressure, and urinary stress incontinence results mechanically if the intra-vesical pressure surpasses the intra-urethral pressure.[5] After weight loss the incidence fell significantly to 12% without any surgical intervention for it.

INFERTILITY

Anovulatory cycles and infertility have been found to be associated with obesity. The correlation between obesity and oligo-ovulation has been confirmed.[4] Our study found that 25% of 115 morbidly obese patients had infertility problems. However, after substantial weight loss, all nine women who tried to conceive were successful.[1] The polycystic ovary syndrome, characterized by oligo-amenorrhea, hirsutism and infertility, is also associated with obesity.[6]

PREGNANCY AND OBSTETRIC COMPLICATIONS

Those obese women who are able to conceive are at higher risk for developing obstetric complications. The three main antenatal complications in obesity are pre-eclampsia, hypertension and diabetes.[7] A threefold increase in the incidence of deep venous thrombosis in obese pregnant women was also reported.[7] In a 10-year review in Minnesota, pulmonary embolism was shown to be a leading cause of maternal mortality in the obese; this risk was found to be more than twice that in the non-obese women.[8] In our series,[1] hypertension with incidence 27%, pre-eclampsia 13%, diabetes 7% and venous thrombosis 7% were found in morbidly obese pregnant women. In subsequent pregnancies after weight-loss stabilization, none of these complications occurred.

The issue of cesarean section in obese patients is controversial. While most authors deny significant increase,[9,10] others note two to fourfold increase in cesarean section rates in obese patients.[7,11]

The infants of morbidly obese women were on average 400 g heavier than those delivered after weight loss.[1,7,9] Edwards et al[10] found that the infants of massively obese women, although proportionally larger at birth (but not obese), became obese at age 12 months.

Pregnancy following bariatric surgery is advised beyond the malnutrition stage and after weight-loss had stabilized.[12] Weight-loss usually plateaued 18 months after jejunoileal bypass[13] and 12 months after gastric restrictive operations.[14]

MALIGNANCIES

Obese women, especially in the postmenopausal stage, have an increased incidence of breast carcinoma and endometrial carcinoma.[15]

SEX HORMONAL ABNORMALITIES ASSOCIATED WITH OBESITY

AN OVERVIEW OF SEX HORMONES AND SEX HORMONE-BINDING GLOBULIN (SHBG)

ANDROGENS. Small amounts of androstenedione, dehydroepiandrosterone sulfate (DHEAS) and testosterone are secreted in females from the ovaries and adrenal glands. Androstenedione, a weak androgen, is a precursor of testosterone or estrone. DHEAS is also a precursor which arises almost exclusively from the adrenals and can be converted to androstenedione and then, testosterone or estrone. In women, almost two-thirds of circulating testosterone, the major androgen, is bound to SHBG, while most of the rest is bound to albumin and corticosteroid-binding globulin, and only 1.3% is free. Androgens except testosterone are mainly converted to 17-ketosteroids and excreted in the urine. A small amount is converted to estrogens (testosterone to estradiol; androstenedione and DHEAS to estrone) through the process of aromatization, which occurs in muscle and in adipose tissue and its stromal cells.[16–18]

ESTROGENS. Among the three estrogens present in the circulation (estradiol, estrone and estriol), estradiol is the major component and the most potent. Estrogens are secreted by the theca interna and granulosa cells of the ovarian follicles, by the corpus luteum, by the placenta and in small amounts by the adrenal cortex. They are also formed by aromatization of androgens (see above). Only 3% of the circulating estradiol is free, while 60% is bound to albumin and 37% to SHBG. Estrogens are metabolized in the liver and excreted in the urine.

Despite the small proportion of free sex hormones, it appears that it is this and not the bound fraction which is biologically active.

SEX HORMONE-BINDING GLOBULIN. SHBG is a beta-globulin probably produced by the liver and acts as a plasma transport protein for androgens and estradiol. It has a high affinity for testosterone and less so for weaker androgens and estradiol. Estrone and estriol do not bind to it. SHBG reduces the metabolic clearance rates of sex-steroid hormones and thereby prolongs their effective half-life in blood. Changes in SHBG levels regulate the proportions of sex hormones in plasma: its concentration correlates directly with bound sex hormones and inversely with free sex hormones. SHBG increases in cirrhosis of the liver, pregnancy and after the administration of estrogens; SHBG decreases after the administration of androgens, growth hormone and glucocorticoids, in thyroid hormone deficiency and in obesity. Serum SHBG can be measured by a number of immunochemical techniques such as radial immunodiffusion, electroimmunoassay, radioimmunoassay, enzyme immunoassay and immunoradiometric assay. Because of the instability of pure SHBG and problems associated with the production, purification and storage of radiolabelled tracer, the immunoradiometric method is probably the most advantageous.[19]

SEX HORMONES IN OBESE FEMALES

It has been difficult to document sex hormonal changes in premenopausal females,[20,21] since functioning ovaries produce massive amounts of estrogens, compared to the contribution from the adrenal glands and from aromatization of androgens in muscle and adipose tissue. However, it is this latter contribution which increases with degree of obesity. In massive obesity, we found high serum levels of estrogens and androgens together with low SHBG,[22] explaining the clinical features associated with obesity mentioned above. The hormones and SHBG normalize with weight loss.

Postmenopausally, the changes in estrogens are seen more clearly, likely because of lack of cyclic ovarian function. In our study of morbidly obese females, markedly elevated estradiol and DHEAS were documented, both of which returned to normal with adequate weight loss.[22]

It is known that estrogens stimulate the growth of mammary ducts and endometrium. The high estrogenic state associated with obesity is believed to be responsible for the increased incidence of endometrial hyperplasia, endometrial cancer and breast cancer in these individuals.[15]

Most women with the polycystic ovary syndrome are obese, but the actual cause of the syndrome is not known.* On the other hand, only a small percent of morbidly obese women have the polycystic ovary syndrome. The polycystic ovary syndrome and hyperprolactinemia have been suggested as responsible for anovulation and infertility in obese women. However, several studies have failed to consistently demonstrate an abnormal luteinizing hormone (LH) to follicle stimulating hormone (FSH) ratio and increased LH secretion (characteristics of the polycystic ovary syndrome) or increased serum prolactin.[23–25] In our study, FSH, LH and prolactin did not change significantly with weight loss in the 17 premenopausal morbidly obese females.[22] On the other hand, a significant decrease in estrogens and androgens and a significant increase in serum SHBG were found. This suggests that sex hormonal abnormalities, rather than polycystic ovary syndrome or hyperprolactinemia, are the primary cause of infertility in morbidly obese women.

EXPLANATION FOR SEX HORMONAL ABNORMALITIES IN THE OBESE

A scheme describing endocrinologic disturbances and their clinical effects in obese females is shown in Fig. 30.1. The markedly increased adipose tissue leads to various metabolic abnormalities including increased cortisol metabolism, increased aromatase activity and changes in estrogen metabolism.

*Studies suggest estrogen as a trophic agent on adipocyte replication and differentiation.

Cortisol metabolism can occur in white fat tissue and increases with degree of adiposity.[26] White fat is the regular fat found mostly subcutaneously and in the omentum, unlike brown fat* which is located around the kidneys, adrenals, pericardium and large vessels of the mediastinum and neck. Accelerated catabolism of cortisol tends to decrease plasma cortisol and results in an increased production of ACTH.[27] Fat tissue also has a marked capacity to oxidize cortisol to cortisone[28] which is a weaker suppressor of ACTH compared to cortisol. This contributes to excessive secretion of ACTH.

The increased ACTH as a consequence of this feedback mechanism maintains normal plasma cortisol. However, increased ACTH also stimulates the adrenal glands to produce androgens, reflected by elevated urine androgen metabolites (17-ketosteroids).[29] Elevated androgens account for the hirsutism and partly for the amenorrhea and infertility in obese females.

Androgens are converted to estrogens through the process of aromatization in adipose tissue and skeletal muscle.[16–18] In obese individuals as a result of increased adiposity, aromatase activity is increased. High levels of serum androgens have also been found to be associated with a decrease in SHBG, resulting in decreased bound sex hormones and increased free sex hormones.[30,31]

It has also been found in obese females that

*The greatest amount of brown fat is found in infancy and decreases with age, and has a function of heat generation.

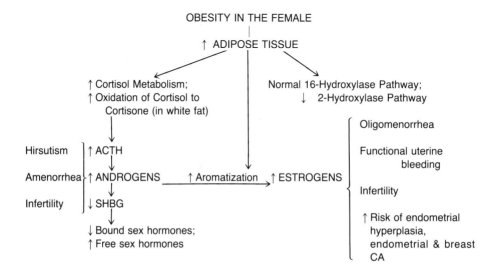

FIGURE 30.1. Endocrinological disturbances and their clinical effects in obese females.

the catabolism of estrogens is altered in such a way that the 16-hydroxylase pathway (which produces estriol, a weak estrogen) is maintained and favored, whereas the 2-hydroxylase pathway (which produces 2-hydroxyestrogens which are non-estrogenic metabolites) is decreased.[32] Thus, more estriol is produced, giving more estrogenic activity. High, unopposed (i.e. persistently elevated) estrogens explain the gynecologic-obstetric abnormalities discussed above.

CLINICAL FEATURES AND SEX HORMONAL CHANGES IN THE OBESE MALE

Generally speaking, markedly obese men are able to maintain normal reproductive function. However, the weight of the body, dyspnea on exertion in intercourse, and inability to penetrate due to fat-folds make the sexual act difficult. Obese males have normal volume of ejaculate, number and motility of sperm, potency, nocturnal penile tumescence and libido.[33]

Elevated serum estrogens, low total testosterone and low SHBG were found in obese males.[22,34,35] Androstenedione and DHEAS, on the other hand, were found to be high.[22] This suggests adrenal hyperactivity secondary to the same mechanism described above in females, and explains the elevated serum estrogens (aromatization). After adequate weight loss, these values returned towards normal with a decrease in estrogens, androstenedione and DHEAS and an increase in total testosterone and SHBG.[22,35,36] Circulating free testosterone was found to be normal in obese men[34] and remained unchanged with weight loss,[35] suggesting no abnormalities in androgenic activity and reproductive function. However, in some massively obese men, low free testosterone with inappropiately low 24-hour mean serum LH was reported.[33,34] This suggests a mild form of hypogonadotrophic hypogonadism, possibly due to feedback suppression by high plasma estrogens found in these individuals.[33]

Sporadically, a decrease in libido has been claimed after loss of massive excess weight, with no biochemical or nutritional explanation. Generally however, libido improves or remains unchanged.

CONCLUSION

The biochemical and clinical gynecologic-obstetric abnormalities associated with obesity are reversible. With adequate weight loss following dietary control or bariatric surgery, sex hormones and SHBG return to normal and in the female are reflected in a correction of the clinical disorders.

REFERENCES

1. Deitel, M, Stone E, Kassam HA, et al: Gynecologic-obstetric changes after loss of massive excess weight following bariatric surgery. J Am Coll Nutr 7:147–153, 1988.
2. Rogers J, Mitchell G: The relation of obesity to menstrual disturbances. N Eng J Med 247:53–55, 1952.
3. Mitchell G, Rogers J: The influence of weight reduction on amenorrhea in obese women. N Eng J Med 249:835–837, 1953.
4. Hartz AJ, Barboriak PN, Wong A, et al: The association of obesity with infertility and related menstrual abnormalities in women. Int J Obes 3:57–73, 1979.
5. Mattingly RF: Stress urinary incontinence, urethrocele and cystocele. In Mattingly RF, Thompson JD (eds): Telinde's Operative Gynecology. Philadelphia: J.B. Lippincott, 1977, pp 531–550.
6. Goldzieher JW: Polycystic ovarian disease. Fertil Steril 35:371–394, 1981.
7. Oats JN, Abell DA, Andersen HM, et al: Obesity in pregnancy. Compr Ther 9:51–55, 1983.
8. Maeder EC Jr, Barno A, Mecklenbutg F: Obesity: a maternal high-risk factor. Obstet Gynecol 45:669–671, 1975.
9. Gross T, Sokol RJ, King KC: Obesity in pregnancy: risks and outcome. Obstet Gynecol 56:446–450, 1980.
10. Edwards LE, Dickes WF, Alton IR, et al: Pregnancy in the massive obese: course, outcome and obesity prognosis of the infant. Am J Obstet Gynecol 131:479–483, 1978.
11. Roopnarinesingh SS, Pathak UN: Obesity in the Jamaican parturient. J Obstet Gynecol Br Commonw 77:895–899, 1970.
12. Wong KH, Leader A, Deitel M: Maternal nutrition in pregnancy. Part II: the implications of previous gastrointestinal operations and bowel disorders. Can Med Assoc J 125:550–552, 1981.
13. Deitel M, Bojm MA, Atin MD, et al: Intestinal bypass and gastric partitioning for morbid obesity: a comparison. Can J Surg 25:283–289, 1982.
14. Deitel M, Jones BA, Petrov I, et al: Vertical banded gastroplasty: results in 233 patients. Can J Surg 29:322–324, 1986.
15. Siiteri PK: Extraglandular estrogen formation and serum binding of estradiol: relationship to cancer. J Endocrinol 89 Suppl:119p–129p, 1981.
16. Perel E, Killinger DW: The interconversion and aromatization of androgens by human adipose tissue. J Steroid Biochem 10:623–627, 1979.
17. Longscope C, Pratt JH, Schneider SH, et al: Aromatization of androgens by muscle and adipose tissue in vivo. J Clin Endocrinol Metab 46:146–152, 1978.
18. Cleland WH, Mendelson CR, Simpson ER: Aromatase activity of membrane fractions of human adipose

tissue stromal cells an adipocytes. Endocrinology 113:2155–2160, 1983.

19. Hammond GL, Langley MS, Robinson PA: An immunoradiometric assay for human SHBG. 2nd Joint Meeting of British Endocrine Societies. 5–8th April, 1983, York. Abstract 89.

20. Zumoff B, Strain GW, Kream J, et al: Obese young men have elevated plasma estrogen levels but obese premenopausal women do not. Metabolism 30:1011–1014, 1981.

21. Zumoff B: Relationship of obesity to blood estrogens. Cancer Res 42 (8 Suppl): 3289S–3294S, 1982.

22. To TB, Deitel M, Stone E, et al: Sex hormonal changes after loss of massive excess weight. Surgical Forum 38:465–467, 1987.

23. Laatikainen T, Tulenheimo A, Andersson B, et al: Obesity, serum steroid levels, and pulsatile gonadotropin secretion in polycystic ovarian disease. Eur J Obstet Reprod Biol 15:45–53, 1983.

24. Kopelman PG, White N, Pilkington TR, et al: The effect of weight loss on sex steroid secretion and binding in massively obese women. Clin Endocrinol 15:113–116, 1981.

25. Zhang YW, Stern B, Rebar RW: Endocrine comparison of obese menstruating and amenorrheic women. J Clin Endocrinol Metab 58:1077–1083, 1984.

26. Glass AR, Burman KD, Dahms WT, et al: Endocrine function in human obesity. Metabolism 30:89–104, 1981.

27. Slavnov VN, Epshtein EV: Somatotrophic, thyrotrophic and adrenocorticotrophic functions of the anterior pituitary in obesity. Endocrinologie 15:213–218, 1977.

28. Raith L, Steiner R, Karl HJ: Metabolic transformation of ^{3}H-cortisol to tetra- and hexahydrated derivatives in obesity. Acta Endocrinol (Suppl) (Kbh) 152:97, 1971.

29. Simkin B: Urinary 17-ketosteroid and 17-ketogenic steroid excretion in obese patients. N Engl J Med 264:974–977, 1961.

30. Anderson DC: Sex hormone-binding globulin. Clin Endocrinol (Oxf) 3:69–96, 1974.

31. Lindstedt G, Lundberg P, Hammond GL, et al: Sex hormone-binding globulin—still many questions (Editorial Review). Scand J Clin Lab Invest 45:1–6, 1985.

32. Schneider J, Bradlow HL, Strain G, et al: Effect of obesity on estradiol metabolism: decreased formation of non-uterotropic metabolites. J Clin Endocrinol Metab 56:973–978, 1983.

33. Strain GW, Zumoff B, Kream J, et al: Mild hypogonadotrophic hypogonadism in obese men. Metabolism 31:871–875, 1982.

34. Glass AR, Swerdloff RS, Bray GA, et al: Low serum testosterone and sex-hormone-binding-globulin in massively obese men. J Clin Endocrinol Metab 45:1211–1219, 1977.

35. Stanik S, Dornfeld LP, Maxwell MH, et al: The effect of weight loss on reproductive hormones in obese men. J Clin Endocrinol Metab 53:828–832, 1981.

36. Deitel M, To TB, Stone E, et al: Sex hormonal changes accompanying loss of massive excess weight. Gastroenterol Clin North Am 16:511–515, 1987.

31

Plastic Surgery After Massive Weight-Loss

ARNIS FREIBERG

Few, if any, massively obese patients can benefit from body sculpting plastic surgical procedures alone, mainly because large amounts of fat cannot safely be removed without removing the overlying skin. Although some improvement in functional symptoms, such as intertrigo, may be achieved by a lipectomy alone, the relatively minimal improvement does not warrant the magnitude of the surgery. With the development of improved operations for morbid obesity, the need for plastic surgery following extensive weight-loss in these patients has increased. This chapter discusses the surgical procedures, techniques, indications, postoperative care and prognosis.

GENERAL INDICATIONS

A. INDICATIONS FOR LIPECTOMIES WITHOUT PREVIOUS WEIGHT-LOSS SURGERY

1. Older patients not suitable or fit for weight-loss surgery, with functionally disabling symptoms, e.g., symptomatic, large abdominal pannus.
2. Reduction mammaplasty in patients whose breasts do not respond to general body weight-loss.

B. INDICATIONS FOR LIPECTOMIES AFTER SURGERY FOR MORBID OBESITY AND AFTER EXTENSIVE WEIGHT-LOSS

Ideally, plastic and reconstructive procedures should be considered only when most of the following criteria have been fulfilled:

1. Significant weight-loss has occurred following surgery, exercise programs, diets, etc., or a combination of these.
2. The patient's weight has stabilized, or an ideal weight has been reached *and maintained* FOR A SIGNIFICANT PERIOD OF TIME (usually 6 to 9 months).
3. The patient has identified definite symptoms or complaints, e.g. upper back pain, submammary or subabdominal pannus intertriginous dermatitis which can be cured or improved by a surgical procedure.
4. The patient has a thorough understanding of the scope of the procedure and "trade-offs," e.g., scars, loss of waistline, etc.

RELATIVE INDICATIONS

1. In selected individuals, a lipectomy may provide a desirable moral boost or stimulus to lose more weight. Although this type of individual is difficult to select, one who has a positive previous record of weight-loss may warrant serious consideration.
2. In selected individuals a reduction mammaplasty can improve respiratory function by removing weight from the chest wall.

CONTRAINDICATIONS

A. DEFINITE

1. Because the skin has the ability to stretch and subcutaneous tissue can reaccumulate fat, surgery to remove both skin and fat without other weight reduction methods should rarely be considered. An exception may be the elderly patient whose excess skin and fat interfere with daily activities, e.g., abdominal pannus with walking. Obese patients are often poorly motivated and thus may seek methods of weight-loss that can be performed by others (e.g., the surgeon) on their behalf.
2. Most fat or skin reduction procedures, with the exception of rhytidectomies (face-lift), should be considered as major surgical procedures, performed under general anesthesia. Serious cardiovascular or pulmonary disease should be considered as contraindications to this surgery.

B. RELATIVE

1. Psychologically unstable patients or those in acute social and interpersonal relationship crises, e.g., separation, divorce, new boyfriend, etc., are rarely good candidates for reconstructive or purely esthetic surgery.
2. For optimal results following surgery, a certain amount of patient cooperation is essential. Those with a poor compliance record should be selected cautiously.

SURGICAL PROCEDURES USED AFTER MASSIVE WEIGHT-LOSS

1. Rhytidectomy (face-lift)
2. Arm lipectomy (correction of "batwing" deformity)
3. Reduction mammaplasty
4. Abdominal lipectomy (panniculectomy)
5. Thigh lipectomy
6. Other "lipectomies," e.g., buttocks, flanks, etc.

1. RHYTIDECTOMY

Requests for a face-lift for lower facial and neck skin redundancy are relatively rare among "post morbid obesity" patients. One suspects that other areas of the body take precedence, especially in view of functional symptoms and altered body image. Standard face-lift procedures are adequate for the post morbid obesity patient, and discussion of these procedures is beyond the scope of this chapter. Redundant skin in the face and neck area rarely causes functional symptoms; therefore, a face-lift is performed for purely esthetic purposes.

2. ARM LIPECTOMY

The so-called "bat-wing" deformity is very common after massive weight-loss. Surgery in this particular area, in the author's experience, is seldom indicated, for several reasons:

1. There are few, if any, true functional complaints.

2. The major complaint is the inability to wear short-sleeved blouses, dresses or shirts. Regardless of the procedure performed, noticeable scars are the rule rather than the exception. Following this procedure, the patient is likely still unwilling to wear the above-described garments.

3. Since the procedure is performed for purely cosmetic purposes, it is seldom covered by third-party insurance.

3. REDUCTON MAMMAPLASTY

A variety of procedures have been described, and each plastic surgeon has a favorite procedure, with or without modifications. For the past 10 years, the author has used the technique described by Robbins[1] with several modifications[2] which will be

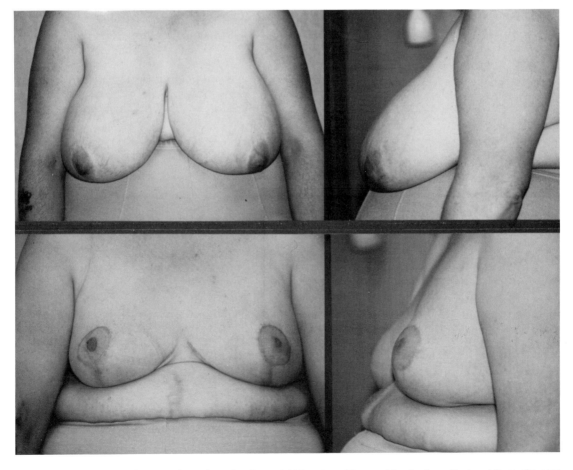

FIGURE 31.1. Mammary hypertrophy and ptosis after weight-loss in a 40-year-old patient pre (top) and 8 months post reduction mammaplasty (bottom).

briefly discussed. This procedure has been used because:

1. Nipple sensation and function are preserved and often improved. Several patients have successfully breast-fed following this procedure.

2. There is no limitation to breast size. The procedure is equally suitable for the ptotic as well as the gigantic breasts.

3. Simplicity.

4. Nipple and areola blood-supply safety—dual blood supply.

5. Good cosmetic results (Fig. 31.1).

The following modifications to the standard Robbins procedure have been beneficial in reducing complications, common with massive reductions:

1. Modification of the Wise pattern[3] markings. In the initial stages of a series of breast reductions, the Wise pattern was used to mark the definitive nipple-areola placement. During follow-up, it was noted that the nipples were placed too high, in time causing pseudoptosis of the breast in a significant number of large reductions (Figure 31.2). Presently the nipple-areola portion is marked out but not cut (Figure 31.3 A and B). Breast reduction is completed and the final nipple placement calculated with the patient in a semi-sitting position. The lower border of the areola should be no higher than 4 cm above the original inframammary skin crease (Figure 31.4 A to C).

2. Intra-operative use of local vasoconstrictors has almost completely eliminated blood transfusions and decreased postoperative morbidity. After induction of general anesthesia, the previously marked areas are injected with a dental syringe using a #30 4-cm needle, and 2% lidocaine with epinephrine cartridges. Approximately 16 to 18 1.9-mL cartridges are used in large reductions. Injections are carried out before the patient is prepared with appropriate antiseptics, allowing 5 to 10 minutes for the epinephrine to take effect. Careful hemostasis is obtained and drains are seldom necessary.

3. The use of a small triangle at the center of the pedicle-flap (Figure 31.5) decreases tension at the three-point closure—a site for delayed healing common to all types of reductions using the method of the "inverted T" closure. Care must be taken to observe the 4.0-cm distance between the inferior portion of the areola and the inframammary skin crease.

4. The use of simple interrupted sutures, instead of the "corner stitch" subcuticular suture, has further decreased local flap necrosis and delayed healing (Figure 31.6 A and B).

5. A continuous intracuticular polyglycolic acid suture (4–0 Dexon) closure along the in-

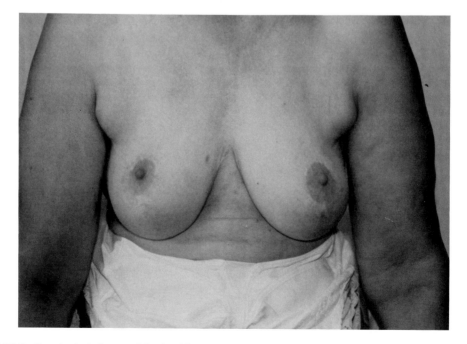

FIGURE 31.2. Pseudoptosis 2 years following bilateral reduction mammaplasty. The nipple-areola complex had been placed too high above the inframammary skin crease.

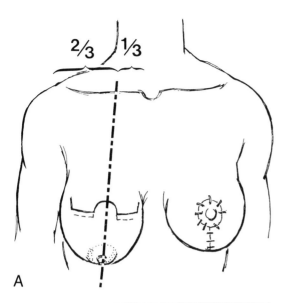

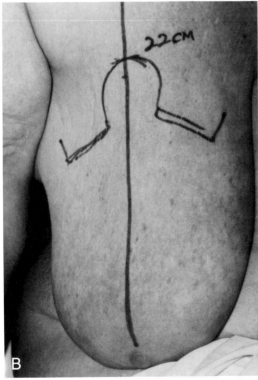

FIGURE 31.3 A and B. A vertical line is drawn from the clavicle to the nipple. A transparent Wise pattern is used to outline the proposed flaps. For larger breasts the medial and lateral flaps are extended to allow for closure without tension. The semicircular nipple-areola part is marked but not incised.

cision has eliminated cross-hatching scars and painful suture removal. Interrupted 5–0 nylon sutures are only used around the areola.

Tapes and bandages have been eliminated by the use of the patient's bra following the operative procedure. This has eliminated painful tape removal and occasional "tape-blisters."

Indications (Table 31.1)

A. ESTHETIC. The body image of the patient following massive weight-loss is often described as repulsive and ugly. Almost all patients following weight-loss desire improvement in cosmetic appearance in many parts of the body. Since the breasts symbolize femininity, the desire to have improvement in this area is often stronger than in other parts of the body. Difficulty in finding clothing seems to be an almost uniform complaint in these patients.

When considering reduction mammaplasty, the patient must be warned about unavoidable scars. Most obese patients tend to minimize or ignore this problem, because they feel that they will not be attractive without clothing anyway.

B. FUNCTIONAL. Improvement in most breast-related symptoms following reduction mammaplasty can almost be guaranteed in a large percentage of patients.

1. Submammary Intertrigo. Severe ptosis is common in all "post weight-loss" patients. Removal of excess skin and fat provides an excellent improvement in this complaint.

2. Upper Back and Neck Pain. Although some patients have, over a number of years, developed poor posture and early degenerative changes in the cervical and thoracic spine, improvement in these symptoms can be anticipated following large reductions.

3. Shoulder Strap Marks and Grooves. Significant improvement can be promised in all patients following significant reductions or correction of severe ptosis.

Before considering breast reduction, it is important to establish the patient's weight gain/loss pattern, which falls into three categories: 1) weight can be gained in breasts easily, but no loss occurs with weight-loss elsewhere; 2) weight is lost from breasts, but not regained with weight-gain elsewhere; 3) breast weight fluctuates in accordance with the rest of the body. These three points should be discussed with the patient pre-operatively, to avoid disappointment following surgery or weight changes.

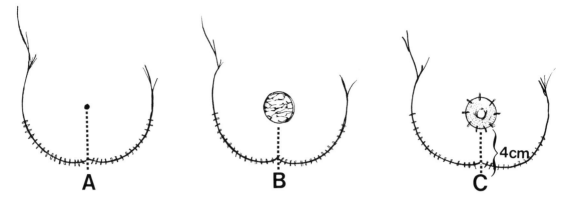

FIGURE 31.4 A–C. A. The breast mound is temporarily formed. B. The new nipple-areola site is estimated and marked using a transparent medicine glass. The circle is then excised or de-epithelialized to obtain better projection. C. Care must be taken to make sure that the lower portion of the areola is no higher than 4.0 cm above the *actual* inframammary skin crease.

4. ABDOMINAL LIPECTOMY (PANNICULECTOMY)

Several problems, both functional and esthetic, face the weight-loss patient (Table 31.2).

A. Functional Problems

As a result of weight-loss, tissue laxity and gravity, the abdominal skin and soft tissues sag, producing the following symptoms:

1. Intertrigo is the most common complaint of all "post-morbid obesity" patients.

2. Difficulties in interpersonal relationships, especially sexual intercourse.

3. Difficulty in physical exercises, e.g., running, swimming. A loose overhang is frequently a deterrent to these activities. The well-motivated patient is anxious to rebuild body shape, and thus exercise becomes a very important aspect of the total rehabilitative process.

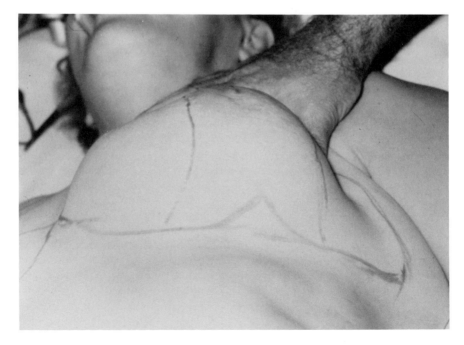

FIGURE 31.5. A small triangle in the center of the pedicle decreases tension at the three point closure, thus minimizing delayed healing. Care must be taken to remember that the inframammary skin crease has been artificially raised and the new areola location should be measured from the *base* of this triangle.

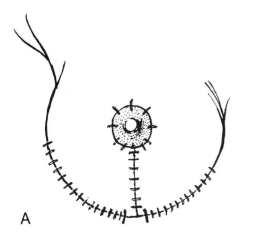

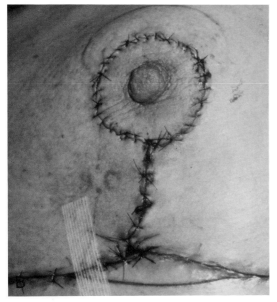

FIGURE 31.6 A and B. To avoid flap tip necrosis the usual "corner stitch" is omitted. Simple interrupted sutures are used near but *not* at the tip of the flaps to minimize delayed healing in this area.

4. Difficulty in reaching the lower extremity, e.g., trying to tie shoes or washing lower extremities.

5. Lower back pain. Part of the problem may be longstanding, and irreversible changes in the lower thoracic and lumbar spine may have already occurred. An abdom-

TABLE 31.1. INDICATIONS FOR REDUCTION MAMMAPLASTY

A. Esthetic
B. Functional
1. Submammary intertrigo
2. Upper back and neck pain
3. Shoulder strap marks

TABLE 31.2. ABDOMINAL PANNUS—PROBLEMS

A. Functional
1. Intertrigo
2. Interpersonal relationship difficulties
3. Difficulties in physical activities
4. Difficulty in reaching lower extremity
5. Lower back pain
6. Pain in knees
7. Urinary stress incontinence
8. Ventral hernias and diastasis recti
9. Tight abdominal scars
B. Esthetic
1. Difficulty in obtaining clothing
2. Striae and loose abdominal skin
3. Abdominal scars
4. Altered body image—embarrassment

inal lipectomy will improve or prevent some of these symptoms.

6. Pain in knees. Older morbid obesity patients may have early degenerative changes in the knees, and the loss of extra weight in the lower abdomen may improve these symptoms.

7. Urinary stress incontinence may be aggravated by the extra lower abdominal weight and may be improved following lipectomy.

8. Ventral hernias due to previous surgical procedures or diastasis recti are relatively common in the obese patient. Both conditions should be corrected at the time of abdominal lipectomy.

9. Tight abdominal scars. Most of the operative incisions to correct morbid obesity are vertical midline. Occasionally a tight sensation with hyperextension is present and needs correction.

B. Esthetic

1. Difficulty in obtaining adequate clothing is a universal complaint. Some patients can wear only pants with a central zipper. The lower part of the abdomen is frequently out of proportion with the rest of the body, requiring expensive tailor-made clothing.

2. Striae and loose abdominal skin. Although definite improvement can be promised by excision of loose skin, the patient must be warned that some of the striae will still be present following abdominal lipectomy.

3. Abdominal scars. Due to weight-loss and gravity, some of the previously relatively acceptable surgical scars may become more noticeable and occasionally symptomatic. Most of the scars between the umbilicus and the pubis can be removed with an adequate lipectomy.

4. Altered body image. Most patients are extremely self-conscious and will not wear

bathing suits or shorts. Significant improvement can be provided, while leaving patients with an acceptable scar which can be hidden by usual garments.

SURGICAL TECHNIQUES

Although numerous abdominal lipectomy procedures have been described, most have dealt with purely cosmetic problems. Few authors have concentrated on techniques especially designed for large lipectomies.[4-8] The technique most commonly used by the author, which is simple, safe, efficient and has produced satisfactory results over the past 10 years, will be described.

If correction of a large ventral incisional hernia is required, the patient is dealt with by a two-team approach with a general surgeon. Combined pre-operative planning is important. The procedure is started by the plastic surgeon, the hernia repaired by the general surgeon, and the procedure completed by the plastic surgical team. The postoperative care is shared by the two teams, with responsibilities for each team outlined before surgery to avoid oversight or overlap in total patient care.

Essentially three types of lipectomy have been used:

1. *Transverse abdominal suprapubic closure,* using a "lazy W" design, has been used most commonly (Figure 31.7 A to E).

2. *Vertical T-shaped closure* (Figure 31.8 A and B) is used where: a) the vertical midline scars are unacceptable and can be improved, and b) the re-creation of a "waistline" is important for the patient (usually lost by the more standard lower transverse approach).

3. *Central or upper abdominal lipectomy* (Figure 31.9) is sometimes indicated where most of the loose skin and striae are confined to the upper and mid abdomen. This procedure is rarely indicated in "post massive weight-loss" patients.

The Lower Abdominal Suprapubic Technique

The incisions (Figure 31.7A) are marked in the suprapubic area, extending laterally beyond the anterior superior iliac spines. The incision can be curved, superiorly or inferiorly in a "lazy W" fashion from the horizontal, depending on the amount of fat present over the hips. The lateral limits of the incision are dictated by the operating-room table. "Dog-ears" can be corrected at the time of wound

closure or as a minor surgical procedure later. To minimize intraoperative bleeding, vaso-constrictors are used as described in the reduction mammaplasty procedures.

The superiorly based flap is developed by both sharp and blunt dissection in the relatively bloodless supra-aponeurotic plane. Large perforating blood vessels should be tied; smaller vessels can be controlled by cautery. It is not essential to remove all the fat from the aponeurosis; this minimizes some of the bleeding from the smaller vessels.

Elevation is carried out to the level of the umbilicus. The umbilicus is preserved by cutting a circle around the stalk in an "apple-coring" fashion, making sure that the stalk and its blood supply are preserved. A #11 blade is useful for cutting the relatively loose skin.

At this point the flap is split in the midline to facilitate dissection superiorly (Figure 31.7B). The undermining is carried cephalad to the lower costal margins and xyphoid process. Care must be taken while undermining the midline scar to make sure that the peritoneal cavity is not entered. Small incisional hernias, when present, are identified at this time and repaired. Diastasis recti can also be corrected at this time, using heavy polypropylene sutures.

After careful hemostasis is obtained, the operating-room table is flexed to obtain maximum laxity of the abdominal skin to be removed. The two flaps are advanced inferiorly, marked and cut. The two sides are weighed to ensure symmetry.

If a decision has been made pre-operatively to remove the vertical scar above the umbilicus, a triangular wedge is estimated and excised. A central marking suture is placed in the midline at the midpubic area (Figure 31.7C). Appropriate adjustments are made laterally to correct "dog-ears" as required.

Since the skin of the abdominal flap is usually thicker than the skin in the inguinal regions and suprapubic areas, the excess fat is removed in a tapered fashion. The skin is closed by a continuous intracuticular 4–0 polyglycolic acid suture to eliminate cross-hatching (Figure 31.7D). A few interrupted 4–0 nylon sutures are used to reinforce the suture-line. These latter sutures are removed in 3 to 4 days, before discharge from hospital, to minimize scarring.

Drains are used only if excess oozing occurs during the procedure. In our experience this

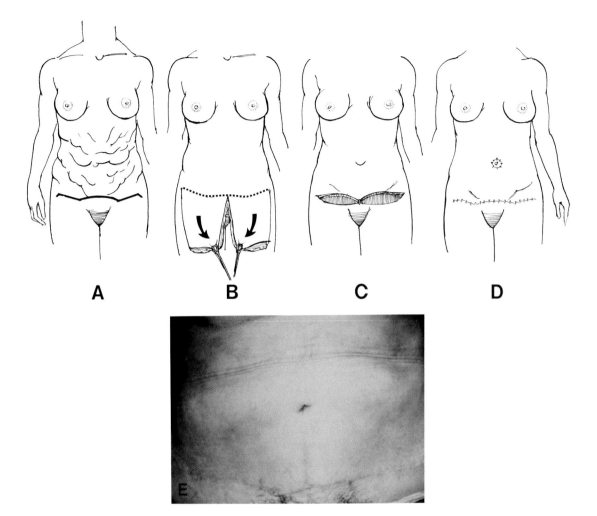

FIGURE 31.7 A–D. A. Suprapubic incision is marked usually in the natural crease, at the base of the apron. B. The flap is split in midline and each section weighed to assure symmetry. C. The flap is advanced inferiorly with the operating-room table in a flexed (jack-knifed) position. D. Repair is accomplished by the use of a continuous subcuticular 4–0 Dexon suture. A 2-layer closure of interrupted sutures is used to suture the "neo-umbilicus." E. Clinical picture showing scars 1 year after abdominal lipectomy using the technique described in Fig. 31.7 A–D.

is rarely necessary (approximately 5% of cases).

CARE OF THE UMBILICUS. The umbilicus should be preserved whenever possible, as it is a significant factor in maintaining a relatively normal body image and esthetic appearance. Several methods of umbilical reconstruction have been described; however, this appears to be more important in a purely cosmetic abdominoplasty.

Two simple methods of umbilical reconstruction have been used by the author. The procedure chosen depends on the thickness of the abdominal wall at the level of the umbilicus. In patients with a relatively thick abdominal wall, the umbilicus is brought through the transverse incision and sutured

with 4–0 polyglycolic acid sutures for the subcutaneous tissues and interrupted 5–0 nylon sutures for the skin. A circular umbilicus is thus placed in a transverse incision, producing a close resemblance of a normal umbilicus (Figure 31.10).

In patients with a thin abdominal wall, the umbilical stalk is too long. The excess tissue is amputated and the remaining tissue sutured to the abdominal wall skin, as described above.

Only in cases requiring repair of a large ventral hernia is the umbilicus sacrificed. This possibility must be discussed with the patient pre-operatively.

POSITION OF THE UMBILICUS. For esthetic purposes, it is important that the umbilicus

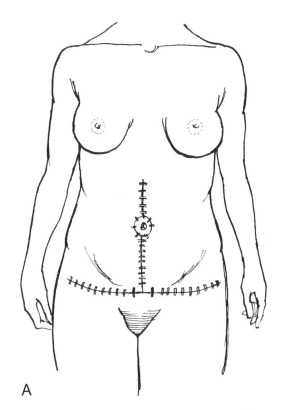

A

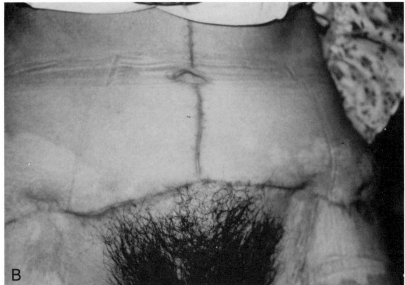

B

FIGURE 31.8A. Vertical T-shaped closure to improve unsightly midline scars and improve waistline. B. Clinical picture 10 weeks after lipectomy, using this technique (2 years after gastric partitioning). Scars are still hypertrophic and are expected to improve.

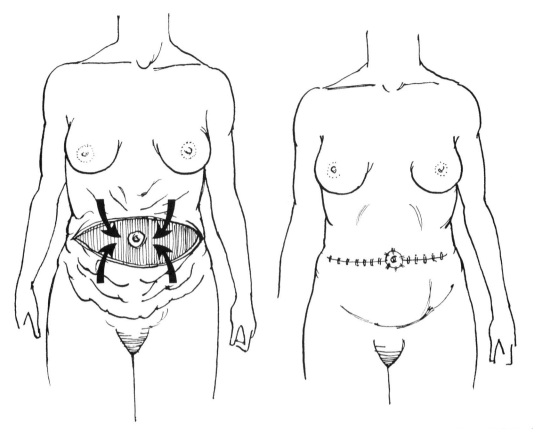

FIGURE 31.9. Central abdominal lipectomy technique used in selected cases where most of the skin redundancy is located in the peri-umbilical area. Seldom suitable for patients after massive weight-loss.

is in the midline. It should be placed along a vertical line, marked between the xyphoid and the central part of the pubis. The horizontal level of the umbilicus is determined by placing it approximately 2.5 cm above the anterior superior iliac spines. The level is often best determined by simply placing the stalk at right angles to the temporarily sutured abdominal flap.

POSTOPERATIVE CARE. The suture-lines are covered with 1.25-cm "steri-strips," Jelonet and wet saline-soaked dressing pads. Following the operative procedure, the table is gently leveled and the patient transferred to his or her own bed, with a many-tailed abdominal binder on the bed. The binder is tied tightly and secured with a safety pin, and is left in place for 24 hours. The patient's bed is flexed to reduce tension on the suture-line. Complete bed rest is advocated for 24 hours. The first dressing change is accomplished at that time, and the patient allowed bathroom privileges in a semi-flexed position.

A shower or bath is allowed by the third or fourth postoperative day, and the patient is usually discharged between the fourth and sixth postoperative days. A girdle or tight pantyhose is advocated for the next 14 to 21 days. Umbilical sutures are removed between the tenth and twelfth postoperative days.

Prophylactic antibiotics have not been used routinely. Blood transfusions are seldom required because of the use of intra-operative vasoconstrictors and careful hemostasis. Drains, if used, are removed 48 hours postoperatively. Nasogastric tubes are rarely necessary postoperatively, as ileus is uncommon unless a ventral hernia repair was done in conjunction with the lipectomy. Only mild postoperative analgesics are required, as the flaps are temporarily denervated and subcuticular sutures minimize wound discomfort.

COMPLICATIONS

1. Hematoma. Rare.

2. Seroma or Fat Necrosis is a Relatively Common Complication. It is believed that this can be partially minimized by the use of an abdominal binder and later a girdle support, thus minimizing the shearing forces between the abdominal wall and the abdominal skin.

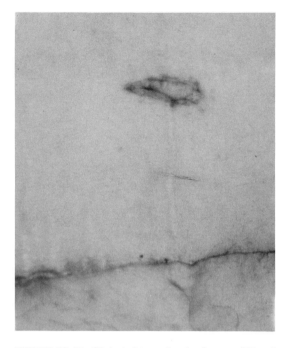

FIGURE 31.10. Clinical picture showing "neo-umbilicus" 5 weeks postoperatively.

3. Delayed Wound Healing. Minor wound healing problems are encountered as in other types of surgery for obese patients. Significant skin loss, requiring secondary skin grafting or closure, has not been required for the past 10 years (>100 patients). Occasional delayed wound breakdowns can be treated by dressings on an outpatient basis.

More prolonged healing is seen most commonly in the vertical excision lipectomies (Figure 31.11). This complication can be minimized by: a) removal of the thin skin in the region of the previous umbilicus excision site; b) a vertical triangle of skin from the pubic area minimizes the tension at the three point closure site (Figure 31.12). The flap can also be de-epithelialized to: a) minimize delayed healing and b) correct the commonly seen depression in this area.

4. Wound Infection. No serious infections have been encountered in uncomplicated lipectomies without large ventral hernia repairs. Infected hematomas, requiring hospitalization, are rare and usually seen in the grossly obese patient and in those in whom a ventral hernia repair has also been performed at the time of lipectomy.

5. Loss of Waistline. Since most patients have excess skin and fat over the hips pre-operatively, a definite although not necessarily pleasing waistline is present. In the individual

with excess fat over the hips, a successful lipectomy may lose the apparent waistline. After an adequate resection with extensive undermining, the waistline often disappears. For some patients this is very important, and this potential problem must be thoroughly discussed pre-operatively to avoid disappointment and patient dissatisfaction. If a waistline is very important to the patient, a vertical wedge excision, as described previously, must be considered. The patient must realize that the "trade-off" may be delayed healing at the lower T portion of the closure, as described above.

Unsatisfactory Umbilicus Location or Appearance. Since in most patients the umbilicus is placed in a lower portion of the vertical scar used for morbid obesity surgery, there is little chance for late changes in position. The scar is mature and protects migration as the abdominal skin sags due to gravity and aging of the skin.

a. Umbilicus too High. "Rain-catcher deformity" is perhaps the most obvious and least acceptable deformity. As the superior border of the umbilicus is sutured to unyielding scar and the inferior border to sagging loose skin, a "rain-catcher deformity" may result. This can be avoided by making sure that the umbilical stalk is at right angles to the temporarily sutured abdominal skin flap.

b. Umbilicus too Low. This is very seldom a complaint (Figure 31–13). It is esthetically more acceptable to have a low rather than a high umbilicus.

c. Bulging or "Swollen" Umbilicus. This deformity (Figure 31.14) is usually caused by a discrepancy between the size of the umbilicus and the slit made in the abdominal flap. To avoid this deformity the umbilicus must fit loosely in the "buttonhole" made in the abdominal flap. This deformity can also result from a stalk which is too long for the thickness of the abdominal flap. Partial amputation will result in a shorter stalk.

d. Umbilicus too Small. This deformity usually results from a too generous amputation of the umbilicus stalk. If recognized, this deformity can be corrected by: a) enlarging the recipient defect, or b) placing a superiorly based triangular skin flap in a slit made in the umbilicus; the base of the triangle increases the diameter of the "neo-umbilicus."

e. Asymmetrical Placement of the Umbilicus. The umbilicus should be placed on a vertical line drawn between the xyphoid processes and

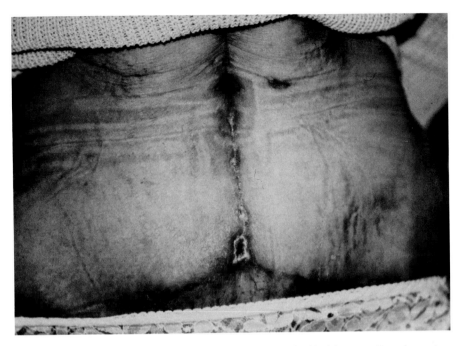

FIGURE 31.11. Delayed healing of the vertical component of the abdominal incision seen 6 weeks postoperatively.

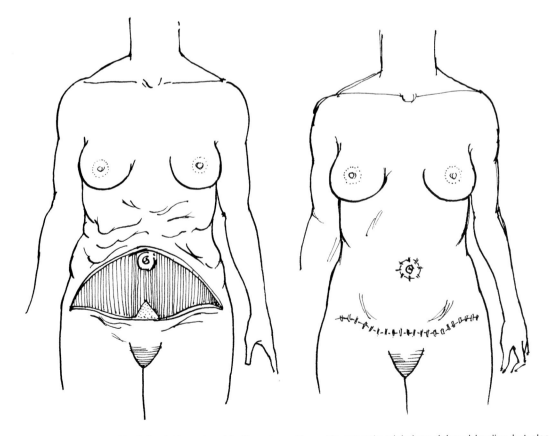

FIGURE 31.12. A de-epithelialized triangular skin flap above the pubis not only minimizes delayed healing but also improves the often encountered suprapubic depression.

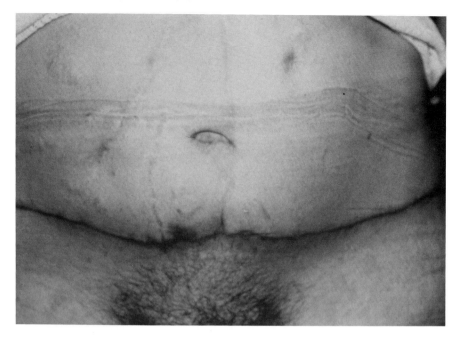

FIGURE 31.13. Umbilicus placed too low—patient 8 weeks postoperative.

midline of the pubic escutcheon or in line with the superior pole of the introitus.

7. Recurrence of Abdominal Pannus and Related Symptoms. The laws of gravity and elasticity of skin cannot be avoided. In order to minimize this complaint, the abdominal lipectomy should be properly timed:

1) The procedure should only be considered after stabilization of weight-loss—at least 6 to 9 months post-stabilization.

2) The patient must be warned preoperatively that the lipectomy does not prevent weight gain, nor does it delay the increasing laxity of the skin caused by generalized aging process.

8. Loss of Sensation Below the Lower Incision.

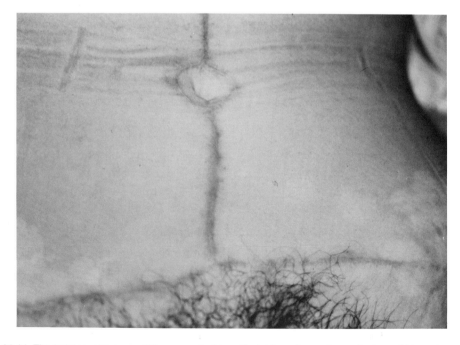

FIGURE 31.14 The bulging, circular umbilicus seen in this patient 10 weeks postoperatively could have been improved by simple amputation of the tip of the stalk or by making a longer transverse donor incision.

This is common, if tested for, but the patient is often unaware of this occurrence. This sequela can be at least partially minimized by preserving the perforating neurovascular bundles in the lower abdominal flap during elevation of the flap.

9. Swelling Above the Suprapubic Incision. Some temporary edema of the flap occurs in all lipectomies. This problem can be minimized by tapering the lower portion of the abdominal flap by excising some of the fat from the flap. It is important that the thickness of the flap matches the thickness of the skin over the pubis, and most importantly, the usually thinner skin in the inguinal regions.

10. Suprapubic Edema. This deformity is often seen preoperatively and usually cannot be satisfactorily corrected at the time of the abdominal lipectomy. This should be pointed out to the patient pre-operatively. Secondary correction is sometimes necessary at a later date.

11. Unacceptable Scars. The patient's ability to scar can usually be estimated by observing pre-existing abdominal scars. Scarring must be discussed with the patient in the initial interview. Since lipectomies are usually performed for mainly functional problems, e.g., intertrigo, complaints about the scars are rare postoperatively. Scar revisions are only occasionally necessary to correct "dog-ears" in both flanks. Intracuticular closure has completely eliminated cross-hatching, commonly seen in other abdominal scars. *Spread scars* are common due to increased tension at the time of closure but are seldom a major concern to the patient.

5. THIGH LIPECTOMY

Almost all "massive weight-loss" patients complain of some problems related to inner thigh skin redundancy. Not every patient, however, is a candidate for surgery in this area. The most common complaint deals with the esthetic appearance of the thighs and inability to wear dresses, shorts or bathing suits. A significant scar along the medial aspect of the thigh is required to correct the deformity and may not be acceptable to the patient.

Other, more functional complaints are rubbing of the thighs with irritation and difficulties with interpersonal relationships. Surgery for this type of patient is more successful than for the former.

With regard to patterns of thigh fat and skin distribution, there are three patient types:
1) involvement of the entire inner thigh;
2) involvement of the upper one-third of the thigh;
3) local involvement of the upper one-third of the thigh but sparing the inguinal region.

For the type 1 patient, to correct the problem, a vertical skin ellipse with extension into the inguinal area, superiorly and posteriorly, is essential. This procedure requires extensive undermining, large flaps, and a T-shaped closure in the groin. All three factors predispose to potential hematoma and seroma formation, infection, and occasional delayed healing. Dressings and immobilization in this area are difficult; therefore, patients require prolonged periods of bed rest and hospitalization, significantly increasing the cost of these procedures. Because of these factors, and often unacceptable scars, the author has limited experience with this procedure.

Type 2 and 3 patients are more suitable operative candidates because: a) the problem may be solved by a "mini" lift consisting of removal of excess skin and fat from the inguinal area following undermining of the thigh (Figure 31.15); and b) the procedure avoids the three-point closure often complicated by skin necrosis and delayed healing, and leaves easily concealable scars in the groin. Postoperative care consists of no dressings, complete bed rest for 3 or 4 days and gradual mobilization. Tight support by a pantyhose type of garment is worn for another 2 to 3 weeks.

6. OTHER "LIPECTOMIES"

Almost every part of the body can be involved in skin redundancy and "lipodystrophies" following massive weight-loss. The most common areas, other than those discussed above, are hips, flanks, buttocks and calves. The complaints in these areas are chiefly esthetic in nature. Many procedures to correct these deformities have been described, and the discussion of these procedures is beyond the scope of this chapter.

SUMMARY AND CONCLUSIONS

Massive weight-loss usually leaves the patient with varying amounts of loose skin in different areas of the body. The skin redun-

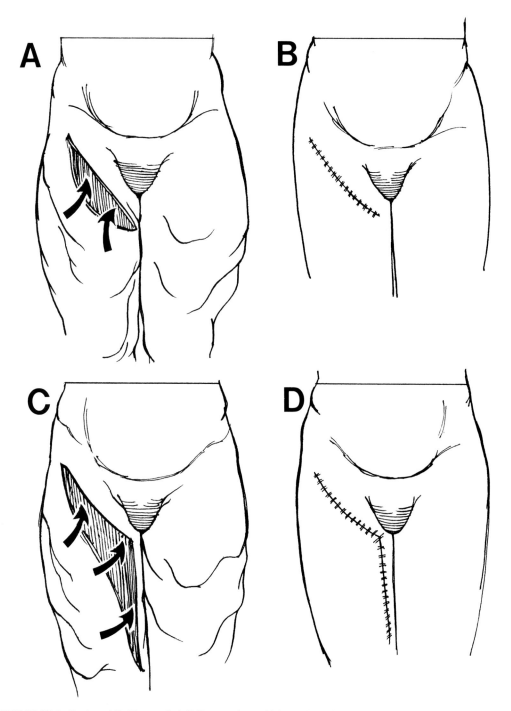

FIGURE 31.15 A–D. A and B. Show a "mini" lift procedure which carries a low morbidity and leaves acceptable scars. C and D. Show a more extensive procedure with a longer medial thigh incision. A larger amount of skin can be removed, but this procedure carries a higher risk for delayed healing and leaves a less acceptable scar.

dancy can not only aggravate the preweight-loss problem, e.g. subabdominal pannus intertrigo, but also increase the patient's dislike for his or her body image. Plastic surgery can produce, in carefully selected patients, improvement in symptoms and body image. The most satisfying results can be obtained from abdominal lipectomies, breast reduction and localized thigh lipectomies. Other areas are less satisfactory because of the magnitude of surgery (total thigh lipectomy) and permanent scarring (upper arm lipectomies). Important points are:

1. "Post weight-loss" surgery should only be considered when the patient's weight has remained stable for at least 6 to 9 months.

2. Each proposed procedure should be discussed in detail, stressing the magnitude of the procedure and potential complications, realistic expectations, scars, and cost of not only direct medical expense but also time off work.

3. Some procedures, e.g. abdominal lipectomies in some individuals, are "trade-offs." Elimination of uncomfortable inguinal intertrigo may lose a previously acceptable waistline.

4. Correction of ptotic breasts by a reduction mammaplasty will create a much more youthful appearance, but does leave significant scars.

In some areas the "trade-off" in the author's opinion may not be worthwhile; e.g., correction of "bat-wing" deformities in the arms will leave the patient with visible scars, and short sleeves may not be worn even after the surgery. In spite of some of the shortcomings and "trade-offs," plastic surgical procedures in the patient after massive weight-loss can be a worthwhile and satisfactory adjunct

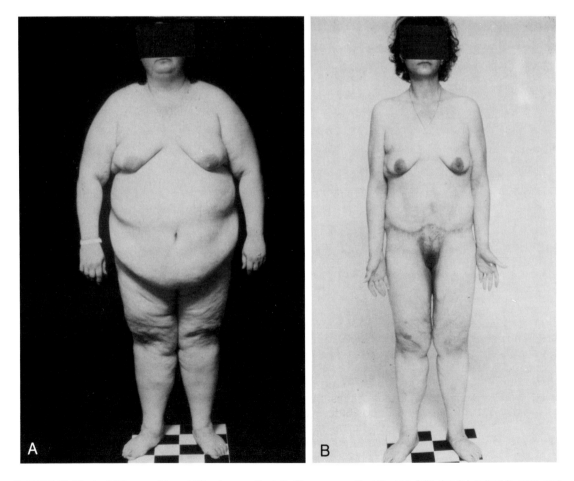

FIGURE 31.16. A. A 38-year-old morbidly obese patient. B. The same patient 3 years following jejunoileal bypass and one year following abdominal lipectomy.

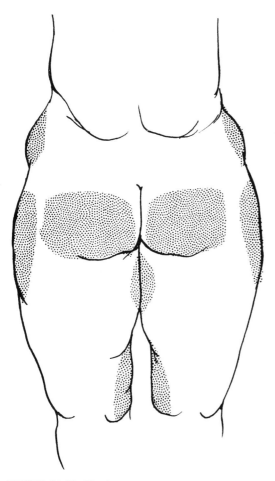

FIGURE 31.17. Lipodystrophy sites suitable for suction lipectomy.

to the total rehabilitation of the obese patient (Figure 31.16 A and B).

LIPOSUCTION AS APPLIED TO THE PROBLEM OF OBESITY

WILLIAM R.N. LINDSAY

Liposuction (also called suction assisted lipectomy) is a surgical technique which was originated in Europe in 1977 by Parisian and Swiss plastic surgeons. There has been a rapid increase in knowledge about the technique and equipment, and the procedure is used worldwide. The technique is designed to remove subcutaneous fat deposits to give improved body contour.[9–12] This permits the removal of deep, excess subcutaneous fat through 2-cm incisions, and is performed with a blunt cannula attached to a suction source of approximately one atmosphere. The cannula is passed throughout the loose sub-

cutaneous fat and suctions out fat with approximately 15–18% blood content. The fibrous connections between skin and deep fascia, often containing blood vessels, remain intact. The chief problem relates to removing the desired amount of fatty tissue and leaving a smooth body contour.

The procedure was originally designed as a cosmetic procedure, most ideally suited for patients under age 50 who had a satisfactory body contour except for excess fat in the trochanteric, lower flank, buttock, upper inner thigh or inner knee area (Figure 31.17). The operation is now being used in patients over age 50 with excess subcutaneous fat in the central abdominal area, or large amounts of fat in the lower torso region. These patients must be realistic in their expectations of the result to be obtained. A reasonable amount of subcutaneous fat may be removed from the most obvious area of abnormal body contour, i.e. the trochanteric area (commonly called "saddlebags") or the front of the thigh or inner thigh regions. Considerable improvement may be obtained in obese patients, although the amount of fat removed seldom reaches the expectations or wishful hopes of the patient. Secondary procedures can be carried out a few months later to improve residual pockets of fat.

In obese patients, the amount of fat removed requires hospitalization and may cause enough change in the hemodynamics of the body to require a blood transfusion. Experience has shown that the skin does not become loose or sagging, but tends to flatten into the area from which the fat was removed. The skin is often firmer and flatter after surgery.

Based on established procedures for recontouring the body surface, one might expect that complications such as infection, hematoma, collection of fluid serum, or even major problems with skin breakdown and skin loss and grafting might occur. Theoretically all these complications are possible, but the record after several thousand cases suggests that these complications are not being seen.

Although suction lipectomy for small localized deposits of fat may be performed on an outpatient basis, the surgery in the obese patient is carried out in the hospital under general anesthesia. The hospital stay is usually 3 days. The areas treated are firmly taped to give support and prevent fluid collection, and the patient is encouraged to remain fairly quiet in bed for 3 to 4 days except for getting up for bathroom and meals. The taping is changed at 5 days, and the patient is encouraged to increase activities to reach a stage in 10 to 14 days where he or she is walking 2 miles each day. The treated areas are given good support with an elastic girdle.

Most patients experience very little pain postoperatively, except in the case of the abdomen, which tends to be quite tender. Massage to the treated areas is of help. There is a varying amount of swelling, with some temporary minimal skin numbness. Results are not obtained for at least 3 months. A considerable number of patients have experienced continuing weight-loss for several months.

Suction lipectomy is not a new answer for the patient with morbid obesity or the patient who has experienced major weight-loss and is left with large amounts of redundant skin and excess fat. However, it is proving to have a place in improving body contour in selected patients to give them more freedom to choose clothes and more satisfaction with their body image. Suction lipectomy may be combined with skin tightening surgery to remove excess skin.

REFERENCES

1. Robbins TH: A reduction mammaplasty with the areola-nipple based on an inferior dermal pedicle. Plast Reconstr Surg 59:64–67, 1977.
2. Freiberg A, Schlosser H: A critical look at the Robbins' reduction mammaplasty technique. Transactions of the Seventh International Congress of Plastic Surgery, Montreal, June 26–July 1, 1983, pp 551–553.
3. Wise RJ: A preliminary report on a method of planning the mammaplasty. Plast Reconstr Surg 17:367–375, 1956.
4. Kamper MJ, Galloway DV, Ashley F: Adominal panniculectomy after massive weight loss. Plast Reconstr Surg 50:441–446, 1972.
5. Palmer B, Hallberg D, Backman: Skin reduction plasties following intestinal shunt operations for treatment of obesity. Scand J Plast Reconstr Surg 9:47–52, 1975.
6. Shons AR: Plastic reconstruction after bypass surgery and massive weight loss. Surg Clin North Am 59:1139–1152, 1979.
7. Savage RC: Abdominoplasty following gastrointestinal bypass surgery. Plast Reconstr Surg 71:500–507, 1983.
8. Foged J: Operative treatment of abdominal obesity, especially pendulous abdomen. Br J Plast Surg 1:274–284, 1948.
9. Illouz Y-G: Body contouring by lipolysis: a 5 year experience with over 3000 cases. Plast Reconstr Surg 72:591–597, 1983.
10. Fournier PF, Otteni FM: Lipodissection in body sculpturing: the dry procedure. Plast Reconst Surg 72:598–609, 1983.
11. Hallock GG: Fat suctioning. Contemp Surg 29:21–27, 1986.
12. Mantse L: Liposuction: a new body sculpturing procedure. Can Med Assoc J 135:975–976, 1986.

ADDITIONAL BIBLIOGRAPHY

1. Baroudi R, Keppke EM, Netto FT: Abdominoplasty. Plast Reconstr Surg 54:161–168, 1974.
2. Castanares E, Goethel JA: Abdominal lipectomy: a modification in technique. Plast Reconstr Surg 40:378–383, 1967.
3. Davis TS: Morbid obesity. Clin Plast Surg 11:517–524, 1984.
4. Delerm A: Refinements in abdominoplasty with emphasis on reimplantation of the umbilicus. Plast Reconstr Surg 70:632–638, 1982.
5. Pitanguy I: Abdominal lipectomy: an approach to it through an analysis of 300 consecutive cases. Plast Reconstr Surg 40:384–391, 1967.
6. Psillakis JM: Plastic surgery of the abdomen with improvement in body contour: Physiopathology and treatment of the aponeurotic musculature. Clin Plast Surg 11:465–472, 1984.
7. Rich JD, Gottlieb V, Pagadala S: A precise method of locating the umbilicus during abdominoplasty. Ann Plast Surg 10:397–399, 1983.
8. Savage RC: Abdominoplasty combined with other surgical procedures. Plast Reconstr Surg 70:437–443, 1982.
9. Mason EE: Panniculectomy. Surgical Rounds April 1985, pp 17–24.
10. Borges AF: W plastic dermolipectomy to correct "bat wing" deformity. Ann Plast Surg 9:498–501, 1982.

32

The National Bariatric Surgery Registry

EDWARD EATON MASON

GENERAL PLAN
ORGANIZATION
QUESTION FORMULATION
DATA COLLECTION AND
    MANAGEMENT
ANALYSES BY PARTICIPANTS
CENTRAL REGISTRY ANALYSES
REPORTING OF RESULTS
COMMUNICATION
FUNDING
SUMMARY

The surgical treatment of obesity has progressed rapidly during the first 30 years since the introduction of intestinal bypass. Operative procedures have become much more standardized with results that are more predictable. However, there remain questions that require a surgeon to compare the results of his operation, and techniques used, with the experience of other surgeons using different operations and techniques. This requires a pool of data from a larger number of surgeons and a much larger number of patients than has been available to date. The National Bariatric Surgery Registry (NBSR)* is a cooperative study designed to assist in the collection, pooling and analysis of data from a large number of surgeons so that existing questions may be answered and new questions stimulated.

GENERAL PLAN

Surgeons have always learned from review of their personal experience and by comparisons with the experience of others, but most surgeons do not have the time and the computer programs to make these studies on a recurring basis. It is the aim of the NBSR to provide all participating bariatric surgeons with the ability to review and compare their experiences in a way that requires insertion of the information about each patient's encounter into the NBSR data base only once. This capability, together with the opportunity to exchange information rapidly with others who have similar interests, will help in the provision of optimum care for extremely heavy patients.

Great care has been taken to maintain confidentiality. The NBSR will make comparisons of the effects of different operations, operative techniques and methods of patient care but will not make comparisons between the results of individual surgeons. If any surgeon wishes consultation about differences observed between his results and the pooled results, this can be provided, but only to the surgeon who provided that set of exclusive data and requested the consultation.

There are many existing questions that the NBSR may be able to answer. For example, we all want to know if in fact our operations do restore a normal mortality rate and what the effect is upon the quality of life. Other sample questions might relate to the best and most effective operations, or how equipment and techniques of performing these operations can be used to minimize complications or how to reduce the rate of reoperation. It is of concern to know whether the prophylactic use of antibiotics is cost effective. Should we use mini-dose heparin? Is heparin as effective as intermittent venous compression? What regimens are the best for perioperative care? Does the use of a histamine (H2) blocker to decrease acid secretion in the stomach decrease the incidence of aspiration pneumonitis? Does it increase the incidence of wound infection? What is the cost-benefit, considering these two possible effects of H2 blockers?

It is the nature of clinical research to look for partial answers or trends and then to use that information to design specific prospective randomized studies to confirm or further test the hypothesis. The NBSR will provide a better basis for designing such studies.

The use of standardized, central analyses allows surgeons to make comparisons of their data with a larger pool while using only data from well defined operations and operative techniques. It will be possible to obtain types of analyses which will allow reliable comparisons with the experience of others. This has not always been the case in the past. For example, weight loss is often presented without indicating either the mean or the variability of the initial weights of the patients under study. Marked variation in initial weight has a very significant influence on the final weight regardless of the operation used, and must be controlled before valid comparisons between operative procedures can be made.

Covariance analysis, using the initial weight as the covariant, is one approach to the solution of this problem. A useful but somewhat less exact approach is to divide patients into only two groups, the morbidly obese (160 to 225% of ideal weight) and the super obese (above 225% of ideal weight) on the basis of their initial weight. We will be able to make studies of more than one analytical method in any one problem and to develop a better understanding of the effects of the method(s) selected. We should, as a result, become more aware of the risks of inappropriate selection of methods of data management and statistical analyses and the need for appropriate application of analytic approaches before attempting to interpret results.

Of great help in deciding when to change

---

*National Bariatric Surgery Registry, Department of Surgery, The University of Iowa Hospitals and Clinics, Iowa City, Iowa 52242, U.S.A. (Phone: 319-356-3996)

abandon an operation in the University of Iowa experience over the last 20 years has been the actuarial analysis of the rate of revision. The first gastric bypass, with divided stomach and a loop gastroenterostomy, had a reoperation rate of 5% per year. During the first three years of use of horizontal gastroplasty, with a seromuscular Prolene suture for reinforcement of the stoma, the reoperation rate was 15% per year. Vertical banded gastroplasty, with the outlet of the small meal-sizing-pouch stabilized by a Marlex mesh collar, has a reoperation rate of 1.7% per year. This rate will undoubtedly be lowered as a result of the decrease in pouch volume, the use of smaller collars (5.0 cm), and the introduction of a four row stapler, for stapling-in-continuity.

Actuarial analyses were originally developed for calculating survivorship of patients, usually following treatment for cancer, and had the advantage of allowing use of all patients even though they had been followed for different lengths of time. Presently, actuarial analyses are used by the NBSR for calculating the "survivorship" (without revision or reversal) of different operations, so that comparisons between operations can be made using a single rate of reoperation for each operative type. The NBSR will use this same approach when comparing the obese patient's length of life, as influenced by the different operations, but this will take more data and more years of follow-up.

This is an appropriate time to begin the NBSR because of recent developments. A major development was the organization of the American Society of Bariatric Surgery (ASBS) in 1983. All of the more than 200 members have committed a significant portion of their professional lives to the care of the morbidly obese and are interested in the kinds of questions that the NBSR is designed to study. Another facilitating development is in personal computers which are now available at relatively low cost and with the speed and storage capacity to handle the job. Also available are data transmission programs that enable the user to send and receive data by telephone across long distances at great speed and at very little cost. The presence of knowledgable and experienced personnel at the University of Iowa, along with the necessary mainframe computer equipment and programs, permits the establishment of the NBSR central office without any major investment in equipment. A data base from over 1600 patients with a

variety of gastric reduction operations followed for up to 20 years provides a template for creation of the NBSR. All of this permits each participating surgeon to enter data and obtain reports in a way that simulates access to the experience of hundreds of surgeons with thousands of patients in a system that represents thousands of man-hours of effort.

ORGANIZATION

The NBSR is organized under a part-time bariatric surgeon director and a full-time manager. There are two committees, medical advisory committee (MAC) and technical advisory committee (TAC), that provide expert advice. The MAC is composed of surgeons who have a special interest in bariatric surgery, computer applications and related data analysis. The TAC is made up of people from industry and the University, each of whom has some special expertise pertinent to the project. Part-time supporting staff include a secretary, a statistician who assists in the planning and execution of the mainframe analyses, and a computer programmer who writes programs for use in the surgeon's offices. As of March 1988, there were 52 surgeons in 45 practices who had joined the NBSR and were collecting data. We are actively recruiting new members with the hope of involving between 200 and 300 surgeons by the end of 1990. The aim is not merely to obtain a sample of information about the surgical treatment of obesity but to attempt to include all of the patients who are being treated in the United States and even in other countries. This may not be realistic but it is theoretically possible, with the use of modern data processing capabilities, and it is a worthwhile goal.

QUESTION FORMULATION

Questions to be answered through use of the NBSR will usually be formulated as null hypotheses. Questions for analysis can be formulated by anyone who is a NBSR member The proposed methods of answering questions are to be written up as one would for a formal grant proposal. The required data must be specified so that it can be found in the existing NBSR data base or can be added to a new field for data collection. Any proposal for a special study must state who will be responsible for coordinating the study and whether the data is to be collected by a specific subset of surgeons or the entire membership of the NBSR. The study's goals, time frame, level of confidence and end-point must all be specified. A solid plan for data management and analysis is required.

DATA COLLECTION AND MANAGEMENT

Each surgeon joining the NBSR receives the same specially designed data collection program. At the present time, the program runs only on an IBM PC or IBM PC compatible computer. Also available is a special program that can be used to schedule appointments, identify patients who missed their appointments and create letters for notification of patients of new appointments. Data collected are consistent with recommendations of the American Society for Bariatric Surgery. Data transfer, analysis and return of reports is on a regular schedule for the general data and as requested for special projects. The technical committee will review requests for addition of new data fields to the main data collection program. Biannual updates and enhancements of software are planned.

ANALYSES BY PARTICIPANTS

Data analysis programs running on the office PC will be available from the NBSR for the individual surgeon's use. These programs will allow tabulation and analysis of the data in his own data base. The statistics will include mean, standard deviation and range. Since the data base runs under Knowledgeman™, an information management system, the data base is accessible to the surgeon. If the member wishes to either add additional variables to his own data base or write programs to manipulate his data, he may do so through the use of the Knowledgeman program which is supplied as a part of the membership materials. Customized programming for individual surgeons can be provided by NBSR but only for a fee that covers the development of such software.

CENTRAL REGISTRY MAINFRAME ANALYSES

The NBSR will perform all group analyses on a mainframe computer (an IBM 4381). The analyses will include time analyses of weight loss, actuarial analyses of reoperation rates and general statistical analyses. There will

also be confidential analyses of each surgeon's data with comparisons of the pooled data. These analyses will be returned to the surgeons in report form for their review. Analyses conducted on the mainframe will allow special studies using the pooled data to answer questions that require a great deal more data than can be obtained by any one surgeon. The mainframe has available a large library of analytical programs so that special requests can be met with very little programming beyond that needed to assemble the data and the programs.

REPORTING OF RESULTS

Each member will be able to use the analyses of his own data by the NBSR for publication. Any publications that involve NBSR analyses of the pooled data must first be approved by the NBSR. This approval step should prevent publication of conflicting interpretations of the pooled data analyses that might arise from some misunderstanding and should prevent duplicate publication of results. When results of analyses of the pooled data are published, the source is to be acknowledged.

In each special project adequate planning at the outset is essential. At the conclusion of a project's data gathering, a clear and concise plan of action will facilitate rapid completion of analyses and an efficient use of the results, with proper assignment of work and acknowledgement of credits.

The NBSR is a resource available to all participants. Those responsible for the running of the registry will make every effort to see that it is not used for selfish purposes or to the benefit of individuals who have not made a major contribution to the study involved.

It is hoped that the planning at the beginning of each special study will prevent conflicts from arising. The medical advisory committee will recommend ways of resolving any conflicts of interest. We know that the NBSR cannot succeed without the enthusiastic cooperation of its members. Each member will need to give up some autonomy in the use of results from the pooled data in order to have available the extensive resources of the Registry. This is a cooperative venture that depends upon mutual trust and the integrity of the members in their relationships with NBSR.

COMMUNICATION

Communication is the glue that holds all of this together. A quarterly Newsletter provides information about Registry activities and in addition notes about bariatric surgery literature and special problems that are commonly met in the care of the extremely obese surgical patient. The Newsletter is intended also to be a forum for presentation of questions, opinions and proposals regarding the search for better answers to questions.

FUNDING

Adequate financial support is essential for success. A major source of funding for the first two years has been provided by a one time grant. While participating surgeons have had to provide equipment and people to collect the data in their offices, the NBSR has been able to provide a data collection program at a fraction of the usual cost by purchasing a large lot of the supporting software and by use of central programming. Members will be asked to provide their proportion of the budget for running of the NBSR (charter members will not be charged a membership fee for the first two years). The more members the NBSR has, the less it will cost per member and the larger and more variable and valuable, will be the data pool. The members should encourage their colleagues in the practice of bariatric surgery to join the NBSR. Support for special projects will be requested in grant applications.

SUMMARY

The National Bariatric Surgery Registry will facilitate the gathering, analysis and dissemination of information about the care of morbidly obese patients. The NBSR was developed from the belief that in the experience of hundreds of surgeons, with many thousands of patients, there are answers to questions about unusual situations that arise and that there is also information about selection of patients, operations, operative techniques, perioperative care, quality of life and longevity that will further improve the management of extreme obesity. Many people have contributed to this new, cooperative study of the surgical care of the morbidly obese. Their efforts are greatly appreciated.

AFTERWORD

It has been an honor and a privilege to work with the distinguished co-authors and to be a part of the bariatric surgical community. Some of the chapters in this book have presented operations which have been superseded by other operations. However, there are principles to be learned from every procedure. Some operations are no longer performed, because good results could be reproduced in only a few expert hands. Other procedures are being performed on a large scale—vertical gastroplasties with reinforcement of the outlet, Roux-en-Y gastric bypasses, gastric restrictive procedures with distal Roux-en-Y, gastric banding, biliopancreatic bypasses and modifications of the malabsorption operations. Thanks to free-enterprise technology, the sophisticated materials vital to perform these procedures are available. The bariatric surgeon requires greater than average surgical knowledge, technical ability, and commitment.

Public health estimations indicate that more than 14 million people in the U.S.A. are >45 kg (100 lb) overweight and that 300,000 are super-obese (>225% above ideal weight). In carefully selected and informed morbidly obese patients who have failed to sustain weight loss on extensive conservative regimens, the only effective treatment is surgery. These operations require indefinite follow-up, so that the loss of massive excess weight can be achieved safely and also for assessment of the ultimate long-term results. The substantial health risks of a large population of morbidly obese patients in our society can be reduced. With respect to physical and psychological consequences of massive obesity, the rehabilitation of these patients following bariatric surgery is usually gratifying. Most of these individuals are enabled to come out into the world and make a positive contribution to society. No other mode of therapy has been found to be as effective in these patients.

Mervyn Deitel, M.D.
Toronto, Canada

INDEX

Page numbers in *italics* indicate figures; numbers followed by "t" indicate tables.

393